Hans-Joachim Mörsdorf

Sleep related Breathing Disorders and Sleep Stages from ECG Signals

Hans-Joachim Mörsdorf

Sleep related Breathing Disorders and Sleep Stages from ECG Signals

Applying Pattern Recognition Methods to ECG Signals to detect Sleep related Breathing Disorder Events and Sleep Stages

Südwestdeutscher Verlag für Hochschulschriften

Impressum/Imprint (nur für Deutschland/only for Germany)
Bibliografische Information der Deutschen Nationalbibliothek: Die Deutsche Nationalbibliothek verzeichnet diese Publikation in der Deutschen Nationalbibliografie; detaillierte bibliografische Daten sind im Internet über http://dnb.d-nb.de abrufbar.
Alle in diesem Buch genannten Marken und Produktnamen unterliegen warenzeichen-, marken- oder patentrechtlichem Schutz bzw. sind Warenzeichen oder eingetragene Warenzeichen der jeweiligen Inhaber. Die Wiedergabe von Marken, Produktnamen, Gebrauchsnamen, Handelsnamen, Warenbezeichnungen u.s.w. in diesem Werk berechtigt auch ohne besondere Kennzeichnung nicht zu der Annahme, dass solche Namen im Sinne der Warenzeichen- und Markenschutzgesetzgebung als frei zu betrachten wären und daher von jedermann benutzt werden dürften.

Coverbild: www.ingimage.com

Verlag: Südwestdeutscher Verlag für Hochschulschriften GmbH & Co. KG
Heinrich-Böcking-Str. 6-8, 66121 Saarbrücken, Deutschland
Telefon +49 681 37 20 271-1, Telefax +49 681 37 20 271-0
Email: info@svh-verlag.de

Approved by: Erlangen, Friedrich-Alexander-University, Diss., 2011

Herstellung in Deutschland:
Schaltungsdienst Lange o.H.G., Berlin
Books on Demand GmbH, Norderstedt
Reha GmbH, Saarbrücken
Amazon Distribution GmbH, Leipzig
ISBN: 978-3-8381-2482-7

Imprint (only for USA, GB)
Bibliographic information published by the Deutsche Nationalbibliothek: The Deutsche Nationalbibliothek lists this publication in the Deutsche Nationalbibliografie; detailed bibliographic data are available in the Internet at http://dnb.d-nb.de.
Any brand names and product names mentioned in this book are subject to trademark, brand or patent protection and are trademarks or registered trademarks of their respective holders. The use of brand names, product names, common names, trade names, product descriptions etc. even without a particular marking in this works is in no way to be construed to mean that such names may be regarded as unrestricted in respect of trademark and brand protection legislation and could thus be used by anyone.

Cover image: www.ingimage.com

Publisher: Südwestdeutscher Verlag für Hochschulschriften GmbH & Co. KG
Heinrich-Böcking-Str. 6-8, 66121 Saarbrücken, Germany
Phone +49 681 37 20 271-1, Fax +49 681 37 20 271-0
Email: info@svh-verlag.de

Printed in the U.S.A.
Printed in the U.K. by (see last page)
ISBN: 978-3-8381-2482-7

Copyright © 2012 by the author and Südwestdeutscher Verlag für Hochschulschriften GmbH & Co. KG and licensors
All rights reserved. Saarbrücken 2012

Abstract

The society becomes more and more aware of sleep disorders. This is mainly due to two reasons: first, the media companies attempt to attract attention by publishing topics everyone is interested in. And second, it is in fact true that more and more people become affected by sleep disorders. This is mainly due to the way of living in the industrialized nations characterized increasing levels of stress and Body Mass Index (BMI).

"Sleep disorders" is a pretty broad term, i.e., it summarizes completely different types of disorders, mainly physiological and psychological ones. The physiological disorders are caused by organic failures and the psychological disorders result from stress and anxiety.

This work deals with the so called "Sleep Related Breathing Disorders" (SRBD). These disorders are characterized by a sleep induced breathing failure which usually can not be observed during the wake state. The latter makes it hard to diagnose the disease as those affected are generally not aware of their critical health condition. The immediate consequences of this disease are fatigue and a reduced daytime efficiency which is often made responsible for car accidents and severe accidents in operating machines. Leaving this disease untreated affects the cardiac system and may lead to heart failure and cerebral insult.

The diagnosis of the sleep related breathing disorders is a complicated procedure which requires the evaluation of up to 25 vital parameters by especially trained personal in sleep laboratories.

The approach which is pursued in this work aims at reducing the required sensor set to just an electrocardiogram (ECG). The missing information is thought to be retrieved from this vital signal by signal processing algorithms which consider the heart rate as well as the shape of the ECG signal. If possible, this approach would yield not only the option to detect sleep related breathing order events, but to trace potential cardiac sequel as well with just one measurement. Long term ECG recordings are widely applied in today's cardiological diagnosis.

The electrocardiogram signal is processed according to two different approaches: The first approach considers only the current heart rate and feeds it into a model of the autonomous nervous system. The second approach seeks the morphological side effects of cardiac load fluctuations on the ECG wave due to changes in the sleep stages or during the compensation phase following a SRBD event. Along with the most important morphological markers, e.g., the R-peak or the T-wave, approaches like the Independent Component Analysis and the Fourier transformation are evaluated.

The evaluation comprises the selection of the best classifier for each feature set and the determination of the achievable classification rates for each single event type. On the training data set classification rates of up to 86.4% for the obstructive and up to 22.2% for the central apneas were achieved. For the sleep stage classification the achieved results over all sleep stages range from 74.7 - 99.0%. On the test data set 79.2 - 98.9% of all SRBD events were detected. Considering the sleep stage classification, the detection rate for wake state was up to 94.4%, for light sleep up to 69.4%, for deep sleep up to 29.3%, and for REM up to 35.5%.

Kurzfassung

Die Gesellschaft wird zunehmend für Schlafkrankheiten sensibilisiert Dies hauptsächlich aus zwei Gründen: erstens versuchen die Medien Aufmerksamkeit auf sich zu ziehen, indem sie Themen publizieren, für die sich viele interessieren. Und zweitens entspricht es auch den Tatsachen, dass immer mehr Menschen von Schlafkrankheiten betroffen sind. Dies wird hauptsächlich durch den Lebensstil in den Industrienationen verursacht, der durch zunehmenden Stress und ungesunde Leibesfülle gekennzeichnet ist.

"Schlafstörungen" ist ein sehr weit gefasster Begriff, d.h. er fasst komplett verschiedene Krankheitsbilder zusammen. Die physiologischen Krankheiten werden durch organische Defekte und die psychologischen Krankheiten durch Stress und Angst hervorgerufen.

Diese Arbeit beschäftigt sich mit den so genannten "Schlafbezogenen Atmungsstörungen". Diese Krankheiten werden durch Atemaussetzer charakterisiert, die im Wachzustand nicht beobachtet werden können. Dieser Umstand erschwert die Diagnose der Krankheit, da die Betroffenen sich ihres kritischen Gesundheitszustands im Allgemeinen nicht bewusst sind. Die unmittelbaren Konsequenzen dieser Krankheit sind Müdigkeit und eine reduzierte Leistungsfähigkeit am Tage, die häufig für Autounfälle oder schwere Unfälle bei der Bedienung von Maschinen verantwortlich gemacht werden. Bleibt diese Krankheit unbehandelt, führt sie zu Belastungen des Herz-Kreislauf-Systems und schlussendlich zu Herzinfarkt und Schlaganfall.

Die Diagnose schlafbezogener Atmungsstörungen ist ein kopmpliziertes Prozedere, welches die Auswertung von bis zu 25 Vitalparametern durch spezielll ausgebildetes Personal in Schlaflaboren erfordert.

Der Ansatz, der in dieser Arbeit verfolgt wird, zielt darauf ab, die Anzahl erforderlicher Sensoren auf lediglich das EKG zu reduzieren. Die fehlende Information soll dabei durch Signalverarbeitung aus dem EKG-Signal gewonnen werden. Berücksichtigt werden dabei die Herzfrequenz und die Gestalt des EKG-Signals. Dieser Ansatz bietet nicht nur die Möglichkeit schlafbezogene Atmungsstörungen zu erkennen, sondern auch kardiologische Folgeerkrankungen mit nur einer EKG-Langzeitmessung zu verfolgen. EKG-Langzeitmessungen sind heute Standard in der kardiologischen Diagnostik.

Das EKG wird mittels zweier verschiedener Ansätze ausgewertet: Der erste Ansatz berücksichtigt nur die aktuelle Herzfrequenz und deren Änderung und speist diese in ein Modell des autonomen Nervensystems. Der zweite Ansatz sucht die morphologischen Nebeneffekte der kardiologischen Laständerungen auf die EKG-Kurve. Die Laständerungen werden z.B. von Wechseln der Schlafstadien bzw. der Kompensationsphase nach Auftreten von schlafbezogenen Atmungsssstörungen verursacht. Zusätzlich zu den markanten morphologischen Markern, z.b. der R-Zacke oder T-Welle, werden Ansätze wie die Independent Coponent Analysis und die Fourier-Transformation zur Charakterisierung der EKG-Kurve als Ganzes ausgewertet.

Die Auswertung umfasst die Auswahl des besten Klassifikators für jeden Merkmalssatz und die Bestimmung der erreichbaren Klassifikationsraten für jedes einzelne Schlafstörungsereignis. Auf den Trainingsdaten wurden Klassifikationsraten von bis zu 86,4% für obstruktive und von bis zu 22,2% für zentrale Schlafstörungen er-reicht. Für die Schlafstadienklassifikation bewegen sich die Erkennugsraten über alle Schlafstadien zwischen 74,7 und 99,0%. Auf den Testdaten wurden bis zu 98,9% der obstuktiven Schlafstörungen erkannt. Die Schlafstadienklassifikation betreffend lag die Erkennungsrate für den Wachzustand bei bis zu 94,4%, für Leichtschlaf bei bis zu 69,4%, für Tiefschlaf bis zu 29,3% und für REM-Schlaf bei bis zu 35,5%.

Acknowledgment

This work would not have been possible without the support from persons guiding and supporting me. I would like to thank them heartedly and personally:

I would like to thank Prof. Dr.-Ing. Elmar Nöth, University of Erlangen, for his assistance concerning pattern recognition technologies and his suggestions of improvement for this work.

Next, I want to express my gratitude to Prof. Dr. Penzel, Charite, Berlin, for the fruitful discussions about the physiology of the sleep apnea syndrome and its correlations to the ECG.

Further on, I am indebted to the clinical partners who recorded and annotated the data namely OA Dr. Herold, Klinikum Nord, Nuremberg, and Dr. med. Sebastian Canisius, University of Marburg. The later one I thank for his lectorship as well.

For creating the circumstances which allowed to finish my work, I want to thank Prof. Dr.-Ing. Heinz Gerhäuser, Fraunhofer IIS, Erlangen.

Apart from these mainly scientific supporters, I would, of course, like to thank my family who gave confidence and kept patient with me.

Hans-Joachim Mörsdorf

About this Work

References

The following conventions are applied for flagging references to Figues, Tables, equations, and across Sections:

- References to Figues and Tables don't have any symbol around them, as they are usually headed by "Figure" or "Table".

- Numbers in braces, e.g., (1.1), refer to equations.

- Numbers in braces headed by "p.", e.g., (p. 11), refer to pages.

- Numbers and text in brackets, e.g., [AU06], refer to literature.

- Numbers in slashes, e.g., /1.1/, refer to Sections.

Abbreviations used in this Work

A remark concerning the abbreviation "SRBD" as this is used quite often. As reading it is somewhat "cumbrous", I read it in plain text. That's why the combination with the indefinite article is spelled "*a* SRBD event" instead of "*an* SRBD event".

The following Table introduces the abbreviations used in this work, their plain text and where to find them.

Abbrev	Meaning	Page
AASM	American Academy of Sleep Medicine	7
AHI	Apnea-Hypopnea-Index	15
AM	Autonomous Model	76
ANS	Autonomous Nervous System	34
ARFF	Attribute Relation File Format	63
ASCII	American Standard Code for Information Interchange	198

Continued on next page

Abbrev	Meaning	Page
AV	Atrio-Ventricular (Node)	27
BMI	Body Mass Index	18
bpm	Beats per Minute	31
BtB	Beat-to-Beat	159
CHD	Coronary Heart Disease	1
COPD	Chronic Obstructive Pulmonary Disease	1
CPAP	Continuous Positive Airway Pressure	24
CR	Classification Rate	159
CSAS	Central Sleep Apnea Syndrome	13
DCT	Discrete Cosine Transformation	132
DGSM	Deutsche Gesellschaft für Schlafmedizin	26
DP	Diseased Patient	159
ECG	Electrocardiogram	27
EDF	European Data Format	62
EEG	Electroencephalogram	21
ELR	Euler-Liljestrand-Reflex	33
EMG	Electromyogram	1
EOG	Electrooculogram	1
EVA	ECG Evaluation Application	1
FM	F-Measure	159
GMM	Gaussian Mixture Model	204
GUI	Graphical User Interface	197
HMM	Hidden-Markov-Model	1
HP	Healthy Patient	159
HR	Heart Rate	31
HRV	Heart Rate Variability	31
ICA	Independent Component Analysis	205
ICSD	International Classification of Sleep Disorders	7
NREM	Non-REM Sleep	9
OSAHS	Obstructive Sleep Apnea Hypopnea Syndrome	13
OSAS	Obstructive Sleep Apnea Syndrome	13
pdf	probability density function	206
PNS	Parasympathetic Nervous System	34
PSG	Polysomnography	21

Continued on next page

Abbrev	Meaning	Page
RaK	Rechtschaffen and Kales	159
REM	Rapid Eye Movement (Sleep stage)	9
RLS	Restless Leg Syndrome	8
RRZE	Regionales Rechenzentrum Erlangen	63
SHM	Sleep-Home-Monitoring (device)	59
SNS	Sympathetic Nervous System	34
SRBD	Sleep Related Breathing Disorders	5
SWS	Slow Wave Sleep (Sleep stages 3 and 4)	9
VCO	Voltage Controlled Oscillator	76

Table 1: Abbreviations used

Contents

1 Introduction   **1**
   1.1 Sleep, Breathing, and the Focus of this Work 1
   1.2 Motivation 2
   1.3 Hypothesis 3
   1.4 Overview of this Work 3
   1.5 Summary and Preview 4

2 Sleep related Breathing Disorders   **5**
   2.1 Prevalence and Incidence 5
   2.2 Classification of Sleep Disorders 7
   2.3 About Breathing 7
   2.4 About Sleep 8
     2.4.1 Entering Sleep 8
     2.4.2 Sleep Architecture 9
     2.4.3 Influences on Sleep 11
   2.5 Types and Severity of SRBD Events 11
     2.5.1 Snoring 12
     2.5.2 Hypopnea 12
     2.5.3 Apnea 13
     2.5.4 Obstructive and Central Events 13
     2.5.5 Mixed Sleep Apnea 14
     2.5.6 Quantity 15
   2.6 Course of Events during an Apnea – A vicious Cycle 16
   2.7 Symptoms, Risk Factors, and Medical Risks 17
     2.7.1 Symptoms 18
     2.7.2 Risk Factors for SRBD 18
     2.7.3 Medical Consequences of OSAHS 19
   2.8 Diagnostic Procedures 19
     2.8.1 Cardio-respiratory Polysomnography 21

	2.9	Therapeutic Procedures	23
		2.9.1 Sleep Hygiene	24
		2.9.2 CPAP Therapy and its various Manifestations	24
	2.10	Facilities, Institutions and other Resources	26
	2.11	Summary and Preview	26
3	**Medical Introduction to the Heart**		**27**
	3.1	The Heart and the Electrocardiogram	27
		3.1.1 Recording an Electrocardiogram	29
		3.1.2 Influences on the Recording of an ECG	31
	3.2	Heart Rate and its Variability	31
		3.2.1 Introduction	31
		3.2.2 HR and Sleep Apnea	32
		3.2.3 Euler-Liljestrand Reflex	33
	3.3	The Antagonists Sympathetic and Parasympathetic Nervous System	34
		3.3.1 Activity of Sinoatrial Node	35
		3.3.2 Wake-Sleep-Influences	39
		3.3.3 AV-Blocks	40
	3.4	Reactions to different Load Conditions	41
		3.4.1 P-Wave	41
		3.4.2 Amplitude of the R-Peak	42
	3.5	Myocardial Ischemia	43
		3.5.1 ST-Segment and Ischemic Influences	44
		3.5.2 ST-Segment Depressions	44
		3.5.3 ST-Segment Elevations	45
		3.5.4 T-Wave	45
	3.6	Summary and Preview	46
4	**State of the Art**		**47**
	4.1	Deriving Autonomous Activity from the Heart Rate	47
		4.1.1 Quotient of the SNS and PNS Energies	47
		4.1.2 Power Law Slope and Poincare Plots	49
	4.2	Physionet Database	50
	4.3	Methods and Classification Rates	51
	4.4	Summary and Preview	57
5	**Acquiring Medical Data**		**59**
	5.1	BFS Project "Sleep Home Monitoring"	59

	5.2	Overview over the Data Flow Chain	60
		5.2.1 Sleep Laboratory – Recording Data	60
		5.2.2 Clinical Data Evaluation – Annotations	62
		5.2.3 Data Export – From Proprietary to Raw Data	62
		5.2.4 Feature Extraction – From ECG to Features	63
	5.3	Consistency of the Medical Annotations	64
	5.4	Summary and Preview	66
6	**Detecting SRBD Events and Sleep Stages from an ECG Signal**		**67**
	6.1	Preprocessing of the ECG	68
		6.1.1 Mains Supply	68
		6.1.2 DC-Shifts	69
		6.1.3 General Noise	71
		6.1.4 Compensating Filter Delays	72
	6.2	ECG Distinctive Point Detection	72
		6.2.1 Labeling the Distinctive Points in the ECG	73
		6.2.2 R-Peak Detection	74
		6.2.3 Detection of the Remaining Distinctive ECG Points	74
	6.3	Autonomous Model	76
		6.3.1 Technical Description of the Model	76
		6.3.2 Model and Physiology (Hypothesis)	77
		6.3.3 Implementation of the Autonomous Model	79
	6.4	Morphological Features	91
		6.4.1 Common Features of the Morphological Functions	91
		6.4.2 P-Wave	95
		6.4.3 R-Peak	98
		6.4.4 ST-Segment	101
		6.4.5 T-Wave	105
		6.4.6 Timing	111
		6.4.7 Overall Shape: Deviations	114
		6.4.8 Overall Shape: Independent Component Analysis	119
		6.4.9 Overall Shape: Spectral Transformations	132
		6.4.10 Overall Shape: Differences of Spectral Transformations	146
	6.5	Summary and Preview	149
7	**Experimental Results**		**151**
	7.1	ECG Distinctive Points Detection	151
		7.1.1 Types of Artifacts in the recorded ECGs	151

	7.1.2	R-Peak Detection	153
	7.1.3	Remaining Distinctive Points Detection	153
7.2	Running the Feature Extraction		156
7.3	Selection of the Appropriate Classifiers		158
7.4	Evaluation of the different Feature Sets		159
	7.4.1	Autonomous Model	163
	7.4.2	P-Wave	165
	7.4.3	R-Peak	166
	7.4.4	ST-Segment	167
	7.4.5	T-Wave	168
	7.4.6	Timing	169
	7.4.7	Overall Shape: Deviations	170
	7.4.8	Overall Shape: Independent Component Analysis	172
	7.4.9	Overall Shape: Spectral Transformations	174
	7.4.10	Overall Shape: Differences of Spectral Transformations	175
	7.4.11	Detection of Artifacts	176
	7.4.12	Concluding the patient-dependent Classification Rates	176
7.5	Patient-independent Evaluation		179
7.6	Discussion		182
7.7	Summary and Preview		185

8 Outlook 187

9 Summary 189

10 Appendix 195

10.1	Criteria for Rating the Concordance	195
	10.1.1 Kappa Coefficient	195
	10.1.2 Modified Kappa Coefficient	196
10.2	Introduction to EVA ml	197
	10.2.1 The GUI of EVA ml	197
	10.2.2 Processing Configurations	199
	10.2.3 EVA ml processing Vital Data	199
10.3	ECG derived Respiration	201
10.4	Principle of the Gaussian Mixture Model Approximation	204
10.5	Independent Component Analysis – ICA	205
	10.5.1 Introduction	206
	10.5.2 Basic mathematical Principle	206

10.6 Definitions of applied Means 209
10.7 Applied Classifiers 209
    10.7.1 Bayes Networks 209
    10.7.2 RBFNetwork and MultilayerPerceptron 210
    10.7.3 IBk and KStar 210
    10.7.4 Bagging 210
10.8 Detailed Classification Results 211
    10.8.1 Autonomous Model 212
    10.8.2 P-Wave 214
    10.8.3 R-Peak 216
    10.8.4 ST-Segment 218
    10.8.5 T-Wave 220
    10.8.6 Timing 222
    10.8.7 Overall Shape: Deviations 224
    10.8.8 Overall Shape: Independent Component Analysis 226
    10.8.9 Overall Shape: Spectral Transformations 228
    10.8.10 Overall Shape: Differences of Spectral Transformations 230

List of Figures   **233**

List of Tables   **237**

Bibliography   **239**

Index   **245**

Chapter 1

Introduction

1.1 Sleep, Breathing, and the Focus of this Work

"Death is a long sleep - Sleep is a short death" - at least this is what Joseph Haydn[1] believed. This hints on what people thought of sleep in former times: death's little brother. Today, on contrary, we know that sleep is essential for life – even though we do not know yet, why humans and animals sleep at all. Even though humans spend approximately one third of their lives asleep, sleep medicine is a quite young branch of medical research. This is partly because the topic is very complex and there was no appropriate medical equipment to perform reliable measurements, and partly because the sleeper him/herself usually is not able to describe the course of events as sleep "steals" the consciousness.

A well-known experience is that a reduced amount of sleep leads to reduced efficiency. But, usually, the body retrieves the required amount of sleep during the next night. If a subject is prevented from sleeping over a long period by a disease, however, the negative effects accumulate. A direct consequence of extreme fatigue is the impairment in vigilance. Vigilance means the subject's ability to keep attention to monotonous tasks like driving cars on highways. The likeliness of being involved in a car accident increases threefold in patients with SRBD. In detail, fatigue appears to be the main reason for 3% of car accidents with material damage, for 20% causing injuries and for 50% entailing death. According to a study mentioned in [HUK 94] about 25% of all lethal car accidents account to a vigilance impairment. In [Penz 05] the authors claim that there is a larger number of serious car accidents under the influence of hypersomnia than under the influence of alcohol or drugs, and that even mild forms of SRBD increase the risk of being involved in a car accident by a factor of six.

---
[1]Haydn, Joseph (31st March 1732 - 31st May 1809): Austrian Composer

Likewise, the lack of vigilance impairs subjects when it comes to operating dangerous machines or supervising critical processes, e.g., in nuclear power stations, because sleep onset in these subjects can be abrupt and imperative.

There are many diseases interfering with sleep which have their causes in e.g., drugs, stress, organic or psychic diseases (see (2.4.3). From all of these diseases this work focuses on the SRBD (see /2/). The SRBD are grouped around a phenomenon, which is called "apnea". The word "Apnea" derives from a Greek word meaning "lull"[Air 06] or "no air": it means the unintentional ceasing of the subject's breathing *only* during sleep for from ten seconds up to three minutes. A (limited) number of short apneas occurs in healthy people several times a night as well. But if these events last longer than ten seconds and reoccur over and over again, i.e., more than five times a night, they threaten the subject's health. The ceased breathing only restarts after an arousal (see /2.5.3/), which means that the patient wakes up just below consciousness, i.e., the sleep interruption goes unnoticed. Generally, an arousal is accompanied by a loud snore, which is why most patients are sent to see a physician by their spouses in the first place.

SRBD do not only affect the quality of sleep, but have severe side effects: headaches, excessive tiredness with an almost overwhelming urge to sleep, daytime fatigue, testiness, and concentration dysfunction. As SRBD usually go unnoticed by the subjects, they do not consider an illness the reason for their indisposition which is why many cases of SRBD are not diagnosed.

In addition, sleep deprivation shows an impact on the subject's mental power which prevents them from achieving their personal ambitions in the private and business field. This does not only greatly limit the subject's quality of life, but quite often triggers depressions.

However, sleepiness and reduced efficiency are only the short term consequences and the ones the patient is aware of. They are only the tip of the iceberg, as among the long term consequences there are a degraded immune system, severe damages to the cardio-vascular system like hypertension, arrhythmias, and eventually heart attacks and cerebral insults.

Affected by sleep disorders in general is every tenth to fourth male aged 30 - 60 years. The percentage in the females is about half of the males at younger ages but assimilates from about 60 years onwards. About 20% of the male population snore and the percentage in the obese males is threefold higher [Lasc 06]. According to another survey, about 25% of the adult population suffer from sleep disorders, and more than 10% of them experience their sleep "often or constantly as being non-restorative". This statement is supported in [Fisc 05], where the authors claim that in Germany there are about 8 Mio. people (10% of the population) who suffer from non-restorative sleep. More details on the prevalence of sleep apnea in the population can be found in /2.1/.

The highlighted consequences for the individual show a strong impact on the overall economy. The economical impact (car accidents, loss of productive machine usage) is estimated to reach 10 Million Euro in Germany and all sleep disorders together produced costs of 700 Mio. Euros in the year 2002 as claimed in [Penz 05].

1.2 Motivation

As with most diseases the expectations for therapy are best, if the disease is diagnosed as early as possible. This requires a systematic screening of the population as is demanded by many physicians. This, however, is hardly possible with today's "Gold Standard" for diagnosing SRBD: the cardio-respiratory polysomnography /2.8.1/. This examination is expensive, time-consuming, and requires highly educated personnel. Subjects suspected to suffer from SRBD often have to wait a long time to get an appointment in one of the diagnostic facilities, i.e., sleep laboratories.

The aim of this work is to evaluate, whether today's diagnostic procedure can be simplified by means of using a simple single lead ECG. If so, screening for SRBD could be performed by every physician and the percentage of successfully treated subjects may be increased.

1.3 Hypothesis

Among sleep medicine experts (somnologist), there is an ongoing discussion, whether the evaluation of an ECG signal alone allows detecting respiratory events and, hence, diagnosing sleep apnea. The supporters of the "ECG derived OSAS diagnosis" fraction claim that the ECG is such a central vital signal that all important physiological variations *must* be visible. The opposite fraction says exactly the same, meaning that because every physiological variation affects the ECG, the changes caused by SRBD events are drowned in all the other influences and, therefore, *can not be* visible, i.e. distinguishable.

The technical ancillary conditions for the evaluation of this criterion are not perfect. The ECG signal which is recorded during the subject's sleep does not provide the highest quality. Usually, there is only one ECG lead in stead of the twelve channels which are used in a "true" cardiological examination and the signal is distorted due to the patient's unintentional movements during sleep.

Nevertheless, the hypothesis of this work is that it is possible to detect sleep apnea events *and their types* and sleep stages by evaluating an ECG signal alone. This hypothesis is based on the close relationship between heart activity and sleep due to the autonomous system and the morphological influences of mechanical load changes during a SRBD event.

1.4 Overview of this Work

Following this introductory part the subsequent Chapters are organized as follows:

Chapter 2 deals with the SRBD events. It starts with an introduction to the medical aspects of sleep, its possible impairments and their classification. The next Section will illustrate that sleep diseases are really quite common taking into account their prevalence. Next, the reader will be acquainted with some terminology: the terms "apnea" and "hypopnea" will be presented and what role they play in the medical syndromes which have so much impact on the subject's health. Then, means to diagnose the disease and to estimate the severity are introduced. At the end of Chapter 2 today's therapeutic possibilities are given.

Chapter 3 will present the human heart and the measurement of its electrical activity. This will lead to the electrocardiogram (ECG), on which the signal analysis algorithms of this work will operate. Subsequently, one important regulation system of the body will be explained: the sympathetic and the parasympathetic nervous system. Further along this Chapter parameters like heart rate, variations of the shape of the ECG, and their possible reasons will be introduced. This information will be the theoretical basis for the parameters that are extracted for classification.

Chapter 4 presents the state of the art in the field of deriving SRBD events from an ECG signal. It introduces several approaches and their respective classification rates.

Chapter 5 provides some background to this work. It shortly introduces the research project during which the requirements for this work were set. It mainly deals with the way the annotated data was recorded, generated, and preevaluated.

Chapter 6 supplies the argumentation for the extracted features based on the medical knowledge which was introduced in Chapters 2 - 3. It also deals with the implementation and the results of the feature extraction.

Chapter 7 presents the classification rates achieved with the extracted features. A discussion establishes the position of this work in the context of the existing state of the art. In addition to the classification rates the most powerful features are given and related – as far as possible – to their physiological background.

Chapter 8 provides a road-map of future efforts to improve and propel different feature sets which were started with this work.

Chapter 9 summarizes this work and the achieved results in the conclusions of this work.

Chapter 10 contains an appendix which supplies additional background information on some of the principles and mathematical methods used in this work.

1.5 Summary and Preview

This Chapter provided a short explanation of the key words "SRBD", "apnea" and "arousal" along with the medical sequel of this disease: SRBD are characterized by short cessations of breathing during sleep which are called apnea. The apneas are terminated, i.e., normal breathing restarts, after an arousal which is a short awakening.

This Chapter also gave a short overview of the approaches which will be applied to derive SRBD events from the ECG. These approaches are based on the evaluation of the heart rate and the ECG wave shape, respectively.

The next Chapter will provide all the required medical basics concerning sleep and SRBD. It will also introduce the linkage between the sleep stages, arousals, and different resulting load conditions for the heart.

At the end of the next Chapter, there is a short overview of today's diagnostic and therapeutic procedures.

Chapter 2

Sleep related Breathing Disorders

This Chapter is an introduction to the medical basics of the diseases, which are summarized under the term SRBD. They are characterized by the fact that the respiration even in seemingly healthy subjects fails during sleep whereas it works correctly in wake state.

For an assessment of the importance of SRBD this Chapter starts with an introduction to the prevalence of sleep disorders and their classification. Then, it gives some basic insight into sleep, the different sleep stages, and their arrangement in the so called sleep architecture. Further on, various influences on the sleep quality like diseases and personal habits are discussed.

The next Sections explain the disease in detail: First, there is an explanation of what happens during an apnea and the apnea itself is split into its various manifestations leading to measures for the severity of the disease.

At the end of this Chapter, the symptoms, risk factors, and possible sequels of SRBD along with today's methods of diagnosis and therapy will be introduced.

This Chapter is mainly based on [Virc 04], [Hade 04], [Psch 98], [Grot 96], [Pete 95], [Pete 91], [Fisc 05], [Temm 06], [Penz 05].

2.1 Prevalence and Incidence

This Section is to state the necessity of dealing with sleep disorders as they are much wider spread than commonly assumed.

Prevalence and *Incidence* are both termini of medical statistics. Prevalence reveals the number of people presently suffering from a specific disease in a given population. When dealing with relative numbers, the used terminus is *prevalence rate*. Incidence, however, reveals the number of people sickening anew each year from a specific disease. Both values are derived from epidemiological surveys.

Snoring is considered a possible early clue to breathing disorders during sleep. It is more likely to happen in the male population (25% male and 15% in females) and the likelihood increases with age – in the range from 41 - 64 years 60% of males and 40% of females snore. After 65 years of age the levels of male and female snorers assimilate.

Sleep disorders are quite common. In [Noel 97] the author states that 31% of the population from 16 years of age onwards claim to suffer sometimes or even frequently from an unspecified sleepiness. This is in perfect concordance with the authors of [Grot 96] who claim that in the western industrial nations 20 - 30% of the population suffer from sleep disorders.

The high rate of fatigue in youngsters is mainly explained by their usually bad sleep hygiene (see /2.9.1/). 16 hours of accumulated sleep deprivation have the same impact on mental and physical efficiency like two nights of complete sleep deprivation.

Asked for their personal experience with fatigue, the sensation of strong fatigue prevails in 27% of the female and 14% of the male population. Other studies say that females seem to suffer more frequently from insomnia than males. Taking into account that the prevalence for SRBD is 2.5 times higher in males [Penz 05], it can be assumed that in females stress is more likely to be a trigger for insomnia complaints than organic diseases.

In [Temm 06] the authors claimed that at least 3% of the adult population are suffering from manifest sleep disorders. The ratio male to female patients is said to be 2 : 1, but converges after the menopause. In the group of the 30 - 60 years old 16% of male and 22% of the female confess daytime fatigue/sleepiness, 24% of male and 9% of female have an AHI^1 higher than 5, taking both criteria there are 4% of male and 2% of the female population suffering from sleep apnea. The percentage of people snoring and suffering from daytime fatigue is shown to be ten times higher. The risk increases with age and the Body Mass Index (see p. 18), which is of pronounced interest, when recalling that the population is becoming older and older and increasingly obese.

Summing up all facts so far, the typical patient for obstructive sleep apnea (see /2.5.4/) is male, older than 40 years, overweight and suffering from hypertension. In the group of the 30 - 60 year olds, 9% of the female and 24% of the male show first indicators [Virc 04].

---

[1] Measure for the number of sleep disturbances per time unit, e.g., one hour, affecting sleep quality, /2.5.6/

The prevalence for central sleep apnea (see /2.5.4/) is lower, but increases with age. Thus, subjects younger than 45 years show symptoms only seldom, in the group of the 45 - 64 years of age a prevalence of 0.4% was found, which rose to 1.1% in subjects older than 65 years [Penz 05].

In [Air 06] the author claims that 90% of all people in Germany who suffer from sleep apnea are untreated. According to this publication there are 250.000 patients currently in therapy, but there is supposed to be a total of 2.5 Million. This suits perfectly to claims in [Pete 95] that many patients suffering from SRBD are falsely treated for cardiovascular diseases, because the true underlying reason is not diagnosed.

The big variations of the different studies result from three main reasons: the selected set of patients, the variability of the measurement equipment, and the fact that the definitions of the different types of sleep events are not standardized.

The DGSM (Deutsche Gesellschaft für Schlafforschung und Schlafmedizin, German Sleep Society) estimates that only about 1% of all patients complaining about their sleep quality suffers from SRBD [Penz 05]. Other authors claim that SRBD is found in 8% of the male subjects aged 40 - 60 years. The main group is obese middle-aged males exhibiting loud and irregular snoring. Moreover, patients with hypertension and cardio-vascular diseases are very likely to suffer from an undetected sleep disease which worsens the medical condition or even creates it. Apart from the snoring hypersomnia[2] is also a significant signpost, as it is found in about one third of the patients [Pete 95].

Even though mainly adults from midlife onward suffer from SRBD, children and babies may suffer from it as well. Medical issues found in this group are for example babies dying of sudden infant death syndrome (SIDS) and children with growth retardation.

2.2 Classification of Sleep Disorders

In 1979 a first attempt to classify sleep diseases and concurring impairments was conducted. This classification was based on the observed symptoms which led to a reoccurrence of the same pathological reasons in several groups of symptoms [Grot 96].

Therefore, in 1990 the former "American Sleep Disorders Association", now the "American Academy of Sleep Medicine", revised this classification system and introduced some updates to it. This renewed release was named "International Classification of Sleep Disorders" (ICSD) [Hade 04].

---

[2] Hypersomnia is a physiological state where patients experience a strong urge to sleep.

Insomnias	Primary Insomnias, Insomnias due to environmental conditions, Insomnias due to other existing diseases
SRBD	The different types of SRBD /2.5/
Hypersomnias without SRBD	Narcolepsy, lack of sleep hygiene, hypersomnias due to existing diseases, drugs
Disturbances of the circadian rhythm	Jet-lag, shift working
Parasomnia	Sleep walking, teeth grinding (bruxism), head banging, talking in sleep; usually they do not affect the quality of sleep
Sleep related Movement Disorders	Restless Leg Syndrome (RLS)
Other sleep disturbances	Normal variants and sleep disorders due to other diseases, proposed disorders

Table 2.1: ICSD-2

In 2005 the new ICSD-2 was introduced. Even though a few new classes were defined and some diseases were regrouped to reflect new research results, the old classification system can still be used. The ICSD-2 consists of the classes mentioned in Table 2.1. According to this classification pattern the SRBD belong to the class of the *intrinsic sleep disorders*. In [Pete 87] the authors proposed a more differentiated classification which allows assigning observed symptoms to different subgroups to account for the wide variety of sleep disorders.

Some of the risk factors introduced beforehand, e.g., alcohol and medication, can be grouped into *Hypersomnias without SRBD* as they are mainly due to a lack of sleep hygiene, i.e., due to "bad habits". Likewise, jet-lag and shift working could be assigned to this group, but usually these are not "voluntary". Accordingly, these influences are considered separately during the diagnosis (see /2.8/).

2.3 About Breathing

Breathing[3] is a compound mechanism. The respiratory center in the brain gathers the gas partial pressures from different chemoreceptors for oxygen (O_2) and carbon dioxide (CO_2) in order to "compute" a respiratory drive, which varies in frequency and intensity. On the intake of air the respiratory center has to trigger different muscle groups in a well-defined order: First, the muscles dilating the pharynx and the upper airways have to be put into action. Second, the muscles of the chest (thorax) and the belly (diaphragm) have to be driven in order to widen the lungs which finally entails the ventilation. Expiration is accomplished in a simpler way, as it usually just means releasing the muscle tone and, the higher pressure in the lungs compared to the environment will do the rest. (In the case of forced expiration the muscles of the thorax and diaphragm have to be triggered.)

Usually, breathing is under autonomous control, thus, it happens "automatically". Nevertheless, it provides a "manual override mode", which means it can be influenced deliberately through the cortex to speak, cough, and while diving.

2.4 About Sleep

Sleep is not just a period of doing nothing with eyes closed. It is essential for physiological and mental recreation, i.e., during sleep a lot of processes to keep the body and soul intact are accomplished like repairing cells, the operation of the immune system, and a "garbage collection" of psychological stressors. All evolutionarily higher species are known to implement a sleep procedure.

2.4.1 Entering Sleep

How is it possible that the subject's breathing works perfectly while awake, but fails while asleep? This Section is meant to supply a short answer to this question.

During the process of entering sleep the set points of the autonomous (respiration, circulation, and digestion), the endocrine (hormonal), and the temperature control system are modified according to the different sleep stages (see /2.4.2/). This results in a lower respiratory drive and, important for later considerations, lower muscle

---

[3]Under special circumstances, there is a differentiation between the terms "Breathing" and "Respiration". Breathing means only the ventilation of fresh air into the lungs, whereas respiration includes the gas exchange in the lungs down to single cells as well. This differentiation is of importance for discussing lung diseases, but for the purpose of this work there is no need to differentiate between them. Hence, both terms are used synonymously throughout this work in accordance with the literature concerning sleep diseases.

tone as well. Moreover, the respiratory pump tends to hypoventilation in horizontal position, which is the usual sleep position.

The activity of the brain is modified as well. This can be observed in an electroencephalogram (EEG) which is the recording of the electrical activity of the brain. During wake state the frequency of the recorded waves is high and the waves look a little "messy", as each area of the brain operates independently. Falling asleep the frequencies drop significantly and the EEC amplitude rises as the different areas of the brain synchronize with one another. The patterns shown in the EEG define the subject's sleep stage (see /2.4.2/).

If breathing fails due to respiratory instabilities during sleep, the way to restore proper breathing is to wake up the subject and reset the respiratory set points to their wake state condition. Waking up is performed by issuing an arousal (see /2.5.3/). This is something to keep in mind as it is of essential importance for SRBD.

2.4.2 Sleep Architecture

Sleep has different levels of "deepness" which are called *sleep stages*. The different sleep stages are determined using a combination of the already mentioned EEG, electrooculogram (EOG[4]) and electromyogram (EMG[5]).

Except for the "wake state" there are five sleep stages. The first two are called "light sleep" and the second two "deep sleep"[6]. These sleep stages are numbered from 1 - 4. The fifth sleep stage is called "Rapid Eye Movement sleep" (REM[7]) because of the rapid eye movements occurring in parts of this sleep stage. As REM sleep differs a lot from the other four sleep stages, there exists also a coarse differentiation of the sleep stages into REM and NREM, i.e., "Non-REM", stages.

The process of falling asleep is characterized by dropping frequencies of the brain waves and heart rates accompanied by the relaxation of the muscle tension. The sleep stages can be characterized as follows [Tels 04]:

NREM 1 - 2 The activity of the heart and the respiration is lower and becomes less variable. Skeleton muscles are progressively released. These sleep stages are characterized by a low arousal threshold, i.e., the subject can be woken up easily.

---

[4]EOG is a recording of the movements of the eyes (see /2.8.1/)
[5]EMG is a recording of the electrical activity of the skeleton muscles (see /2.8.1/)
[6]Deep sleep is sometimes called "slow wave sleep" (SWS) in literature because of the low frequencies found in the EEG
[7]Sometimes, REM sleep is also called "dream sleep", as dreams are believed to occur mainly in this sleep stage.

2.4. About Sleep

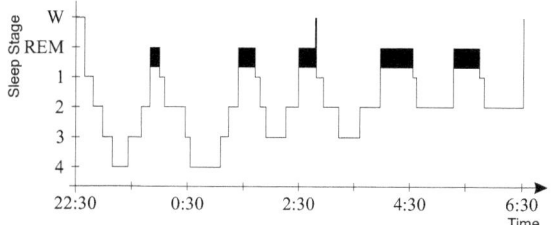

Figure 2.1: A hypnogram is derived from the evaluation of EEG, EMG, and EOG signals (see /2.8.1/) and shows the course of the different sleep stages over the night. This figure shows a hypnogram of a healthy subject. See Figure 2.6 as well.

NREM 3 - 4 During these sleep stages the activity of the heart and respiration drops to the minimum level, and, likewise, the fluctuations of both frequencies. The skeleton muscle tension is further released. Deprivation of these sleep stages results in tiredness and greatly reduced physiological and mental efficiency.

REM Sleep During REM sleep the autonomic system is a "mess", i.e., temperature, blood pressure, and the heart rate show large variations. The respiratory drive is very unsteady. The extensive reduction of the muscle tone hinders the dilation of the upper air way, increasing the respiratory resistance by a factor of two to three compared to wake state. Accordingly, the mechanical load to keep up respiration is elevated[8]. REM sleep exhibits very high mental activity which is attributed to the dream phases. An almost complete paralysis of the skeleton muscles (usually) inhibits the direct bodily reaction to the dreamt motions. In REM sleep the arousal threshold is highest, i.e., the subject can be waken up hardly. Accordingly, an arousal issued by the brain is most likely to fail (see /3.3.1/).

The different sleep stages change cyclically according to a fixed pattern, which is called **sleep architecture**. Usually, such a cycle takes 90 ± 30 minutes. Figure 2.1 shows five repetitions during an approximately eight hour sleep. The illustration of the sleep stages over time is called a *hypnogram*.

As can be seen from the hypnogram in Figure 2.1 the different sleep stages are not equally distributed. NREM sleep makes up 75% of the total sleep time (TST, with NREM 1 - 2 covering about 50 - 55% of the TST and NREM 3 - 4 standing

---
[8]This instability of the life supporting functions and the accompanying physiological strain are the reason why mortality is highest in the early morning hours.

for approximately 20 - 25% of the TST. REM sleep covers the remaining 25% of the TST.

Additionally, the distribution of the sleep stages in each sleep cycle changes over the night: After the onset of sleep the first two sleep cycles are dominated by deep sleep, whereas toward the morning the REM sleep becomes dominant as can be seen in Figure 2.1.

Apart from the variation of each sleep cycle along the night, the pattern and the distribution of the sleep stages additionally undergo some changes in the course of a lifetime, i.e., for example elderly people usually expose shorter overall sleep durations and less NREM 3 - 4 than adolescents.

Each step in the sleep architecture from a deeper toward a lighter sleep stage, e.g., from NREM 4 to NREM 3, the body accomplishes by an **arousal**[9] (see /3.3/). This is meant to say that an arousal is something basically essential for the (healthy) sleep architecture, even though it may appear as something primarily pathologic in the light of an apnea (see /2.6/).

2.4.3 Influences on Sleep

It has already been mentioned that sleep is a central vital function and that there are strong cross-correlations between sleep and other diseases or any other physiological activity. For example, in [Cole 82] the authors evaluated more than 1000 polysomnography (PSG, /2.8.1/) based diagnoses and concluded that from all of the patients suffering from insomnia 34.9% also had psychological problems and another 12.4% were afflicted with alcohol or drug abuse.

The by far largest fraction of sleep diseases is caused by (see /2.1/ as well):

- Psychological diseases, e.g., depressions (24% of insomniac patients suffer from a depression and 53% from another psychological disorder [Char 89].)

- Psychoses, e.g., schizophrenia

- Anxiety Disorders, e.g., phobias

- Organic Sleep Disorders, e.g., Restless Leg Syndrome (movements of the legs during sleep)

- Medication, drugs

---

[9]There exist different definitions for arousals: according to the AASM there are no arousals in NREM, other authors, e.g., C-H Tsai, require them for NREM sleep stage changes as well. In other definitions, e.g., RaK, only an EEG activation for longer than three seconds is given as characteristic [Thom 03].

2.5. Types and Severity of SRBD Events

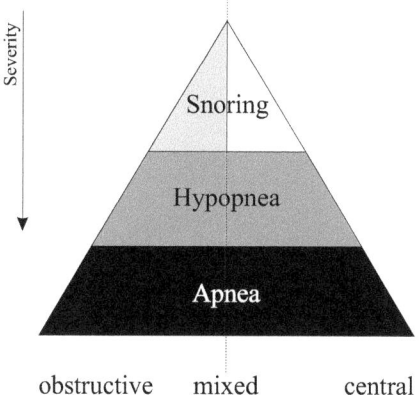

Figure 2.2: "Iceberg" representing the different types of SRBD events: a) Snoring is the one effect which is normally noticed whereas the "real dimension" of the disease is not obvious (Snoring is only half-shaded as a subject suffering from only central SRBD does not snore). b) The disease severity increases from the tip down to the foundation. c) The two types, i.e., obstructive and central, support the iceberg from either side.

- Alcohol

Even though these causes are responsible for the main part of all sleep disorders, they are not in the scope of this work and, therefore, are mentioned only for completeness.

2.5 Types and Severity of SRBD Events

This Section provides an introduction to the different types of SRBD events and the criteria according to which they are classified. An overview is given in Figure 2.2.

Among the SRBD events there are snoring, **hypopnea**, and **apnea**. Each of them can be provoked by an obstruction in the upper airways or by a loss of respiratory drive in the brain's respiratory center.

2.5.1 Snoring

Snoring is the most obvious — and for the spouse the most annoying – symptom of an impairment of the respiratory tract. Snoring is very common in the population. But even though 28% of the female and 44% of the male population claim to snore almost or each night, SRBD were found in only 9% of the females and 24% of the males in polysomnographic examinations. [Penz 05] Therefore, it can be assumed, snoring itself is only a very weak indicator for SRBD. In short: snoring is not sleep apnea, but sleep apnea is often accompanied by snoring (see /2.6/)[10].

Snoring is defined as "the predominantly inspiratoric sound, which is caused by the breathing dependent vibration of the flexible parts of the oropharynx[11]". [Virc 04]

It is more likely to happen during inspiration because of the negative pressure in the respiratory tract. Snoring occurs more frequently in obese people and in dorsal[12] position.

2.5.2 Hypopnea

A hypopnea describes reduced ventilation due to a partial obstruction of the upper airways or a drop of respiratory drive. Its occurrence is more likely in REM sleep.

The criteria for a hypopnea is an air flow reduction of $> 50\%$, on which most laboratories agree, but some of them require an air flow drop of two thirds. Some laboratories require a drop of $PaO_2 > 5\%$ as a consequence of the reduced ventilation, whereas others don't. Accoriding to different difinitions applied the number of annotated hypopneas varies form one sleep laboratory to another.

To make results from different sleep laboratories more comparable, there is a proposed standard which says: A hypopnea is a drop of air flow $> 50\%$ which lasts longer than ten seconds and is terminated by an arousal and/or a desaturation of more than 3% [Penz 05].

If hypopneas occur frequently during the night, the resulting disease is called "Sleep Hypopnea Syndrome" (SHS).

Even though air flow is persisting during hypopnea periods, the resulting hypoxemias and arousals may make the SHS indistinguishable from the Sleep Apnea Syndrome (SAS) where ventilation completely declines. The sequels in either case are just as severe.

2.5.3 Apnea

Apnea means the complete cessation of respiratory air flow because of complete obstruction of the upper airways or a complete loss of respiratory drive.

---

[10]However, new research results hint that the longterm effects of heavy snoring and the collateral ventilation limitations are comparable to those produced by an actual apnea

[11]Medical term for throat

[12]dorsal: on the back

2.5. Types and Severity of SRBD Events

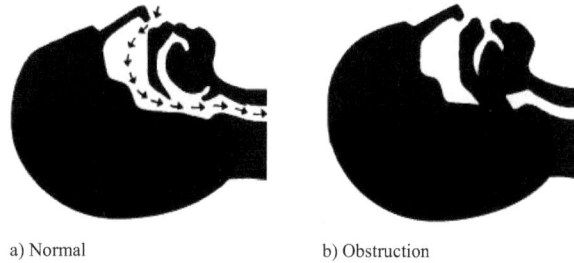

a) Normal   b) Obstruction

Figure 2.3: Genesis of obstructive apnea (Original pictures were taken from www.sleepapnea.org)

The definition of an apnea is less vague. A respiratory event is named apnea, if respiration ceases for more than 10 seconds and is accompanied by a decrease of oxygen saturation > 3 - 4%.
An apnea may last from 10 seconds up to 3 minutes [Lasc 06].

2.5.4 Obstructive and Central Events

This Section will provide a short introduction to the two triggers of sleep apnea events and explain what they have in common and where they differ from one another.

Obstructive Sleep Apnea Hypopnea Syndrome

The Obstructive Sleep Apnea Hypopnea Syndrome (OSAHS) is usually only called "Obstructive Sleep Apnea Syndrome" (OSAS), because a hypopnea may have the same impact on the subject's health as an apnea (see /2.5.2/).
The obstruction of the airways is shown in Figure 2.3. Entering sleep the muscle tone is reduced. Thus, the throat collapses due to the inspiratoric negative pressure or the velum blocks the upper airways due to gravitational effects. The blockage can be complete or partial. It may be accompanied by snoring. Because of the reduced muscle tone in sleep stages NREM 3 - 4 and REM, obstructive sleep apneas are most likely to happen in these sleep stages.

Central Sleep Apnea Syndrome

The Central Sleep Apnea Syndrome (CSAS) is characterized by a temporary loss of central respiratory stimuli leading to a suspension of the *respiratory pump*. In contrast to the obstructive sleep apnea there is no mechanical blockage of the upper airways. Central sleep apneas are rarer than obstructive sleep apneas (see /2.1/). The main group of subjects affected is males of higher age.

Central sleep apneas of 10 - 20 seconds occur in healthy subjects as well, especially during REM sleep and while entering sleep (see /2.4.1/) because of instabilities of the respiratory center. Moreover, central apneas are common in great heights, e.g., during mountain climbing, which is why this type is also called "High Altitude Sleep Apnea".

2.5.5 Mixed Sleep Apnea

Along with the described "pure" apnea types – obstructive and central – combinations of both forms appear in clinical practice which are called mixed apneas.

A mixed apnea arises from an initial disturbance of the respiratory center entailing a central apnea which is followed by an obstructive apnea [Lasc 06]. The obstructive apnea is explained by the loss of muscle tone during the central apnea. The obstructive phase is terminated by an arousal.

Differentiating Obstructive from Central SRBD Events

In the case of an obstructive apnea a blockage entails the cessation of the air flow, while the body still attempts to breathe, i.e., the respiratory effort) persists. This is shown in Figure 2.4 on the right side. In combination with the blockage of the upper airways the persisting respiratory effort entails the so called "inverted or paradox" breathing. It is characterized by anti-parallel thoracic and abdominal breathing excursions. The subsequent increase in intrathoracic pressure swings favors an arousal (via baroreceptors).

In the case of a central apnea there is no blockage of the upper airway, but the respiratory center does no longer issue any triggers to the respiratory muscles. Accordingly, there is no respiratory effort and no ventilation, which is shown in Figure 2.4 on the left.

2.5.6 Quantity

The standard indicator for the severity of SRBD is the so called "Apnea-Hypopnea-Index" (AHI). The AHI counts the number of SRBD events within a defined time period – usually an hour or the complete night.

To give an idea of the degree of severity, Table 2.2 lists the ranges of the AHI and the associated severity level.

2.5. Types and Severity of SRBD Events

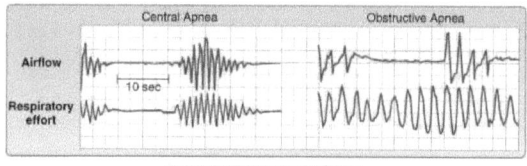

Copyright 2005 by Elsevier Science

Figure 2.4: Comparison between central (left) and obstructive (right) sleep apneas: In the upper panel of either side the respiratory flow, i.e., the degree of ventilation, is shown. In the lower panel the respiratory effort, i.e., the attempt of the subject's body to breathe by contracting and releasing the muscles of chest and belly, is outlined. A comparison of the respiratory effort during the apnea phases reveals the difference between both types: during a central apnea, the subject's body no longer triggers the respiratory muscles, i.e., there is no effort, whereas during an obstructive apnea the subject's body even increases its attempts to breathe over the duration of the apnea (For more details see /2.5/, Figure taken from [Kryg 05])

Events an Hour	Level of Severity
5 - 15	mild
15 - 30	moderate
> 30	severe

Table 2.2: AHI and severity of the SRBD according to ICSD-2

This classification is motivated by the observation that the frequency of the events is correlated to the degree of pathologic impact on the subject's body. Especially in research studies, the AHI is extended by including the duration of the events. Due to the correlation between the event duration and the degree of oxygen desaturation, the duration serves as an additional marker for the impact on the subject's health. In [Temm 06] the authors state that in younger subjects usually the events are of such short duration that there is only a negligible desaturation, whereas in older subjects the durations are remarkably longer, thus, leading to significant desaturation.

Other quantification systems do not count sleep events, but the events of oxygen desaturations of more than 3% and use an AHI > 40 to describe severity degrees [Hade 04].

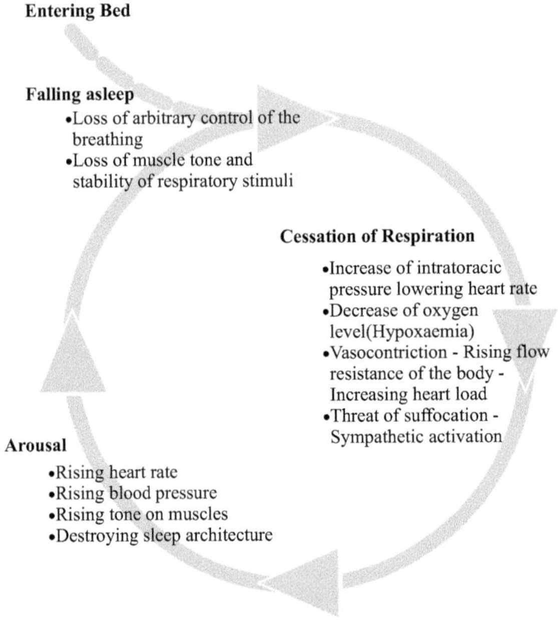

Entering Bed

Falling asleep
• Loss of arbitrary control of the breathing
• Loss of muscle tone and stability of respiratory stimuli

Cessation of Respiration
• Increase of intratoracic pressure lowering heart rate
• Decrease of oxygen level(Hypoxaemia)
• Vasocontriction - Rising flow resistance of the body - Increasing heart load
• Threat of suffocation - Sympathetic activation

Arousal
• Rising heart rate
• Rising blood pressure
• Rising tone on muscles
• Destroying sleep architecture

Figure 2.5: Vicious cycle of (successive) sleep apneas: It starts with the subject entering the bed. When the subject falls asleep, the tone of the muscles which dilate the throat subsides which eventually results in an apnea. Without ventilation the oxygen level drops which finally provokes an arousal to prevent suffocation. The arousal reestablishes proper breathing – and the cycle starts over again. (Analog sequence for the central apnea triggered by a lack of respiratory stimulus)

2.6 Course of Events during an Apnea – A vicious Cycle

This Chapter gives a short overview of the events and their sequence during the occurrence of a sleep apnea[13]. More details will be discussed in later Chapters.

The course of events could be summarized as in Figure 2.5: It starts with the onset of sleep. With the subject diving deeper into the hierarchy of sleep stages and the accompanying loss of muscle tone or respiratory drive, respectively, an obstructive /2.5.4/ or central /2.5.4/ sleep apnea occurs. As a consequence, no more fresh air is ventilated into the lungs and the saturation of the blood oxygen

---

[13]As mentioned there are different types of "sleep apneas" (see /2.5/). Nevertheless, as their common characteristic is the cessation of the breathing, they are referred to by the term "apnea" for convenience reasons.

2.6. Course of Events during an Apnea – A vicious Cycle

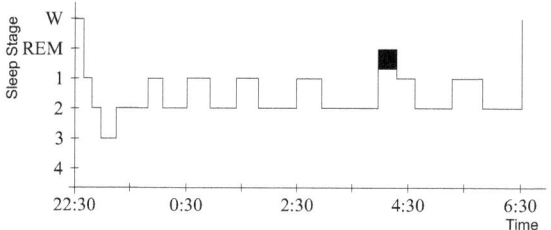

Figure 2.6: Hypnogram of a distorted sleep architecture; see Figure 2.1 as well.

level declines. As soon as desaturation becomes a serious threat, the brain issues an arousal[14] to restore wake state conditions of the respiratory system.

The activations of the central nervous system usually last no longer than five seconds and passes unnoticed by the subject's consciousness. However, in [Blas 03], it is explained that sympathetic activity (see /3.3/) remained at high levels up to 40 seconds after an acoustically provoked arousal. The authors' assumption was that sympathetic activity might accumulate, if apnea events are fired in close succession. Additionally, in [Brin 02], the author claims that the HR at rest is increased depending on the degree of the SRBD. The arousals lead to a sleep fragmentation and a destruction of the healthy sleep architecture. If there are more than 100 arousals a night of prolonged duration, the sleep is non-restorative and daytime efficiency is impaired alike.

In the phase following the arousal the lack of oxygen saturation is quickly compensated by deep breaths at an increased breathing frequency. This process is supported by a faster beating heart, which increases the amount of blood gases (O_2 and CO_2) conveyed.

Figure 2.6 shows an example for a distorted sleep architecture with an increase of NREM 1 and 2 at the expense of NREM 3 and 4 and REM sleep. In the end, it is the destroyed sleep architecture, which is an indicator for the expectable sequels. Or put positively: the sleep architecture is a measure of sleep quality.

In this vicious cycle sleep affects the breathing and the breathing in return affects sleep. It may cycle around up to several hundred times a night.

---

[14] An arousal is a short microactivation of the central nervous system by increasing the sympathetic tone (see /3.3/).

2.7 Symptoms, Risk Factors, and Medical Risks

This Section is an overview over all the symptoms, risk factors and medical risks linked to SRBD.

2.7.1 Symptoms

The most prominent symptoms are *daytime fatigue* and *sleepiness*. A warning signal is when the subject experiences *imperative sleep compulsion* at monotonous tasks like driving a car along a motorway or controlling a machinery plant.

The reduced sleep quality entails *reduced mental and physical efficiency* which is usually accompanied by *forgetfulness* and *poor concentration*. In this state the subjects tend to lose their capability to cope with everyday demands which may lead to *depressions*.

After a prolonged period of suffering from SRBD, *cardio-vascular diseases* will show up. These are usually related to the emerging *hypertension* which persists even during the night as sympathetic activity remains high due to the SRBD events.

2.7.2 Risk Factors for SRBD

Adipositas is the medical term to describe an obese subject. One measure to describe the degree of obesity is the Body Mass Index (BMI[15]). Adipositas with a BMI > 35 (normal range: $20 \leq BMI < 25$) increases the risk of suffering from SRBD. Adipositas is a risk factor in particular for men which is assumed to be rooted in the distribution of body fat.

As SRBD are more likely to happen in the *male* population (see /2.1/), the subject's *gender* has to be considered a risk factor. There are only assumptions for this phenomenon. Possible reasons are the higher percentage of trunk fat and the influences of hormones, as higher levels of progesterone increase the respiratory drive and the tone on the muscles dilating the upper airways, whereas testosterone leads to the opposite effects. Other experts tend to blame it on differences in the oropharyngeal anatomy.

Existing diseases of the lungs serve as a predisposition. Within this group are *Chronic Obstructive Pulmonary Disease (COPD)* and *Asthma Bronchiale*.

Anatomic Abnormalities may be responsible for obstructive SRBD as well, e.g., *large tonsils* and *anatomic abnormalities of the jaw and its position*. These causations are usually treated with surgery.

---

[15]The BMI is defined as: $BMI = \frac{\text{body mass [kg]}}{(\text{height [m]})^2}$.

2.8. Diagnostic Procedures

Alcohol causes vasodilatation on the pharyngeal mucosa, i.e., a widening of the tissue in the throat, narrowing the diameter. Moreover, it leads to a state of relaxation lowering the muscle tone on the pharyngeal dilatation muscles, which makes the airways prone to collapse.

The *Body Position* during sleep also influences the likeliness of suffering from SRBD: Lying on the back is a risk factor, as gravity increases the likeliness that the vellum drops down to block the trachea resulting in an obstruction of the airways (see Figure 2.3).

Cardiac Insufficiency is often found in the context of central apneas.

2.7.3 Medical Consequences of OSAHS

The most obvious impact of SRBD on the subject is *hypersomnia* (also referred to as *hypersomnolence* [Pete 95]). Hypersomnia accumulates to a point, where the subject experiences an "imperative sleep compulsion".

The desaturation of oxygen in the blood – especially when daytime saturation is low as well – leads to *reduced intellectual efficiency* [Temm 06]. Quite often the feeling of no longer being able to cope with everyday challenges and the resulting constant stress and anxiety accumulate to *depressions*.

SRBD are considered an independent risk factor for *hypertension*[16], i.e., *high blood pressure*, by the National Institute for Health (NIH) since May 2003. [Hade 04] Hypertension itself is closely linked to heart attacks and cerebral insults.

The assumption that SRBD leads to *chronic heart disease* (CHD) could be asserted in several studies, while its influence could not be isolated from accompanying risk factors.

All risks can be significantly reduced by applying CPAP therapy (see [Hade 04]) and can even be prevented, when early diagnosis and therapy are provided [Pete 95].

2.8 Diagnostic Procedures

Diagnosing sleep disorders is a complex procedure. And there are two main reasons that add to this complexity. First, the clinical picture itself is multi-faceted, because sleep is affected by many bodily systems. Second, the subject's consciousness is knocked out in sleep. Therefore, the anamnesis provided by the subject

---

[16]This rating is supported by the finding that hypertension in the arterial circulation is found in more than 60% of the SRBD patients. This hypertension is most likely caused by the negative intrathoracic pressures resulting in a higher cardiac preload [Virc 04] and hypoxemia.

himself/herself is only vague, which is why the subject can not contribute to the diagnostic process.

To help physicians along their diagnosis and to ensure a high level of diagnostic quality, the Deutsche Gesellschaft für Schlafmedizin (DGSM, see p. 26) has issued a clinical guideline entitled "Nicht erholsamer Schlaf (engl.: Non-restorative Sleep)". The clinical algorithm mainly consists of a flowchart, which is given in Figure 2.7.

The whole procedure starts with box 0, where the patient enters the medical practice and complains about "having slept badly", i.e., in proper terminology "non-restorative sleep".

Based on the patient's subjective rating[17] or on objective tests[18] the medic personal tries to gain an overview of the patient's efficiency (sleepiness, fatigue, concentration failure, lack of stimuli) (box 1). In case there is no impairment, the patient is given information (box 4) on correct sleep hygiene (p. 24).

In case there is a manifest impairment, the physician has to check the patient's habits concerning sleep (boxes 2 and 3). Among the habits which have an impact on sleep are the usage of alcohol, times and durations of sleep, environmental, and working conditions, i.e., shift work, jet lag, which might be responsible for insomnia. If bad habits are found, the patient is given information on how to improve the sleep circumstances (box 4).

The next step is to find out, whether the patient takes drugs which have an impact on sleep (box 5). Among these are analeptics, barbiturates, antihypertensive drugs, asthma therapeutics, or analgesics. If the patient uses drugs from these groups, the physician will have to find a replacement which affects sleep less or tell the patient to give up on that drug, if possible (box 6).

If the symptoms described by the patient hint on an underlying psychological or physiological disease (box 7), then, these have to be treated at first (box 8).

Finally, if no reason was found along the algorithm, the patient will have to undergo a cardio-respiratory polysomnography (PSG, p. 21) The PSG is conducted at special facilities, the so called sleep laboratories. In Germany, these are called for example "Schlafmedizinisches Zentrum" (SMZ, p. 26).

---

[17]The patient's self-estimation is based on questionnaires like *Stanford Sleepiness Scale* [Virc 04], *Epworth Sleepiness Scale* [Schl 07] (self-test on www.schlaf.de), and *Landecker Inventar für Schlafstörungen* [Hofe 06] and [None 05].
[18]*Multiple Sleep Latency Test* [Rich 78], *Maintenance of Wakefulness Test*, and *Pupillographic Sleepiness Test*

2.8. Diagnostic Procedures

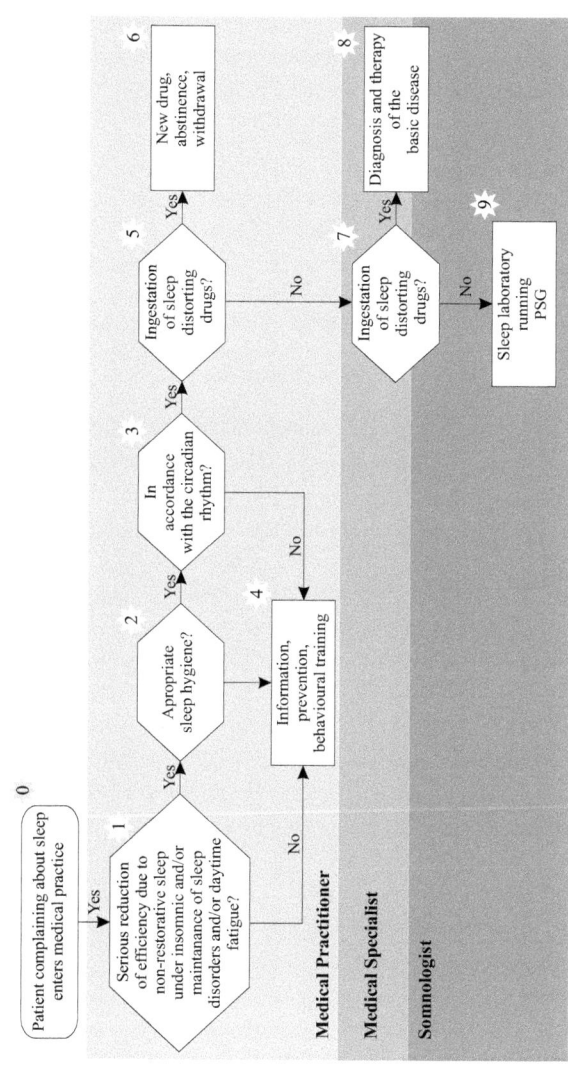

Figure 2.7: Clinical algorithm for diagnosing sleep disorders

2.8.1 Cardio-respiratory Polysomnography

Cardio-respiratory Polysomnography (PSG) is a standardized method of registering sleep, breathing, activity of the heart and movements during sleep. Distortions of the sleep architecture can be retrieved and their possible causes, e.g., disordered respiration and body movements, can be investigated.

Today, Polysomnography is the most reliable method of detecting SRBD. Thus, it is the "gold standard" for the differential diagnosis of sleep disorders. However, it is a complex and complicated examination which is true regarding the technical aspect as well as the medical one. Hence, it has to take place in specialized medical facilities, the so called sleep laboratories. This directly yields three disadvantages:

- Polysomnography is a very costly examination.

- Patients often have to endure long queue times.

- Being torn out of familiar environment might affect – and is assumed to do so – the results. To compensate for this, patients are sometimes obliged to stay two subsequent nights at the sleep laboratory – the first to get acquainted with the situation and the second for the actual measurement.

During visual analysis the recorded data is evaluated in periods of 30 seconds which is the standard interval proposed by Rechtschaffen and Kales [Rech 68]. The complete PSG consists of up to 25 sensors. The most important ones will be explained shortly in the following:

Electroencephalogram The electroencephalogram (EEG) is a recording of the electrical activity of the brain. It is one of the parameters which are recorded to detect the sleep stage.

Electromyogram The electromyogram (EMG) is a recording of the action potentials of the muscles. It is commonly used to diagnose diseases of the peripheral nerves and muscles.

During the PSG the EMG is recorded to measure the muscle tone for two purposes: First, the muscle tone hints on the sleep stages in general and the enervation of the chin is recorded to detect the beginning and the end of the REM sleep phases. Second, the EMG is derived from the legs to detect leg movements during sleep.

Electrooculogram The electrooculogram (EOG) is a recording of the movements of the eyes. The EOG is indispensable for detecting REM sleep.

2.8. Diagnostic Procedures

Electrocardiogram The electrocardiogram (ECG or EKG) is a recording of the electrical activity of the myocardium, i.e., the heart (muscle). During a PSG usually only a one-channel-ECG is recorded. The electrodes are placed corresponding to the bi-polar precordial leads after Nehb (see [Hora 98]). The R-peaks, the P-, and T-waves (see /3.1.1/ and Figure 3.4) are of special importance.

Respiratory Flow The (respiratory) flow is the qualitative measurement of the air flow which passes through nose and mouth during the subject's breathing. The flow is one of the most important vital parameters of the PSG. It is used to detect hypopneas and apneas. Sometimes the parameter "snoring" is derived from this signal as well in order to reduce the number of necessary sensors.

Respiratory Effort In order to breathe, the chest and the belly widen under the effort of the respiratory musculature enlarging the volume of the lungs. The resulting negative pressure in the lungs causes the inflow of air. During the PSG the extensions of the chest (thorax) and the belly (abdomen) are registered separately by elastic belts around the body.

The effort signal is indispensable, because it is required to differentiate obstructive and central apneas. (see Figure 2.4)

Snoring The subject's snoring is recorded by means of a microphone or derived from the flow signal. Evaluating the snoring signal helps to differentiate central from obstructive apneas.

Oxygen Saturation The oxygen level[19] is an indicator for the efficiency of the respiration. Thus, it can be used to detect SRBD events. There are screening devices which evaluate this parameter exclusively. However, according to [Farn 96] the evaluation of only this single parameter is not reasonable, because they found a sensitivity of only 80% and a specifity of 71% in the detection of apnea. They blamed it on the fact that an apnea does not necessarily entail an oxygen desaturation of 4% or more. This is especially true for patients with proper lung function, where sensitivity was even worse. Moreover, in [Schu 06] it is stated that this method is very error-prone, because of internal signal processing in the devices themselves. These devices use low pass filters to calm the displayed value. However, very often the time constant of this filter is too long, thus, preventing the oxygen level from dropping beneath the defined level which conceals the SRBD event.

---

[19] Usually the oxygen saturation is "estimated" using pulse oxymeters. To hint on the measuring method, the value is labeled "SpO_2".

In healthy subjects the oxygen level ranges between 96 - 100%. But during long lasting apneas the level may drop down to 80%. Depending on the literature source, oxygen level drops of more than 3 - 4% are indicators for the occurrence of SRBD events.

Body Position Body position sensors indicate whether the subject lies on the back, the belly, or the sides during sleep.

Video The patient is recorded in his/her sleep for the purpose of verifying visually, whether EEG and/or EMG activity belongs to movements of the patient. This is required for the detection of movement disorders during sleep.

In order not to disturb the patient, the camera and the light are infra-red types, because infra-red light is not visible to the human eye.

Commercially available PSG Devices On the market there are quite a few manufacturers for PSG devices whereof two shall be named: SOMNOmedics for a very compact device and Weinmann for this equipment was used to record the data for this work.

SOMNOmedics markets a device with reduced feature set called SOMNOwatch [SOMN 06b]. This watch-like unit natively detects movements of the subject, but can be extended to measure all relevant vital parameters, e.g., ECG, EEG, and air flow, by attaching external sensors. They also provide a full-featured PSG system called SOMNOscreen [SOMN 06a].

Weinmann also provides a wide range of devices from screening devices, e.g., SOMNOcheck and SOMNOcheck effort, to complete PSG systems called SOMNOlab. The latter is the device which was used for the data recordings for this work (see /5.2.1/). They also market an extensive range of devices for sleep apnea therapy (see /2.9.2/).

2.9 Therapeutic Procedures

For the therapy of SRBD there are different approaches. Most of them do only suppress the occurrence of SRBD events, but do not actually provide healing. The simplest approaches are "oral appliances", e.g., protrusion splints, which aim at preventing the obstruction by shifting and fixing the jaw in a more advantageous position.

Surgery may provide real healing given the appropriate predispositions. Long time success can be achieved in about 20 % of the cases. Standard approaches are

2.9. Therapeutic Procedures

resections of tissue (or bone) in the area of the mouth, jaws, nose, throat, and tonsils, respectively. In severe case a uvulopalatopharyngoplastic surgery may be indicated. Even though the success rate is quite high with 50 %, many patients refrain from it, as it may result in a change of the sound of the patient's voice [Lasc 06].

The next Section hints on measurements which can be taken by everybody to improve the quality of sleep. And, finally, the CPAP therapy which is today's gold standard will be introduced.

2.9.1 Sleep Hygiene

The first step in the therapy of SRBD is to restore proper sleep hygiene. Sleep hygiene consists of promoting habits which support healthy sleep and avoiding those which conflict with it. Some Dos and Don'ts are listed here:

- DOs
    - Establish proper environmental conditions (temperature, no noise)
    - Establish proper daily rhythm, i.e., going to bed at the same time, developing a fixed going-to-bed-ritual, i.e., a fixed order of actions
    - Make sure to get enough sleep
- DON'Ts
    - Overweight
    - Abuse of alcohol and nicotine
    - Dorsal position
    - Extended daytime sleep
    - Largely varying bed times
    - Exciting and extremely emotional activities, e.g., watching horror movies

2.9.2 CPAP Therapy and its various Manifestations

Today's standard therapy is the "continuous positive airway pressure" (CPAP) therapy. It is the "purest" incarnation of the following principle: Before the patient goes to sleep at night, he/she attaches a mask (see Figure 2.8) to his/her face and switches on the pump which supplies the patient with a low positive[20] air pressure via the

---

[20]The air pressure supplied by the mask is "a little higher", e.g., 8 mbar [Jasc 08], than the atmospheric pressure.

30   Chapter 2. Sleep related Breathing Disorders

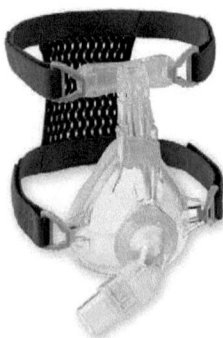

Figure 2.8: CPAP mask (Product Image from Weinmann.de)

mask, which prevents the oropharynx from collapsing during inspiration. Thus, the respiratory resistance of the airway remains low and no obstruction occurs.

While this explanation is quite straight forward for obstructive sleep apnea, it is really astonishing that CPAP often works as well with central sleep apnea, where the reason for the cessation of breathing is a lack of respiratory impulse from the brain.

Under CPAP therapy all vital functions are restored to their normal values, which is especially true, when treatment starts in an early stage. Restored functions are daytime vigilance, blood pressure, regular heart beat (if arrhythmia was SRBD induced), and most important a healthy sleep architecture. In more than two thirds of the patients sleep induced movement disorders vanished under CPAP therapy. Even mortality rate is reduced to average. The patient realizes the success of the therapy in most cases immediately after therapy onset. Just the same, the patient's quality of life is restored.

Because of the high benefit and the overall performance the CPAP therapy has established itself as the gold standard for therapy of the SRBD today. The patients' compliance is about 85%, but may drop to 50 - 80% on the long run.

Despite the benefits quite a few patients (depending on the source 5 - 50%) refuse to start the therapy at all or quit it within the first three months due to a dislike of wearing a mask at all or fear and panic of suffocating. The mask is the Achilles' heel of the CPAP therapy, because it is responsible for skin irritations due to contact pressure, leakage of air causing conjunctivitis or undersupply of pressure to the subject. The main side effects are, however, irritations of the mucosa of the upper air ways due to exsiccosis. The later can be avoided by using humidifiers, which are available from all major producers.

Attempts to improve the quality of the CPAP therapy by supplying oxygen instead of "normal air" to the patient showed that bradycardia during the compensation phase was in fact reduced, but the overall duration of the apnea events was prolonged as the respiratory stimulus was altered [Zwil 82].

For specific patients' needs modifications of the standard CPAP therapy were developed. First, there is the *Bi-PAP therapy* which adjusts the pressure to the patient's inspiratoric or expiratory phase. This is especially helpful for patients with adipositas, who require high CPAP pressures, or those with weak respiratory drive and muscles. The Bi-PAP devices provide the required therapy pressure during the patient's inspiratoric phase, but during the expiratory phase they significantly lower the supplied pressure to ease expiration.

Second, there are the *Auto-PAP devices* which aim at continuously adjusting the supplied air pressure to the patient's current needs in order to reduce pressure-induced sequels. Thus, the pressure follows the varying needs of the different sleep stages and the position of the patient.

2.10 Facilities, Institutions and other Resources

DGSM (Deutsche Gesellschaft für Schlafforschung und Schlafmedizin) provides a lot of information on their homepage on the Internet, which can be accessed via www.dgsm.de.

The DGSM approves facilities which provide a high level of quality and standardized diagnostic methods (see /2.8/) as "accredited by the DGSM". There, the patient can expect to be treated according to the latest developments in the field.

In Germany, there are more than 300 accredited sleep laboratories [Penz 05], where patients can be diagnosed using PSG (see /2.8.1/).

In addition, there are self-help groups, where affected subjects can go to ask others about their experiences with sleep laboratories, CPAP devices, and so on. These groups are quite helpful, because members are usually well-informed and know about the benefits of a certain device because of their own experience.

2.11 Summary and Preview

This Chapter was an introduction to sleep and the SRBD which are the target of this work. It was explained that sleep consists of different sleep stages which can roughly be assigned to three groups: light, deep, and REM sleep. These different sleep stages change according to a pattern which is called sleep architecture (see /2.4.2/). It was mentioned that in the end it is the destruction of the sleep architecture which leads to daytime fatigue, sleepiness, and sequel concerning the cardio-vascular system.

Different types of breathing disorders, i.e., snoring, hypopnea, and apnea (see /2.5/), were introduced by their definitions and explained. There was an explanation of the symptoms caused by those SRBD events and their effect on the subject's health state.

At the end, there was an introduction to the process of diagnosing SRBD. The way of diagnosing SRBD made obvious that sleep apneas are only one disorder of sleep, but there are many others which have to be considered as well.

This Chapter ended with a presentation of different sleep therapy methods including changes of habits as well as technical devices supplying positive air pressure. The latter devices are called CPAP and exist in a variety of flavors.

The next Chapter will be an introduction to the (human) heart. Starting with the blood circulation, the functional principle of the heart will be explained. One of the main points will be the recording and evaluation of the so called electrocardiogram which is the recording of the electrical activity of the heart.

Different influences on the electrocardiogram and how they relate to the SRBD events will be discussed.

Chapter 3

Medical Introduction to the Heart

This Chapter is an introduction to the medical basics of the human heart. It mainly focuses on the genesis of the Electrocardiogram (ECG) and its modulations due to the activity of the autonomous nervous system and varying load conditions.

The medical consequences of SRBD have been discussed in the previous Chapter in common. This Chapter now focuses on their impact on the ECG in detail, as this is the basis for the extracted features.

This Chapter is mainly based on [Hamm 01], [Hora 98], [Habe 03], and [Olsh 96].

3.1 The Heart and the Electrocardiogram

The heart is the blood pump of the body and maintains the blood circulation, whose main purpose is to supply oxygen to the cells of the body. The heart consists of four chambers, thereof two atria and two ventricles. During the diastole, i.e., the rest cycle of the heart, the blood flows from the atria into the dilating ventricles because of relieved muscle tone. During the next systole, i.e., the work cycle of the heart, the heart contracts and the blood is pumped into the body or the lungs, respectively, and the blood returning from there flows into the atria. An schematic of the complete human circulation is shown in Figure 3.1 (Seen from the front, Figure taken form [Psch 98]).

Starting the circulation in the lungs, where the oxygen is gathered from the breathed air via diffusion, the blood arrives at the left atrium. From the left ventricle the oxygen loaded blood is pumped into the organs of the body, e.g., the brain, the liver, and the muscles. The oxygen is burned to maintain the energy processes of the cells. Having unloaded the oxygen and now CO_2 loaded, the desaturated blood flows toward the heart and reaches the right atrium and ventricle. From there the blood flows to the lungs again and the cycle restarts.

34   Chapter 3. Medical Introduction to the Heart

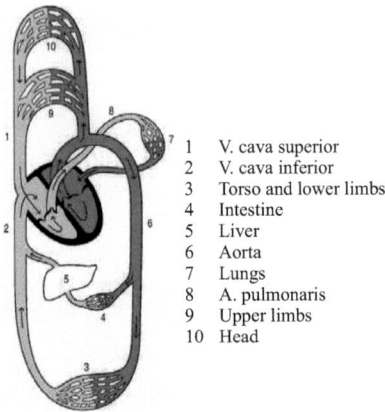

1   V. cava superior
2   V. cava inferior
3   Torso and lower limbs
4   Intestine
5   Liver
6   Aorta
7   Lungs
8   A. pulmonaris
9   Upper limbs
10 Head

Figure 3.1: Schematic of blood circulation in humans in front view (taken from [Psch 98]): the red blood is loaded with oxygen and the cyan blood with carbon dioxide.

The heart can be considered an "electro-mechanical device", i.e., it is controlled electrically to perform a mechanical action. The means of electrical control are depicted in Figure 3.2. All together the black parts constitute the *cardiac conduction system*.

In the healthy heart the main pacemaker is the *sinoatrial node* (SA). In contrary to "normal" nerve or muscle cells, its action potential is not stable (see /3.3.1/) which leads to periodic "shots" triggering the contraction of the heart. From the sinoatrial node the excitation passes along the atria, triggering the left and the right atrium, to the atrioventricular (AV) node.

As shown in Figure 3.2 the AV-node is placed between the right atrium and ventricle which explains the name. The AV-node introduces a deliberate delay into the conduction system. This delay accomplishes two purposes: First, it gives the atria more time to fill the ventricles with blood which increases their output. Second, it is responsible for filtering too high excitation frequencies due to atrial fibrillation, so they can not affect the ventricles. Thus, the AV-node guarantees that the ventricles maintain proper operation.

From the AV-node the excitation spreads along the His[1] fascicles into the Tawara[2] bundle brunches causing the complete myocardium to contract, i.e., the systole.

---
[1] Wilhelm His (born 1863/12/29 in Basel, died 1934/11/10 in Riehen), Swiss internist
[2] Sunao Tawara (born 1873/07/05 in Nakajima, died 1952), Japanese pathologist

3.1. The Heart and the Electrocardiogram

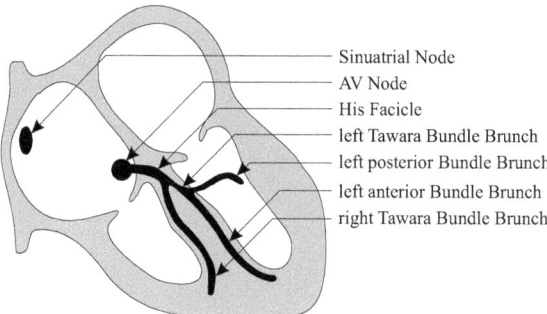

Figure 3.2: Components of the cardiac conduction system

Pacemaker	Eigenfrequency
Sinoatrial Node	60 – 80 bpm
AV-node	40 – 60 bpm
Ventricular Myocardium	20 – 40 bpm

Table 3.1: Cardiac pacemakers and their eigenfrequencies

As can be seen from the position of the conduction system components, the first chamber to contract is the right atrium and the last is the left ventricle.

As the heart is of such importance, the evolution built in redundancy concerning the frequency generation. In case the SA-node fails to trigger the contraction, the AV-node will stand in (at a lower frequency). And if there are no trigger signals at all, the ventricular myocardium starts free-running at an even lower frequency. Even though this multiple redundancy assures that the heart keeps working, the efficiency of the heart is greatly reduced, if the sinoatrial node fails, as the slower frequencies hinder a coping with higher work loads. The different redundant pacemakers and their eigenfrequencies in [bpm^3] are shown in Table 3.1.

The frequencies are adjusted to the subject's current load condition. The adjustment is controlled via two antagonists – sympathetic and parasympathetic nervous system (see /3.3/).

3.1.1 Recording an Electrocardiogram

All the muscle and nerve cells of the human body are operated on the mechanism of the action potential (see /3.3.1/ and Figure 3.10). At rest, the action potential is about -90 mV measured from the inner nerve to the surrounding cover. The action

---
[3]bpm: beats per minute; for details see /3.2/

36   Chapter 3. Medical Introduction to the Heart

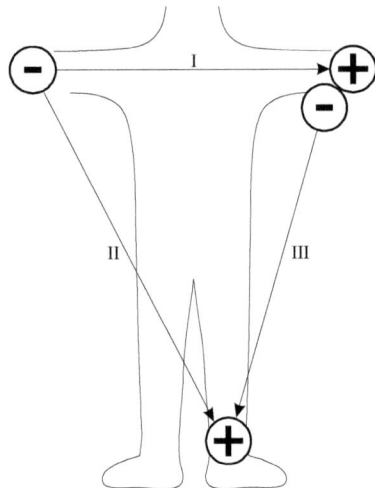

Figure 3.3: Standard pattern of placing the electrodes to retrieve an ECG according to Einthoven which is the most common ECG derivation.

potential is an electrical signal upon which the body's high speed transmission of information between the brain and the sensors, e.g., eyes and ears, or the actors, e.g., muscles, is based. This transmission is a "digital system", i.e., the signal is either on or off. The intensity of a perception is frequency encoded.

The heart is a conglomerate of muscle cells. Accordingly, it is (almost) impossible to measure a single action potential. But, as the electrical fields of all muscle cells add up based on superposition, it is possible to measure the resulting external electrical field, which is "at the heart" of recording an ECG. The electrical field is gathered by placing electrodes around the heart in defined patterns.

There exist different patterns for specific diagnostic questions. The pattern that is shown in Figure 3.3 is called the Einthoven[4] recording. The shape of the recorded ECG depends on the placement of the electrodes. Figure 3.4 shows an ECG wave as seen in Einthoven II (the recording which is used during a PSG (see /2.8.1/). This wave form consists of six distinguishable parts/points – each of them represents a different state of the heart's working cycle.

As already mentioned in Figure 3.4 each of the marked points belongs to a certain phase of excitation and the appropriate state of the work cycle:

---

[4]Willem Einthoven (born on 1860/05/21, died on 1927/09/28 in Leiden) received the Nobel prize for discovery of the mechanism of the electrocardiogram in 1924.

3.1. The Heart and the Electrocardiogram

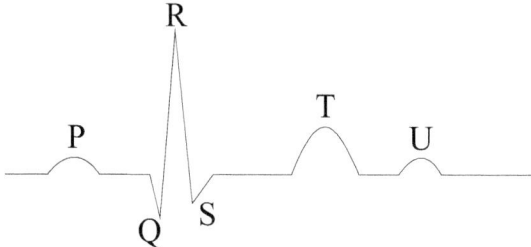

Figure 3.4: Principal morphology of an ECG wave if derived in Einthoven II configuration

- The P-wave is the result of the excitation of the atria.

- The QRS-complex is the representative of the excitation of the ventricles.

- The ST-segment is the phase after the full contraction, where no action potential is present and the segment is iso-electric (in a healthy subject).

- The T-wave is the indicator of the repolarization, the phase of reestablishing the action potential.

- The U-wave is not always visible and is said to be the result of fluctuations during the repolarization phase due to, e.g., electrolyte imbalances (The U-wave is not evaluated in this work and is mentioned just for completeness.).

3.1.2 Influences on the Recording of an ECG

As the ECG signal is a comparatively small voltage, i.e., approximately 1 - 10 mV, it is sensitive to disturbances. The most important non-technical influences are:

Subject's Position   The standard recordings of an ECG which are documented in the literature are recorded with the subject lying on his/her back. This procedure is standardized to have comparable circumstances. If the subject changes his/her position, gravity slightly shifts the heart around in the subject's chest. Hence, the ECG looks different, if the subject lies on his/her back, belly, or the two sides.

Breathing   The size of the lungs varies constantly during the breathing due to the volume of the air which is ventilated. The heart lying next to them is tilted in the chest which changes the direction of the electrical axis of the heart. This can be observed in the ECG as a changing amplitude of the ECG, especially the of the

R-peak (see /10.3/ and Figure 10.3). The influences of the respiratory arrhythmia are discussed in /3.3.1/.

The following technical influences are usually filtered during the preprocessing of the ECG signal (see /6.1/):

- Interferences of the mains supply (50 Hz in Europe)

- Recording device itself

3.2 Heart Rate and its Variability

3.2.1 Introduction

The heart rate (HR) and its variability (HRV) are important indicators for the subject's state – the physiological as well as the autonomous. The HR is the number of heart beats per minute given in the unit "beats per minute" ([bpm]). The HRV indicates the dynamics of the HR and describes its variation with time. Both parameters depend on the subject's current state, i.e., the current level of ANS activity.

The HR reflects the short-term state. For example, during exercise the HR rises and it drops under the lack of oxygen (see Figure 3.11 and explanation). Sleep also influences the set point of the HR (see /2.4.2/).

The HRV hints on both long-term conditions and sudden changes. Among the long-term influences are cardiovascular diseases and chronic stress which entail a low HRV, i.e., a constant HR. Among the ultra-short-term influences are sudden stress conditions, fear, shock, and other impacts on the central nervous activation – like arousals, which may be a result of a sleep apnea.

At rest, the normal heart rate of a human lies between 60 - 80 bpm[5]. Strong deviations from the standard HR are called either *bradycardia* for HRs below 40 bpm or *tachycardia* for HRs over 100 bpm.

Bradycardia may be induced by an SRBD event. In Figure 3.5 a patient with sleep apnea shows prolonged and profound bradyarrhythmias with absence of either atrial or ventricular contraction (see marker). The beat-by-beat blood pressure (BP) recording confirms the absence of any perfusion during the bradycardia.

---

[5]Higher HRs at rest may be found in OSAS (see /2.5.4/) subjects depending on the degree of their disease [Brin 02].

3.2. Heart Rate and its Variability

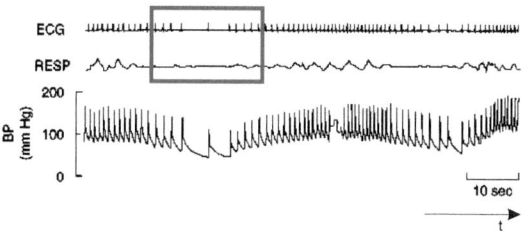

Figure 3.5: Bradycardia during an apnea event

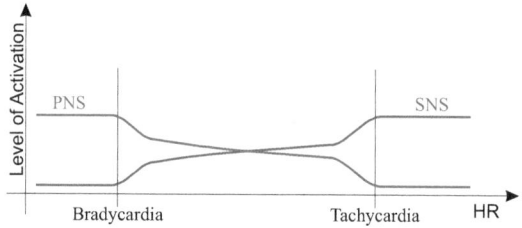

Figure 3.6: Principle of deriving the autonomous nervous activity from the HR: A high HR hints on a dominant activity of the sympathetic nervous system (SNS in the Figure) activity accompanied by a reduced activity of the parasympathetic nervous system (PNS in the Figure) and vice versa. An introduction of these terms is given in /3.3/.

3.2.2 HR and Sleep Apnea

As mentioned in /3.3.1/ the HR and its variability hint on the degree of the subject's autonomous activity. Hence, from the viewpoint of this work, the HR may be an indicator for the subject's sleep state and normal or distorted respiration, respectively. And the HRV suggests sudden changes in the subject's central nervous activity as come along with arousals. This will now be explained to some more detail.

The absolute values of the HR are a sign of the subject's general activation: a low HR is correlated to a dominance of the parasympathetic nervous system, whereas a high HR is driven by the sympathetic nervous system (see /3.3/). Figure 3.6 shows how to retrieve the sympathetic or parasympathetic overall activation from this parameter. A HR below 40 bpm is generally considered bradycardia and above 100 bpm tachycardia.

In a healthy subject, the overall trend of the HR over the night looks like shown in Figure 3.7. The heart rate at rest is mainly governed by a circadian regulation, i.e., on a daily basis under the influence of the intensity of light.

40   Chapter 3. Medical Introduction to the Heart

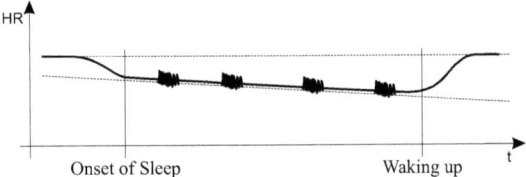

Figure 3.7: Gradient of the HR over the night form the onset of sleep until the waking up the next morning in a healthy subject. The four periods of HR disturbances belong to the REM sleep stages (see /2.4.2/).

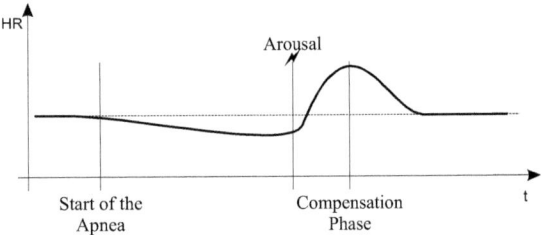

Figure 3.8: Gradient of the HR over an apnea: Due to the diver reflex the HR drops with the occurrence of the apnea. After the arousal entailing the end of the apnea the HR first overshoots to compensate for the lack of oxygen and, finally, returns to the HR before the apnea event (see also Figure 3.11).

It can be seen that the HR drops rapidly with the onset of sleep. Over the course of the night it keeps dropping slowly and rises to normal state with the subject waking up. This overall trend is interrupted by 3 - 4 phases of higher HR fluctuations which relate to the REM sleep state.

If the subject suffers from sleep apnea this standard curve is "speckled" with HR variations that look like Figure 3.8. As a result of intra-thoracic pressure variations and the diver reflex (see /3.3.1/) the HR slowly drops under the impact of an obstructive sleep apnea, until an arousal triggered autonomous activation occurs. As a consequence, under sympathetic control, the HR rises steeply in order to compensate for the reduced oxygen saturation. As soon as oxygen saturation is restored, the HR decays to previous normal state.

3.2.3 Euler-Liljestrand Reflex

The *Euler-Liljestrand-Reflex* (ELR, also known as *hypoxic pulmonary vasoconstriction*) is triggered by hypoxemia. The ELR increases the flow resistance of the vessels by vasoconstriction, i.e., the vessels become tighter, of those areas of the lungs, which are no longer ventilated. This causes those areas to be excluded from the blood circulation, and a deoxygenation of the blood is prevented. But the increased resistance entails a rise of pressure in the pulmonary circulation and the afterload[6] of the heart increases, i.e., the heart has to pump harder. Further details on this mechanism are given in [Psch 98].

As soon as the blood pressure in the right atrium rises, this is registered by pressure sensors which boost the tone of the parasympathetic nervous system which entails a subsequent drop of the HR (see Figure 3.6). Accordingly, the parameter HR should be an immediate indicator to changes in blood pressure.

Another explanation for the dependence of the HR from the current pressure in the pulmonary circulation due to the ELR is that because of reduced circulation the left ventricle is filled much slower. This is registered by pressure sensors in the heart and the adjustment of the HR allows a longer time to fill the ventricles. Thus, the organism saves energy and counteracts hypoxemia.

3.3 The Antagonists Sympathetic and Parasympathetic Nervous System

The sympathetic (SNS) and parasympathetic nervous systems (PNS) constitute the Autonomous Nervous System (ANS) which mostly defies arbitrary control. The balance between the SNS and the PNS regulates the degree of ANS activation (see Figure 3.9).

The SNS and PNS act as antagonists: SNS activity increases the activation of the body and PNS activity decreases it. The SNS pushes all vital functions which are required for physical activity – in former times to counteract a life-threatening situation. Likewise, *an arousal triggers SNS activity* as the body finds itself encountering the risk of suffocation. Among the elevated vital functions are:

- Heart rate

- Blood pressure

- Tone of the skeletal muscles

Likewise, the SNS inhibits all vital functions which hinder physical activity, e.g., the digestion. The antagonists operate at different response times: It is widely

---

[6]The afterload can be regarded as the resistance of the artery, i.e., it counteracts the ventricles ejecting blood into the vessel system.

42   Chapter 3. Medical Introduction to the Heart

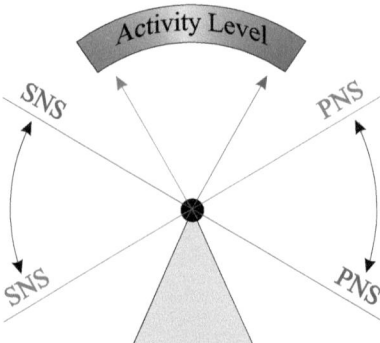

Figure 3.9: This Figure shows how the balance of the ANS results from the respective activity level of either SNS or PNS and how this effects the body's overall activity level: If the PNS activity level is dominant, the resulting body activity is low as well and vice versa for the SNS. The low activity levels may be assigned to NREM 3 - 4, the midlevels to NREM 1 - 2, and the high activity levels may represent REM sleep or an arousal resulting from an SRBD event.

agreed that the HR spectrum in the frequency range from 0.15 - 0.4 Hz is covered by the PNS (see sinus arrhythmia, /3.3.1/). The SNS is said to occupy the frequency range from 0.04 - 0.15 Hz, but discussion is ongoing, whether the PNS contributes to the total energy in this frequency band as well.

3.3.1 Activity of Sinoatrial Node

The ANS (usually) controls the heart rate by means of the sinoatrial node (see Figure 3.2). As this is of importance for later Sections a more profound introduction will be given in this Section.

Repolarization and Funny Current I_f

The current ANS activity level affects the repolarization which manifests in two different ways. First, it changes the speed of the repolarization in the sinoatrial node, thereby the heart rate. Second, it changes the shape of the ST-segment and the T-wave by influencing the repolarization process of the heart muscle.

Usually, the action potential remains stable, until an external event triggers a pulse. As the sinoatrial node acts as a pulse generator, it has to be "unstable", i.e., it triggers itself repeatedly. Since this behavior is unusual, considered "funny[7]", the

---

[7]"Funny" in this context is used to denote an "unusual" behavior.

3.3. The Antagonists Sympathetic and Parasympathetic Nervous System 43

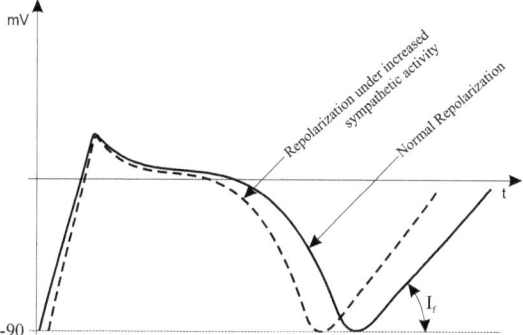

Figure 3.10: Impact of sympathetic activity on the duration of the repolarization

responsible mechanism is called "Funny Channel" or "I_f-Channel". As common in electronics "I" stands for the current – here, the current of repolarization.

Figure 3.10 illustrates one complete cycle of the action potential of the sinoatrial node over time – from repolarization to depolarization. After the depolarization which is only symbolized on the left, the repolarization starts. The dotted line shows the repolarization under the influence of an increased sympathetic activity in comparison to a repolarization under normal sympathetic activity (as continuous line). As displayed, the repolarization under the influence of an increased sympathetic activity occurs faster and, as the depolarization starts immediately after the completion of the repolarization, this entails a higher trigger frequency, i.e., a higher heart rate.

Following the repolarization, which stops as soon as the resting potential of -90 mV is reestablished, on the right side of the Figure, there is a schematic (not to the scale) diagram of the depolarization. The speed of the depolarization, i.e., the steepness of the curve, is parameterized by I_f. And just like for the repolarization I_f depends on the sympathetic or[8] parasympathetic activity: Sympathetic influence increases I_f, parasympathetic influence reduces I_f, i.e., the higher I_f, the higher the heart rate. This parameter is estimated in /6.4.5/.

Hypoxemia, the Diver Reflex, and the Heart Rate

The cessation of respiration during an apnea leads to hypoxemia, i.e., the deprivation of oxygen. Under the influence of hypoxemia, the heart rate drops. This happens for

---
[8] Actually, the heart rate is under sympathetic *and* parasympathetic control at the same time – it's their balance which takes effect. Here, "or" means "the dominant one of the two".

44   Chapter 3. Medical Introduction to the Heart

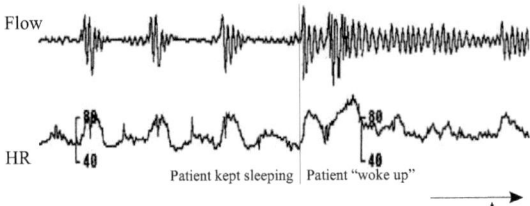

Figure 3.11: Diver reflex in a patient suffering from OSAS: The heart rate (HR) (in the lower panel) directly reacts to the respiratory flow (in the upper panel), with the cessation of the respiratory flow the HR immediately drops, only to overshot the moment respiration restarts. With the onset of constant respiration the HR – after a compensation phase – stabilizes as well. (Figure from the archives of the sleep laboratory of Marburg)

two reasons: First, the heart consumes less energy at a reduced heart rate. Second, the slower flowing blood leaves the oxygen more time to diffuse into the cells of the body. This mechanism is induced by the so called "diver reflex[9]" (see Figure 3.8).

The diver reflex is piped by the PNS. The main reaction to this reflex is a drop of the heart rate between 6 - 15%. The actual degree of the reaction depends strongly on the subject and his/her current condition. The heart rate remains reduced until the next inspiration [Kirs 02]. In Figure 3.11 this effect is shown in a patient suffering from sleep apnea. The upper curve is the respiratory flow and the lower curve is the heart rate.

Actually, Figure 3.11 shows two interesting effects. To the left of the separator (red vertical line) the patient did not wake up and the effect of the diver reflex can be observed. The heart rate jumps directly between tachycardia[10] and bradycardia[11] phases. This is because the arousals do only result in short burst of breathing, but the patient falls into the next apnea immediately afterward. During the bursts of breathing (indicated by the higher activity in the flow curve) the heart rate accelerates in order to compensate for the hypoxemia. But immediately after the anew cessation of the patient's breathing the diver reflex takes over control of the heart rate and, accordingly, it drops significantly. The short heart rate bursts in the bradycardia phases are triggered by the stress which is resulting from the present hypoxemia.

---

[9]The name "diver reflex" is owed to its function principle: it is triggered by receptors placed around mouth and nose, which react upon contact with (cold) water, when *diving*.
[10]Heart rates higher than 100 beats per minute (see /3.2/).
[11]Heart rates lower than 40 beats per minute (see /3.2/).

3.3. The Antagonists Sympathetic and Parasympathetic Nervous System

To the right of the separator the patient finally wakes up or at least retreats to a sleep state, where he manages to breathe constantly. Here, the apnea terminates and after a phase of pronounced superelevation of the heart rate in order to reestablish normal oxygen levels, the heart rate normalizes.

Sinus Arrhythmia

In a healthy person the heart rate varies with the respiratory rhythm which is why this arrhythmia of the sinoatrial node is called *respiratory arrhythmia* as well. The occurrence of the sinus arrhythmia is accounted to four different mechanisms. All of them are based on the assumption of a modulation of the PNS activity [Koep 58].

- The *lung reflex theory* ascribes the RA to the afferent lung vagus[12] which accelerates the heart beat during expansion of the lung and decelerates the heart beat during its shrinkage.

- The *central theory* is based on the assumption that the respiration synchronized central vagal tone is created by direct influence of the vagal kernel area on the neighboring respiratory center via the *cerebro-cardial coupling*, i.e., the synchronization happens directly in the brain.

- According to *Bainbridge*[13] respiration entails an overfilling of the large intrathoracic veins and arteries at each inspiration. Subsequently, his overfilling mechanically triggers the so called Bainbridge-Reflex entailing an acceleration of the heart rate.

- The *pressoreceptor theory* assumes that the respiratory blood pressure waves evoke respiration synchronized modulations of the heart rates by means of the atrial pressoreceptors, i.e., the rise of blood pressure in the atria makes the heart beat faster to lower the pressure overshot.

Some authors ascribe the RA to a combination of these theories. For example [Bren 02] explains that the sympathetic activity changes over time periods of about 10 - 40 seconds, whereas the parasympathetic activity features faster dynamics with time constants of about three seconds. Respiratory oscillations affect both systems, but as the sympathetic system is too slow, changes of the heart rate are driven purely by the PNS tone, which is in perfect concordance with the above statement.

---

[12]The Vagus (vagal nerve) is the biggest nerve of the PNS, hence, the term "vagal nervous system" is sometimes used synonymously for the PNS.

[13]Francis A. Bainbridge, physiologist, London, 1874 - 1921 [Psch 98]

An approach to further differentiate the above influences on the HR generation is presented in [Jo 04]. The authors mainly considered PNS influences represented in the parameters "PNS feedback from lungs stretch receptors ...(and) ...central coupling between respiratory and cardiac drive". The parameter "arterial blood pressure sensors" was intended to reflect SNS influences via the vasoconstriction (see /3.2.3/).

To separate the individual contributing mechanisms, the patients were stimulated by random bursts of CPAP pressure of varying duration according to an experimental protocol. The protocol included daytime and nighttime recordings in W, NREM 2, and REM. The bodily reactions were captured by measuring respiration, HR and blood pressure. Mathematically, their approach was based on a linear autoregressive model. According to their model they computed the impulse responses of the contributing mechanisms. They chose time-domain analysis to apply some restrictions to the processing, e.g., causality.

Their patient collective consisted of nine OSAS and eight healthy subjects of middle age. The impulse responses of healthy and OSAS subjects were compared. The evaluation of the model delivered the following results: first, the authors claimed that their model was capable of predicting 70% of the HRV correctly. Second, the authors found significant differences in the different coupling parameters between healty and OSAS subjects. Third, the complete decay of the impulse responses within 15 seconds hinted on mainly PNS driven processes. Fourth, the authors reasoned that SNS influences may be overlapped by generally higher SNS activity in OSAS patients. These findings are an affirmation of the statements found in the literature.

3.3.2 Wake-Sleep-Influences

During the transition from wake to sleep state the scepter is passed between the two antagonists SNS and PNS. While the SNS influence is dominant in the wake state, this is true for the PNS in sleep state. Vice versa, having determined the activity level of the ANS, this information can hint on the sleep stage (see /2.4.2/).

Recalling the influence of the ANS balance, it is obvious that this transition becomes manifest in some modulations of the ECG:

- The PQ-time is determined by the conduction speed of the AV-node. The higher the sympathetic tone, the lower the conduction delay entailing a shorter PQ-time, i.e., the PQ-time is shorter in wake state.

3.3. The Antagonists Sympathetic and Parasympathetic Nervous System 47

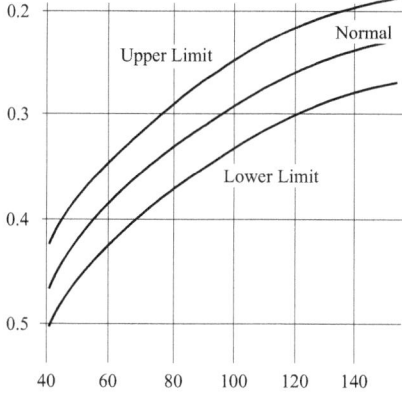

Figure 3.12: Dependency between HR and QT-time

- The QT-time is determined by the duration of the repolarization with the QRS-time being almost constant. However, the repolarization is accelerated under the influence of an increased sympathetic tone. (See Figure 3.10)

- In the wake state, both the HR and the HRV are higher than in sleep state.

Concerning the QT-time, its dependency on the HR has to be taken into account when using it as a marker of ANS activity. There exists a variety of different dependencies of the QT-time from the HR in the literature. The "frequency compensated QT-duration" QT_{comp} according to Bazett[14] is given by equation (3.1).

$$QT_{comp} = \frac{QT_{uncomp}}{\sqrt{\frac{60}{f}}} \qquad (3.1)$$

In Figure 3.12, there is a graphical representation of the dependency between HR and QT-time, which is called a *nomogram*[15] [Habe 03].

[Hamm 01] present a table, which indicates the QT-time depending on the HR. The times given there differ from those in Figure 3.12 in a wider range of acceptable QT-times.

In /6.4.6/ there is an explanation how the timing dynamics of the ECG, i.e., PQ- and QT-time among others, are handled in the scope of this work.

---
[14] Henry Cuthbert Bazett, English-American physiologist, born 1885, Gravesend, England; died July 11, 1950

[15] A nomogram is a graphical representation of a mathematical function that allows to read approximative values from.

48   Chapter 3. Medical Introduction to the Heart

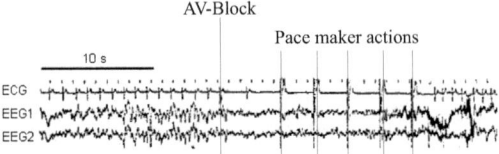

Figure 3.13: AV-blocks during sleep apnea events: This is an extract of a complete PSG and shows only the ECG and some of the EEG channels. At the time index of the first red marker the ECG breaks out of the constant beating and exhibits AV-blocks, i.e., the lack of the ECG working cycle. After about ten seconds, the pace maker steps in and triggers ECG working cycles at a lower frequency (the shorter red markers). (This Figure is supplied by the archives of the University of Marburg.)

3.3.3 AV-Blocks

An AV-block (see Figure 3.2) means that due to a failure of the AV-node the excitation arriving from the atria is not passed on to the ventricles. Thus, in the ECG there is only the P-wave and the rest of the ECG is missing. As no full work cycle is performed, there is no circulation and, accordingly, no palpable pulse in the extremities.

During sleep apnea events – especially in those with deep oxygen desaturations below 80% – AV-blocks are more likely. Their prevalence changes widely depending on the selected piece of literature. [Pete 95] sums up literture and their own studies by claiming that bradycardia with less than 30 bpm occurred in 7 - 36%, sinus arrest lasting longer than 2.5 seconds occurred in 11 - 36% and AV-blocks, 2nd and 3rd order, in 8 - 16% of the patients. The authors explain these wide ranges by the kind of selected subjects for the studies. Blocks are more likely to be reported in subjects suffering from morbid obesity. Due to autonomic deregulation in REM sleep, more than 80% of the block events can be found in this sleep stage. Vise versa, the presence of AV-blocks quite reliably hints on the REM sleep stage which makes it an approach to consider, if aiming at detecting the sleep stage from the ECG.

The periods of third degree, i.e., a complete blockage, AV-blocks can be as long as 14 seconds at the end of an SRBD event with dropping oxygen saturation.

Today, the reason for these blocks is mainly accounted to increased PNS tone due to hypoxemia. But, other explanations shift the responsibility to intrathoracic or intracardiac pressure changes.

In patients with OSAS AV-blocks usually do not appear during daytime. This is to be considered, when evaluating a 24h-Holder-ECG recording to decide, whether or not to implant a pacemaker. If OSAS induced, AV-blocks vanish almost completely (90%) under CPAP therapy (see /2.9.2/).

Figure 3.13 shows the effect of a pacemaker which was implanted into the patient in order to compensate for the AV-blocks which were found in nocturnal ECG recordings. In the end, though, it turned out that this was a wrong diagnosis, because the pacemaker would not have been necessary, as those AV-blocks vanished under CPAP therapy. An example for an AV-block in the recordings analyzed by EVA ml (the feature extractor implemented for this work, see /10.2/) is shown in Figure 7.1d.

3.4 Reactions to different Load Conditions

The human body always strives to balance the current (physical or mental) load and the bodily effort. This compensating effort is reflected in various vital parameters and the ECG is one of the most sensitive of them. The ECG changes become manifest in shape and frequency. Some of these changes are explained in the following as the extracted features (see Chapter 6) are based on them.

3.4.1 P-Wave

The P pulmonary is a high amplitude P-wave. Mainly, it evidences a chronic right-heart load, which results from a pulmonary disease. Variations of the P-wave to thoracic pressure variations are considered subtle, because there is no direct cause-and-effect-chain. Even though the blood pressure increases spontaneously, the P-wave is mainly an indicator for a long-term chronic overload.

However, the P pulmonary is mentioned here because of the ELR (see /3.2.3/). The ELR induced vasoconstriction entails an increase of the pressure in the pulmonary circulation which leads to a higher load. Moreover, the vasoconstriction is taking place anywhere in the body (See /3.3.1/). Thus, with the occurrence of the hypoxemia the flow resistance of the body rises. Consequently, the increased load has to be compensated by an increased heart effort entailing higher amplitudes in both the P-wave and the R-peak.

3.4.2 Amplitude of the R-Peak

Load induced Dynamics

There is the following cause-and-effect-chain: hypoxemia leads to a vasoconstriction via the ELR (see /3.2.3/ and previous Section) which entails a higher afterload to the heart. To compensate for the increased afterload, the heart "reacts" by reducing its residual volume, i.e., it empties itself more completely[16]. The reduced residual volume is accomplished by a powerful contraction which should be registered as a higher R-peak in the ECG. Thus, according to the increased load and the respiration induced R-peak amplitude modulations (see p. 43) the R-peak amplitudes should exhibit the following interplay:

- Obstruction leads to a right-heart overload.

- Futile respiration results in a modulation of the R-peak amplitudes, because the heart is shifted around by the lungs excursions.

- Following the arousal there is an onset of tachycardia with left-ventricular overload. The accompanying deep breaths to compensate for the lack of oxygen result in a high modulation of the R-peak.

This cause-and-effect-chain would be perfectly acceptable, if sleep apnea events were accompanied by direct reactions of the blood pressure. And there is a lot of evidence for this behavior in the literature. For example, in [Pete91], the authors hint on huge fluctuations of the blood pressure which are associated with sleep apnea events. In the group of patients suffering from CHD and SRBD the blood pressure rises as high as 150/300 mm Hg during an apnea event and the repetitive apnea events result in long-term hypertension. At the end of an obstructive apnea the arterial blood pressure may drop to values as low as 40/60 mm Hg. Likewise, the cardiac output drops in the course of an apnea. This process should result in changes of the cardiac load and find its representation in varying heights of the R peak.

And an additional evidence from an experience we had during the development of a photoplethysmograph: Figure 3.14 shows the pulse wave, i.e., the volume changes along a vessel over time due to the pumping heart, recorded at a finger tip photoplethysmographically[17]. Each little peak (of the cyan curve) is a pulse wave, i.e., the direct effect of a heart beat. But what is so interesting about this Figure are the shifts in the DC component[18] of the signal (the red curve), which were provoked by attempting to breathe with nose and mouth blocked deliberately. The DC component being an indirect measure of the diameter of the vessel in the path of

---

[16] This is achieved by the emission of actin and myosin which are shortening the muscle fibers.

[17] "Photoplethysmographically" means that light (being the "photo" part) is used to retrieve volume changes in hollow parts of the body (being the "plethysmography" part), which were vessels in this application.

[18] DC is the abbreviation of Direct Current and means a current which does not change in amplitude and polarization. More commonly, DC is used to separate a slow changing component of a signal from a faster changing one.

3.4. Reactions to different Load Conditions

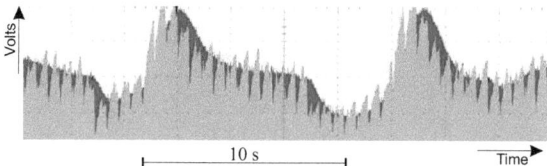

Figure 3.14: Blood pressure changes due to (artificial and deliberate) obstructions: The cyan curve shows the photoplethysmographically recorded pulsations of blood flow at a finger tip. The lowpass filtered pulsation is shown in the red curve. It can be observed that during the periods of deliberate obstructions, there is a significant increase of blood pressure, i.e., an increase of extinction of the light passing through the finger tip (To derive the blood pressure from the photoplethysmographical curve, it has to be logically inverted).

the light from the LED (Light Emitting Diode) to the receiver indicates that the "obstructive" breathing entailed a change of the diameter of the vessel, which is due to a change of blood pressure, as the vessels respond elastically to a change of blood pressure. This observation might serve as an evidence for the previously uttered assertion that a respiratory obstruction entails an immediate rise in blood pressure.

In [Penz 02a], the results of a new sensor which measures the peripheral arterial tone and seems to be similar to the one explained here are presented. The authors claim that this sensor approach delivers additional information (to a PSG, see /2.8.1/) concerning the SNS and PNS activity. The correlation between the sensor measurements and the occurrence of an apnea or hypopnea event is said to be r = 0.66. These findings also support the assumption that a respiratory obstruction directly entails a high load to the heart.

Respiration from the ECG

This Section is mentioned here for completeness concerning the influences on the R-peak amplitude.

Respiration is in principle extractable from the ECG by evaluating a combination of the modulation of the R-peak and the sinus arrhythmia (see /3.3.1/). The principle of this approach is shown in Figure 10.3, a as an example. It can easily be seen that there is a modulation of the R-peaks. Deriving the envelope for the upper and lower peaks[19] and calculating their distance results in the varying amplitude of the R peak. Included in this modulation are breathing, which is desirable, and possible position changes of the subject, which is "noise".

---

[19] Technically speaking, this is an AM-Demodulation.

3.5 Myocardial Ischemia

Ischemia is the interruption of arterial blood circulation with the subsequent drop of oxygen saturation, i.e., hypoxemia. Accordingly, myocardial ischemia affects the heart (muscle) which entails infarction within a short time. Ischemias are caused by constrictions, e.g., arterial stenosis, or blockage, e.g., thrombosis.

As phases of resting respiration, i.e., sleep apnea, entail a decrease of the oxygen saturation, the resulting hypoxemia might be considered an "overall ischemia". As the heart muscle is one of the organs consuming most energy, the ischemia effects on the myocardium should be visible in the ECG.

The evaluation of simultaneous PSG and ECG recordings showed that during the night ischemic phases are found quite often in apnea patients. This is especially true for the REM sleep state where episodes of frequent apnea occurrences led to persisting hypoxemia. This is reasoned to the higher sympathetic activity, increased physiological load, and spontaneous HR fluctuations. As all these effects vanished under CPAP therapy, they must have been SRBD induced.

A problem in diagnosing ischemia is that ischemia – even a manifest infarction – does not mandatorily entail changes in the ECG. The visibility depends on the size and place of the infarct area and the positions of the ECG leads defining the projection direction. Hence, approximately 4% of all infarctions proceed electrocardiographically "silent", i.e., invisible, as [Habe 03] points out.

The next Sections describe shortly the most prominent ischemia markers.

3.5.1 ST-Segment and Ischemic Influences

The ST-segment is extremely sensitive to ischemic influences. Some of the changes of the ST-segment are introduced in this Chapter.

3.5.2 ST-Segment Depressions

ST-depressions in the ECG are common during sleep in apnea patients. Especially horizontal (see Figure 3.15a) and descending (see Figure 3.15b - d) ST-depressions argue for a myocardial ischemia. On the contrary, ascending ST depressions occur even in healthy hearted subjects under higher physiological load and tachycardia and are not pathologic.

The four ST-depressions depicted in Figure 3.15 can not be assigned clearly to a certain cause. Thus, it is possible that each of them represents (a different type of) an ischemia, i.e., the ST-depression may be due to dynamics of the autonomous system or due to changes of physiological load. However, in the scope of this work, this

3.5. Myocardial Ischemia

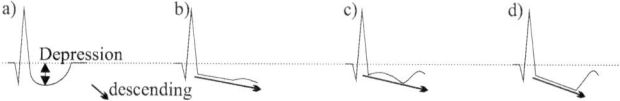

Figure 3.15: Typical shapes of ST-depressions. The arrow indicates the descending behavior.

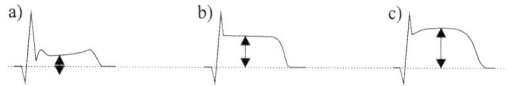

Figure 3.16: Typical shapes of ST-elevations

differentiation is not of importance as SRBD events entail autonomous activation as well as physiological load.

3.5.3 ST-Segment Elevations

ST-segment elevations are mainly indicators for transmural ischemia during transmural heart attack (acute infarct). The infarct starts with an initial negative T-wave. Subsequently, the maximum ST-elevation emerges within 60 - 90 seconds followed by a highly positive T-wave ([Habe 03] and [Hora 98]). Different types of ST-elevations are shown in Figure 3.16.

An ST-elevation can hint on both sympathicotonia, i.e., a dominant activity of the SNS, and parasympathicotonia, i.e., a dominant activity of the PNS. The discrimination between both is based on the T-wave: a flat or negative T-wave points to the first and vice versa. An additional marker of sympathicotonia is an ascending ST-segment starting under the PQ-level.

In addition to the revelation of an ischemia, the dynamics of the ST-segment hint on the physical load which is why it is evaluated during ergometry[20]. If there is something wrong with the efficiency of the heart the tested subjects show a horizontal or even descending ST-segment when the physical load is increased to 75 - 100 W. This is in the range of the work load provoked by an arousal which is estimated to be around 70 W. The dynamics of the ST-segment might even be further increased because in addition to the physical load the occurrence of a SRBD event synchronously entails a lack of oxygen.

---

[20]Actually, ergometry evaluates this parameter in the opposite direction: the subject is exposed to physical load and the reaction of the ST-segment allows to derive information about the subject's cardiac health state.

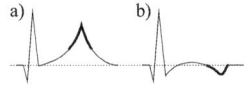

Figure 3.17: At the beginning of an ischemic stroke the T-wave turns into a highly positive peak (a) and during the stroke the T-wave flattens or turns into negative values (b).

3.5.4 T-Wave

The highly positive T-wave in the shape of an isosceles peak is called a "suffocation T" (see Figure 3.17a. It occurs directly at the beginning of a myocardial infarct. *The suffocation T is considered the earliest reaction to ischemia.* Usually, it has already subsided at the time of the ECG registration in a clinic [Olsh 96].

In the focus of this work a "suffocation T", i.e., an increasing positive T-wave amplitude, can be regarded as an SRBD event indicator as it reacts to the apnea driven ischemia.

Negative T-waves occur due to epicardiac or transmural ischemia (see Figure 3.17b. *Within seconds*, i.e., directly related to the onset of a SRBD event, a negative T-wave emerges over the ischemia part of the myocardium, which transforms into the maximum ST-elevation after 60 - 90 seconds accompanied by a highly positive T-wave [Hora 98].

Additionally, the T-wave amplitude varies with the activity of the ANS. Flat or even negative T-wave amplitude may hint on sympathicotonia, whereas a high positive T-wave may relate to parasympathicotonia.

Summarizing this Section, the simple evaluation of the *T-wave amplitude changes* hints on SRBD event occurrences. However, the T-wave is frequently abnormal, as the restitution of the conduction system is sensitive for physiological, pharmacological, and organic changes. Nevertheless, as the reaction to an arousal is a short-time event, the evaluation of the dynamics of the T-wave should yield usable information.

3.6 Summary and Preview

At the beginning of this Chapter the generation and the measurement of an electrocardiogram were explained. The explanation touched the physiology of the heart, the blood circulation, and the genesis of the electrical representation of the heart's activity.

The correlations between SRBD events, the activity of the ANS, and the regulation of the HR were explained. Likewise, the influence of different load conditions or

3.6. Summary and Preview

varying levels of oxygen supply on the morphology of the ECG curve were presented. These physiological basics will drive the cause-and-effect chains which will be used in later Chapters to give reason for the extracted features.

The next Chapter will now give an overview of the State of the Art, i.e., what has already been done in that field of research.

Chapter 4

State of the Art

This Chapter provides an overview of the ongoing work in the field of deriving SRBD events and sleep stages from an ECG signal. It begins with an introduction to some widely applied features and some primary approaches to evaluate the HRV. Likewise, the Physionet database which is almost exclusively used in the various works is shortly introduced.

Subsequently, the various approaches are presented in more detail along with their classification results.

4.1 Deriving Autonomous Activity from the Heart Rate

The HRV is lively discussed in many papers for the detection of autonomous fluctuations. The strong interest in the HR and the HRV derives from the fact that they are under direct control of sympathetic and parasympathetic influences (see /3.3/). This way, by some kind of "reverse engineering", these parameters are not only used to detect SRBD events (because of the striking behavior of the HR during such an event (see Figure 3.8) or sleep stages (see [Blas 03] and [Mali 97]), but also chronic stress and the correlated mortality risk, e.g., in [Wenk 05].

4.1.1 Quotient of the SNS and PNS Energies

The primary idea behind this approach is to compute the energy, i.e., the activity, of each of the two antagonists "separately" and then evaluate their relative contribution to the overall activity of the ANS. The activity of the SNS is separated from the activity of the PNS by means of their respective response times, i.e., the activity of the PNS is mapped to higher frequencies as it is about three to ten times faster.

In the first step, the spectrum of the HR series is computed to retrieve its power spectral density (PSD) according to equation (4.1) where $R_{ECG}(\tau)$ is the autocorrelation of the ECG signal. It describes how the power of a signal or time series is distributed with frequency.

$$S(f) = \int_{-\infty}^{+\infty} R_{ECG}(\tau) e^{-2\pi j f \tau} \, d\tau \qquad (4.1)$$

In the next step, the spectrum is separated into three segments whose exact names and frequency ranges vary slightly from paper to paper. The low frequency (LF) segment ranges from 0 - 0.15 Hz, the high frequency (HF) segment from 0.15 - 0.5 Hz, and the last segment collects any higher frequencies. Only the first two segments are of interest. It is assumed that the LF range represents a mixture of sympathetic and parasympathetic activity and the HF range is dominated by parasympathetic activity.

The overall activity of the ANS, i.e., the balance between the SNS and PNS, is quite often characterized as in equation (4.2), e.g., in [Bren 02] and [Bonn 97]. This method is supported by the results described in [Tels 04]. However, the authors mention that these findings can not be approved for all patients.

$$Activity_{ANS} = \frac{LF}{HF} \qquad (4.2)$$

Typical values for this quotient in relation to different sleep stages are shown in Figure 4.1. These values are the result of a study which is presented in [Vano 95].

In [Khoo 01], the authors extended this activity measure by two additional parameters which consider the respiratory-correlated and the respiratory-independent components, respectively. The correcting factor is computed from the higher frequencies which represent the respiration (see /3.3.1/). These values were found to correlate with the average application duration of CPAP therapy.

In [Vano 95] there is another study concerning the HRV during different sleep stages. Its authors describe a nocturnal increase in the standard deviation of the RR-interval. The authors consider sleep under PNS control which is true for NREM as well as REM sleep, except for the SNS bursts during the phases of high eye movement activity. The authors state that the HR decreased and the respiratory sinus arrhythmia increased during NREM. NREM exposed lower overall HRV, but a higher beat-to-beat variability compared to wakefulness. REM sleep showed contrary behavior with increased overall HRV, but reduced beat-to-beat variability which the authors – in concordance with other publications – attribute to an increased im-

4.1. Deriving Autonomous Activity from the Heart Rate   59

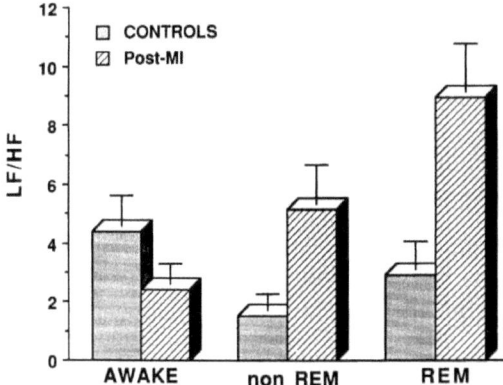

Figure 4.1: Ratio of SNS (LF) and PNS (HF) activity levels during different sleep stages. The LF-to-HR-ratio is given as mean ± SD. The values are computed separately for healthy subjects (left) and for post-MI (myocardial infarct) patients (right) (Figure taken from [Vano 95].

pact of the SNS. The evaluation was based on data intervals of five minutes for the different sleep stages and phases with arousals were explicitly excluded. Figure 4.2 shows an example of a RR-spectrum of a healthy subject during NREM.

4.1.2 Power Law Slope and Poincare Plots

These two approaches are mainly to detect long-term high activity levels of the SNS. This is of interest as elevated SNS activity increases cardio-vascular mortality (which is especially true after an acute myocardial infarction). The main idea of these two approaches is based on the fact that high SNS activity levels bring about a loss of HRV (see [Wenk 05] and [Mali 97]).

The first of these approaches is shown in Figure 4.3a: the power law slope (PLS). Like the former approaches it computes the spectrum, but in the next step approximates the amplitudes by a regression line. The evaluated parameter is its *slope*.

The second of these approaches is a graphical one and is called Poincare Plot (see Figure 4.3b. A Poincare Plot is a plot where the current value of the RR series is plotted over the previous one. Depending on the long-term properties of the HR series the shape varies. The features which are retrieved are the lengths of the principal axes and their quotient.

60   Chapter 4. State of the Art

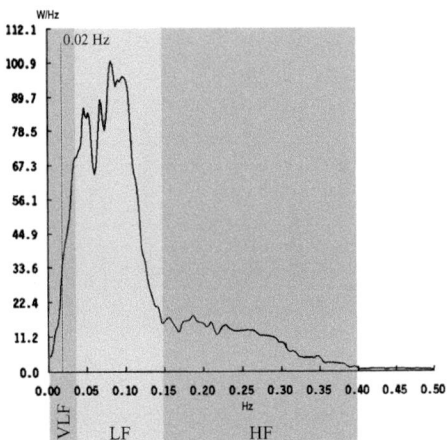

Figure 4.2: Spectral analysis of HRV during NREM sleep in a healthy subject. In OSAS patients the SNS is activated to a higher extent resulting in a reduced power density in the high frequency range. The additional ordinate at 0.02 Hz indicates the "cyclic variation of the heart rate" during subsequent SRBD events which is evaluated by many approaches (see /3.2.2/ and Figure 3.11, original Figure taken from [Vano 95]).

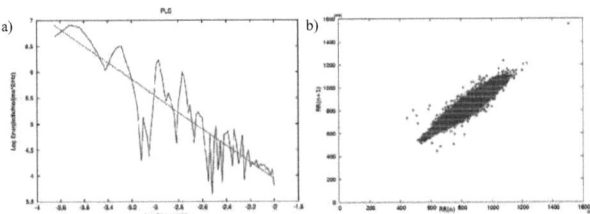

Figure 4.3: Two different approaches of evaluating the HR for estimating the long-term ANS activity (with focus on the SNS, see text): a) PLS and b) Poincare Plot

4.2 Physionet Database

In [Penz 02b], the authors describe the "Computers in Cardiology (CiC) Challenge 2000" which was open for participation between February and September 2000. Many of the studies presented in this Chapter rely at least on the database which was created for this challenge.

The database created for the CiC challenge consists of 70 recordings which are arranged in three groups: the first group are strongly affected, the second group mildly affected and the third group healthy subjects. The total of the recordings was split into two groups for training or testing purposes, respectively.

The recordings included ECG, respiration, oxygen saturation, and SRBD event annotations for the training set. Apnea and hypopnea events were alike considered "SRBD events" and these events were annotated on a minute-to-minute base. Data is available from http://www.physionet.org/physiobank/database/apnea-ecg (see [Phys 04], last visited 02/23/2011).

Two challenges were announced. The aim of the first one was to identify SRBD subjects. The second one went more into detail and aimed at detecting individual minutes of SRBD events. Participants were allowed to submit manifold to improve their results based on an automated feedback. For further details on the organization refer to the mentioned paper itself.

Most of the participants applied HRV features like HRV spectral analysis, Hilbert transformation, time-frequency maps, and spectral power ratios. Some applied morphological features like ECG pulse energy, R-peak duration, S-peak amplitude, T-wave amplitude, and ECG derived respiration.

From the 13 participating approaches, it turned out that the HR based features outperformed the morphology based features, but a combination of both types yielded the best results. The authors conclude that ECG based SRBD detection is feasible. This claim is backed up by classification results of up to 100% for the separation of apneic subjects and up to 92,6% of SRBD event minutes.

This article concludes that algorithms based on frequency domain analysis showed better results than time-domain based approaches. Morphology based features usually increased the classification rate – especially, if the R-peak morphology was considered. The authors summarized the different approaches by pointing out that "the main features are HR derived, but shape based feature may help improve classification rates".

4.3 Methods and Classification Rates

In [Roch 99], the authors described a study to evaluate the reliability of HRV based parameters, i.e., the variation of the RR-interval, for the screening of possible OSAS patients. The complete patient collective was divided into two groups: one for training the algorithm consisting of 91 patients and one for testing it which consisted of 52 patients. The individual health status of each patient was determined by means of a complete PSG recording.

For the aim of their study, the authors evaluated 24 h Holter ECGs. The values of the extracted parameters were computed on a five minutes time base for *daytime* and nighttime, respectively. Starting with a large set of statistical time-domain parameters, the authors purged the parameter set by selecting the most powerful ones and resolving linear dependencies. During the training phase, the optimum threshold for each parameter was found by the CART[1] methodology.

The most powerful parameters were the *mean of the standard deviation of all RR-intervals in the five minutes segments*, the *standard deviation of the RR-intervals during the night* and the *difference between the standard deviation of the RR-intervals during day and night*. They stated that for each parameter the absolute difference between daytime and nighttime values boosted the classification rates.

As a result the authors stated that in patients with an AHI greater than ten a sensitivity of 89.7% and a specificity of 98.1% were achieved in the training group and for the test group the respecive values were 83% and 96.5%. In patients with an AHI greater than 30, the sensitivity increased to 96% and the specificity to 99.7%.

In [Xu 08], the authors recorded 50 PSG of patients suspected of OSAS. The SRBD events were annotated manually. The ECG was evaluated in one minute episodes of RR-intervals aiming at deciding, whether or not there occurred a SRBD event. The ECG signal was evaluated applying the Empirical Mode Decomposition (EMD). This mathematical approach aims at separating the intrinsic oscillations contributing the input signal at a given instant of time which makes it appropriate for non-stationary signals like the ECG. The intrinsic functions are separated by means of Singular Value Decomposition or ICA based methods (Hilbert Spectrum).

According to the authors SRBD events were associated to an additional frequency component of 0.02 Hz. The amplitude of this special frequency rose about five seconds before the actual event. The authors claimed that the algorithms works fine with light to moderate OSAS patients, but needs more refinement to handle severe degrees. For neither group the authors provided classification rates.

---

[1]CART (Classification and Regression Tree) is an algorithm which is used in binary decision trees to find an optimal classification based on the information content.

4.3. Methods and Classification Rates	63

In [Mend 10], the authors evaluated the performance of mainly EMD and Wavelet based features and added the area of the QRS-complex as a measure for respiratory activity and "standard HRV time domain measures". From these features they selected the best performing ones by an automatic feature selection with the sequential feature selection (SFS) method. The selected features were fed into linear and quadratic discriminant classifiers.

They applied their features to 50 recordings from Physionet. They selected a training set consisting of 4950 apneic minutes and 7127 healthy minutes and a test set of 4428 apneic minutes and 7927 healthy minutes. Since they were seeking to detect individual SRBD events, they pointed out the correlation of 95% between the minute based SRBD annotation and the AHI. They achieved an accuracy of up to 89% with the Wavelet features and up to 85% with the EMD features. In any case it was possible to achieve a 100% correct detection of apneic patients by adjusting the appropriate thresholds to the feature extraction method. Their analysis confirmed the SRBD correlated brady-tachycardia oscillation with a frequency of 0.02 Hz, whereas during undistorted breathing the respiration correlated frequency of 0.25 Hz was dominant.

Furthermore, the authors estimated that the maximum detection rate of SRBD events out the ECG signal is limited to about 90% which was true no matter which feature extraction process is applied. The authors stressed that the automatic results depend strongly on the quality of the recorded ECG signal. They suggested that minutes with ten subsequent false R-peak detections should be discarded, even if extensive preprocessing was applied.

In [Shio 97], the authors evaluated the influence of CPAP therapy on several statistical time-domain parameters as well as on frequency-domain parameters. In addition to the previous authors, two extra frequency ranges were considered: the very low frequency range VLF 0.008 - 0.04 Hz and the ultra low frequency range ULF 0 - 0.008 Hz. Compared to [Roch 99] similar statistical parameters, e.g., *mean of standard deviation*, were included, but only the corresponding nighttime parameters.

The authors noticed that under CPAP therapy the powers of VLF and LF dropped significantly, whereas ULF and HF showed no variation. The time-domain statistical parameters were left unaltered. The authors concluded that the evaluation of the frequency-domain features, especially VLF, was helpful for the recognition of OSAS and its appropriate treatment.

In [Khoo 99], the authors used the already well-known frequency ranges to estimate ANS activity. They claimed that the usual LF-to-HR-ratio could be confounded by the respiratory sinus arrhythmia. To overcome this limitation, they established an autoregressive approach which aimed at separating HR influences into one component without respiratory impact and one assuming linear correlation between respiration and HR.

The respiration dependent component was wrapped into a transfer function defining the correlation between the esophageal pressure (see next paragraph) and the RR-interval. Subsequently, this transfer function was used to compensate the already known HF-to-LF-ratio for respiratory impacts.

From their patients collective of six healthy and seven OSAS patients the authors gathered the usual PSG data set (see /2.8.1/). In addition, they applied an esophagus catheter for a precise measurement of the respiratory effort. The esophageal pressure is widely considered as a more reliable measure of respiratory effort, but – being an invasive method – it is not recorded during a PSG in general.

In their results they found an affirmation of their assumption of linearity between the respiratory effort and the respiration dependent component of their transfer function. The transfer function was found to be an order of magnitude larger in healthy subjects compared to OSAS patients which should allow an reliable detection of OSAS patients – but not down to single events. Moreover, they found their corrected ANS descriptors to be indicators of the success of CPAP therapy (which they could measure even in the wake state).

In [Zywi04], the authors followed two approaches: the first one was based on the common "cyclic behavior of the heart rate" (CVHR), i.e., a drop of the HR at the beginning of the SRBD event followed by an increase (see Figure 3.8). These oscillations were tracked by evaluating the different bands in the power spectrum. The authors gave slightly differing definitions of the frequency ranges: ULF 0 - 0.013 Hz, VLF 0.013 - 0.0375 Hz, LF 0.0375 - 0.06 Hz, and HF 0.17 - 0.28 Hz, which means there was a frequency gap which was not considered.

Their second approach consisted in the application of a Discrete Wavelet Analysis (DWT) based on the Battle-Lemarie wavelet for its very good filter characteristics. For classification purposes the wavelet coefficients were described by statistical means, e.g., mean and standard deviation.

Based on the complete Physionet database, the authors claimed an accuracy of 96.7% in the learning set and 93.3% in the test set. In their conclusion the authors pointed out that for a morphological analysis more than one single lead – as used during a PSG – should be available.

In [Mend07], the authors combine HRV and morphological features. From the HRV they computed the power spectral density and they used the area within 200

4.3. Methods and Classification Rates

ms around the R-peak as an indicator for respiration, i.e., ECG derived Respiration (EDR, see /10.3/).

After the automatic R-peak detection the detected peaks were manually corrected. Subsequently, they fed the positions of the R-peaks into a bivariate autoregressive model. The autoregressive model was chosen for its capability of delivering features on a beat-to-beat basis even on non-stationary time series. The spectral density was evaluated in concordance with the standard definitions of the ANS frequency ranges. The time series were normalized to the individual subject to compensate for inter-subject variability.

After a feature preselection which produced a majority of power spectral density related features, the remaining features were fed into a K-Nearest Neighbor classifier (see /10.7.3/).

For their study the authors used 50 recordings from the CiC database, i.e., Physionet, and split them into 25 recordings for training and 25 for testing. They achieved an accuracy higher than 85% in both training and test set and managed a complete grouping of SRBD and healthy subjects. As they examined the frequency produced by repeated events (0.002 Hz), single events were unlikely to be detected by their approach.

In [Byst 04], the authors applied a three step processing. In the first step the following features were extracted:

- RR-interval

- QRS_{dyn}: amplitude of the norm of the first derivative of a five dimensional phase space representation of the QRS-complex

- T-wave area as integral over $[t_{R-peak} + 100$ ms, $t_{R-peak} + 300$ ms$]$

- Jitter: high frequency noise of the spectral power in the frequency band 35 - 45 Hz in the interval $[t_{R-peak} + 50$ ms, $t_{R-peak} + 400$ ms$]$ (which should be approximately the ST-segment including the T-wave) which the authors assumed to be muscular stress

Applying means to these features and evaluating them on different time bases resulted in a total of 15 features which were fed into a neural network in the second step. The neural network assigned each heart beat to one of four consecutive apnea states, e.g., onset and restart of respiration after the SRBD event which allowed to detect the onset and length of an individual SRBD event.

In the third step the neural network output was used as input to a dynamic Markovian state model which made sure that only meaningful sequences, e.g., no second event begins without the end of the current event, were actually produced.

The study was performed on the CiC 2000 database, but the data had to be manually reannotated to provide SRBD event information on a beat-to-beat instead of the standard minute-to-minute base.

The authors claimed an accuracy up to 89.0% in the training set and up to 84.1% in the test set. They pointed out that the deployment of the morphological features improved the accuracy by approximately 7% compared to using only the HRV features.

In [Miet 10], the authors recommended the Hilbert transformation as it was more capable of dealing with "transient, highly nonlinear, and nonstationary" processes than the Fourier transformation or autoregressive models.

The approach described was based on the detection of RR-interval oscillations which are provoked by prolonged periods of subsequent SRBD events. The authors said that the provoked oscillations exhibited a frequency of 0.01 - 0.04 Hz which covered the frequency of 0.02 Hz mentioned by other authors as well.

The signal evaluation operated on intervals of five minutes. During the preprocessing two main tasks were accomplished. First, the suppression of outliers by computing something similar to $m_c(RR, 40)$ and limiting each RR-interval to $m_c(RR, 40) \pm 20\%$. Subsequently, the RR time series was bandpass filtered for assuring a bandwidth limited signal as required by the Hilbert transformation.

Subsequently, the Hilbert transformation was applied to the preprocessed signal to compute the instantaneous amplitudes and frequencies and their means and standard deviations. Additionally, the relative duration of the interval during which these values fell below a fixed threshold were stored as features. During the training phase individual (but fixed) thresholds for all features were iteratively adjusted to yield the best classification results.

Applying this approach to the CiC "Sleep Apnea Test Data" 28 out of 30 (93.3%) recordings, or, on a temporal base, 14591 out of 17268 minutes (84.5%), were correctly classified. The authors admit that only prolonged periods of subsequent SRBD events can be detected, but no short time dynamics or a small number of subsequent events. An introduction to the described software `apdet` can be found in [Miet 00].

In [Miet 06], the authors claimed that SRBD events were associated to 0.01 - 0.04 Hz oscillations in the HR. As these ultra low frequencies (ULF) are hard to handle using standard Fourier transformation, the Hilbert transformation was used

4.3. Methods and Classification Rates

to create an evaluable signal. The achieved classification results were given as 54 out of 60 subjects (90%) and 28576 out of 34313 minutes (83.3%).

In [Miet 06], the authors described an approach aimed at exploiting the cardiopulmonary coupling. It is the basis of the respiratory sinus arrhythmia (see /3.3.1/) and produces high frequencies between 0.1 - 0.4 Hz in the spectrum. Based on the assumption that the SRBD events are represented by low frequencies between 0.01 - 0.1 Hz, the authors implemented a threshold based algorithm which was claimed to allow to distinguish between stable and unstable sleep stages which may hint on SRBD events. The authors did not provide classification results, though.

In [Zywi 02b], the authors recorded a 12 lead ECG along with a standard PSG from nine patients for their evaluation. The 12-channel ECG was acquired using the authors' HES LKG system a description of which can be found in [Zywi 02a]. The morphological features extracted were:

- R-peak amplitude in Einthoven I (see Figure 3.3) and V5 of the Wilson chest wall configuration[2]

- Ratio of R-peak to S-peak amplitude in lead V3 and V4

- STT-integral in V5

- S-peak amplitude in V2

- QRS-complex amplitude and angle in Einthoven I

- T-wave amplitude in Einthoven I

The authors stated that the mean values of the features seemed to be affected only a little by SRBD events, whereas their standard deviations exposed high dynamics correlated with SRBD events. Moreover, they stated that systematic effects on the ST-T-segment could not be found during their study. Summarizing their findings the authors declared that, in general, the morphological ECG clearly hinted on SRBD events, but the patterns seemed to vary widely among patients and leads. As an example the author mentioned the amplitude of the R-peak in Einthoven I which sometimes showed dynamics correlated with the occurrence of SRBD events whereas in other subjects no effects could be observed. Their study must be considered a feasibility study as no classification results were provided.

In [Altu 09], the authors evaluated the morphology of an ECG signal to predict "apnea-bradycardia events in preterm infants" as these events may hint on Sudden

---

[2]Another ECG lead configuration which is usually not available in a standard PSG.

Infant Death Syndrome (SIDS). For their study they compared the behavior of the RR-interval, the R-peak amplitude, and the duration of the QRS-complex under different conditions, e.g., before and during a bradycardia event. Even though the paper focused mainly on the detection of the different ECG phases, it, nevertheless, provided some interesting information about the use of the morphological approach for the detection of SRBD events.

Running their study on 27 preterm infants, the authors were able to show changes in the R-peak amplitude and the duration of the QRS-complex correlated with the onset of the bradycardia event. Even though the detection of SRBD events was not in their focus, it is interesting to mention as bradycardia events precede SRBD events and may, therefore, serve as an indicator of an imminent SRBD event.

In [Penz 06], the authors recorded standard PSGs along with a 12-channel ECG from 56 OSAS patients. From the 12-channel ECG 250 features on a beat-to-beat base were extracted from which five parameters were chosen for further evaluation:

- HR

- Normalized R-peak amplitude

- QRS-complex amplitude, area, and vector angle

All five features showed correlations to the SRBD events and the best two parameters turned out to be the HR with $r = 0.64$ ($p < 0.01$) and the QRS-complex area with $r = 0.61$ ($p < 0.01$). From these results the authors concluded that the inclusion of morphological features in the ECG signal processing may well improve SRBD event classification.

In [Shou 04], the authors focused on the evaluation of the P-wave and its relation to the corresponding R-peak. Their features were the average PP- and PR-interval lengths, respectively. The references for estimating the SRBD event induced dynamics were computed from the interval closest to the onset of an apnea.

In a total, the authors evaluated 28 pediatric subjects' ECG recordings. In their "preliminary work" they provided only a visual evaluation. They found that 21 of 28 subjects showed changes in the PP- and the PR-interval, i.e., the AV conduction delay (see /3.3.3/), lengths. They described an PR-interval oscillation with a period of 10 seconds in severe OSAS patients (AHI > 25).

[Tels 04] evaluated the HRV using a modified Detrended Fluctuation Analysis (DFA) in order to detect sleep stage transitions. The approach proved kind of successful, as transitions toward wakefulness could clearly be detected. The authors believed that transitions from deeper to lighter sleep stages were accompanied by "short intermediate intervals of very strong fluctuations" in the HR, which was due to "short autonomic arousals". They said that correlation time for NREM sleep was about six heart beats, whereas REM sleep showed long time correlations. The later statement contradicted sources saying that during REM sleep there are strong fluctuations of almost every vital parameter – including the HR.

In [Bund 00], the authors attempted to detect the actual sleep stage from the HRV, as the sleep stages differ in parasympathetic activation and, accordingly, the absolute HR and its dynamics.

4.4 Summary and Preview

This Chapter gave an introduction to the many studies which aimed at deriving the properties of sleep from the ECG. Here is now a short review of the state presented.

Many of the studies used the same database – the CiC 2000 challenge accessible via Physionet which makes the results quite comparable. The limitation of this database is that the annotations are on a minute-to-minute base. Therefore, for some of the studies the authors reannotated this database or created one of their own, if higher temporal resolution was required, e.g., for single event detection.

Either driven by the limitation of the used database, e.g., CiC 2000 challenge, or due to the methods applied many of the studies restricted themselves to the minute based temporal resolution, but did not aim at detecting single SRBD events which made it impossible to derive the standard measure for severity – the AHI. Moreover, none of the studies distinguished between any of the different types of SRBD events, e.g., apnea, hypopnea. However, considering that the physiological consequences of the different types do not differ too much, this might be something well acceptable. In some cases the subject him/herself was assigned to one of the states "healthy" or "OSAS", i.e., the SRBD events were not even detected on a one minute basis.

In many of the studies the authors mentioned that they evaluated the power of the frequency band around 0.02 Hz which reflects the brady-tachycardia oscillations of the HRV provoked by *subsequent SRBD events*. Relying on the repetition of SRBD events, the authors mentioned that, accordingly, their approaches failed to detect single events.

In quite a few studies the authors described methods for a feature preselection, e.g., SLS and WRAP, to prevent the curse of dimensionality.

The by far most frequently evaluated feature was the RR-interval, i.e., the HR and the HRV. This is most likely due to the fact that during a PSG only a single-lead

ECG is recorded. Most of the morphological approaches in the studies were usually based on multi-lead ECG records the authors created alongside the diagnostic PSG.

The authors of studies describing morphology based approaches usually mentioned a high inter-subject variability of the computed features. This meant the detection algorithms had to be trained to a specific subject. In general, this prohibits their application in diagnostic devices where the considered subjects are mainly unknown to the algorithm. Nevertheless, the application of morphological features may be useful in devices which support "their" subjects in acquiring a healthier lifestyle.

During the description of their approaches many authors mentioned that they manually corrected the automatically detected R-peaks or excluded artifact loaded data segments from their evaluation. On the one hand, this is truly helpful to assess the power of the applied algorithm. On the other hand, this creates a kind of artificial situation which does not represent everyday reality. This is a kind of limiting factor when most authors claim to ease the SRBD diagnosis by freeing the personnel from the cumbersome task of manually evaluating the recorded data.

The next Chapter will describe the reasons why the Physionet database was not used for this work. It will give an introduction to the project during which the evaluated data was recorded and the way the data was processed to achieve the later on presented results.

Chapter 5

Acquiring Medical Data

5.1 BFS Project "Sleep Home Monitoring"

This work was inspired by the project "Mobile Erfassung, standard-basierte Übertragung und verteilte Verarbeitung medizinischer Messdaten am Beispiel der Schlafmedizin, Kurztitel: Schlaf-Home-Monitoring"[1] which was founded by the Bayrische Forschungsstiftung (BFS, English: Bavarian Research Foundation) between July 2003 and October 2006. The target of the project was to simplify the process of diagnosing OSAS to such an extent that it could be performed by the patient him/herself in his/her own sleeping room. Therefore, the acquisition of vital data, i.e., mainly the application of the sensors, had to be simplified, because trained personnel is required for a full PSG. Moreover, to make the subject's home the practitioner's place, the transmission and the storing of the recorded data were to be addressed. And, finally, to make the system attractive for the clinical partner, the processing of the data to derive a medical conclusion should have been automatized.

The main key to achieving this target was to reduce the number of actually measured vital signals and to compensate for the lost information by algorithms which extract the missing pieces of information from the available vital parameters.

In the end the project partners agreed to create a device (see Figure 5.1) which recorded the following vital parameters:

- Respiratory flow

- Respiratory effort

- SpO_2

---

[1] In English: "Mobile Acquisition, Standard based Transmission, and distributed Processing of Medical Recordings by ways of example Sleep Diagnostic, Short Title: Sleep-Home-Monitoring (SHM)"

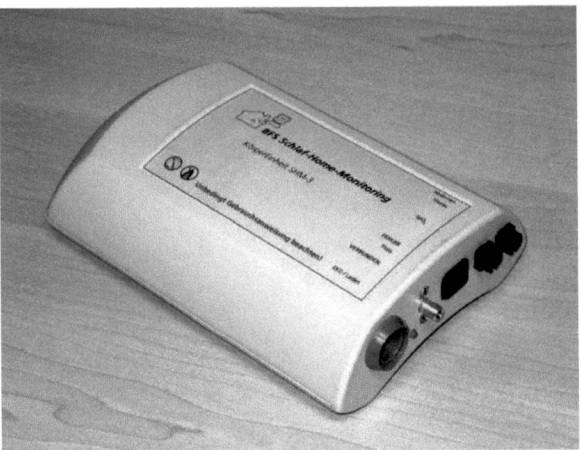

Figure 5.1: The SHM device which was developed during the BFS project (with the sensor connectors)

- Pulse

- Sleeping position (belly, on sides, back)

- ECG

This parameter set is characteristic for the *cardio-respiratory polygraphy* - a reduced PSG (see /2.8.1/). However, driven by the notion to simplify the diagnostic process as much as possible, the idea of abandoning all of the sensors except for the ECG was born.

5.2 Overview over the Data Flow Chain

In Figure 5.2, there is an overview of the complete data flow from the recording of the medical data at the patient's bed to the final evaluation of the extracted features.

In the next Section the data flow chain will be explained stepwise along with the tools which were written or applied, respectively. The two main applications created in the scope of this work are named "EVA" which stands for "**E**CG e**V**aluation **A**pplication.

5.2. Overview over the Data Flow Chain   73

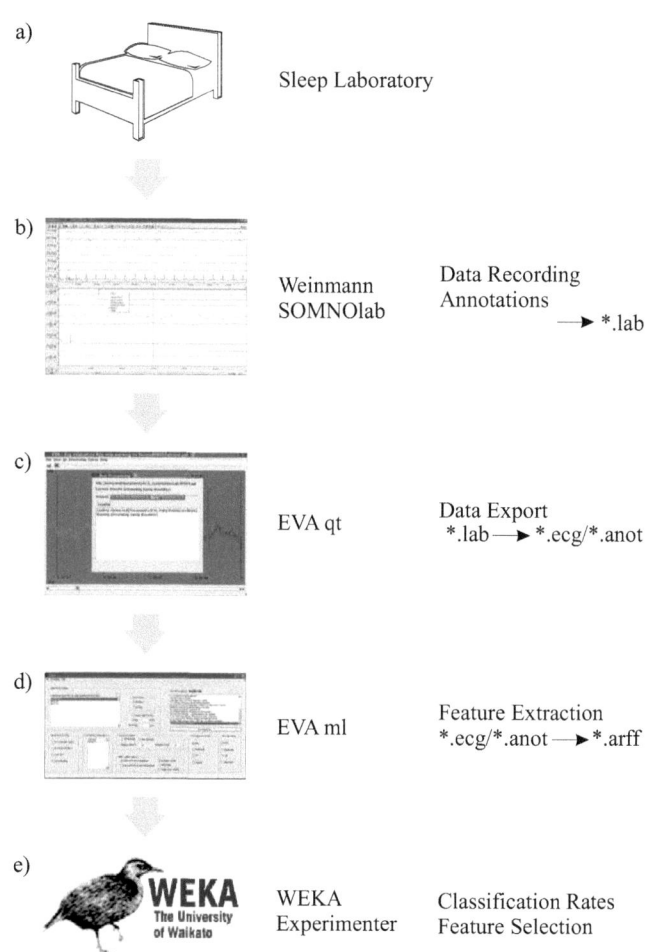

Figure 5.2: Data flow chain from the recording of the vital data (a) to the evaluation of the extracted features (e).

5.2.1 Sleep Laboratory – Recording Data

The initial step (see Figure 5.2a is the actual data recording at the sleep laboratories of the involved clinical partners, Klinikum Nürnberg and the University of Marburg. The data for this project was recorded during their nightly routine.

In total, 58 recordings were made and cross-annotated by both clinical partners. "Cross-annotated" means that after the recording the data files were copied and sent without any annotations to the other clinical partner, where the files were annotated independently. Thus, for each recording, there are two annotations (see next Section). The data recording was done using the Weinmann SOMNOlab PSG system (see /2.8.1/).

5.2.2 Clinical Data Evaluation – Annotations

Each data recording was evaluated by a somnologist for "real-life diagnosis", i.e., as with standard diagnosis all the recorded vital parameters were evaluated to assure high accuracy. During the evaluation process, the sleep stages and SRBD events, e.g., hypopnea and apnea, were annotated (see Figure 5.2b.

Weinmann SOMNOlab writes all the recorded vital data and the expert's annotations to the proprietary file format *.lab which comprises additional data, e.g., the device configuration and patient related data, as well.

5.2.3 Data Export – From Proprietary to Raw Data

For the export (see Figure 5.2c of the proprietary SOMNOlab files, EVA qt was developed. It is written in C++ using Qt 3.0 from Trolltech (see [Trol 05]) – which is where the "qt" derives from – under SuSE Linux 6.3.

The recorded vital data within the SOMNOlab file is stored in the EDF format. EDF stands for "European Data Format" and has become an unofficial standard for persisting physiological data. According to the specification of EDF (see [Kemp 05]), EVA qt exports the recorded vital data as 16 bit RAW data. During the export each data track (ECG, EEG, and so on) is stored to a separate file whose file name equals the name of *.lab file and the extension is derived from the label of the corresponding data track, e.g., BFS2_01.EKG. The ECG signal was sampled with 256 Hz.

EVA qt allows to export all the clinical experts' annotations which relate to SRBD events. The exported annotation file is an ASCII file with the same number of samples as the exported ECG file. Each sample is a character, e.g., "N", "A",

5.2. Overview over the Data Flow Chain   75

SRBD Event	Marker
Normal Breathing	N
Unclassified Apnea	A
Central Apnea	C
Mixed Apnea	M
Obstructive Apnea	O
Hypopnea	H
Artifact	X
Special	S

Table 5.1: The exported SRBD events and their ASCII coded markers

according to the annotated SRBD event. The complete list is given in Table 5.1, along with their corresponding SRBD event.

The event "Artifact" (X) has been included to enable the training of the algorithm for automatic artifact detection.

5.2.4 Feature Extraction – From ECG to Features

The icon of EVA ml (see Figure 5.2d) symbolizes the feature extraction. In this step the ECG data is processed to derive the features (see Chapter 6) for the classification of SRBD events. The "ml" in "EVA ml" indicates that this incarnation of EVA was implemented using Matlab (see /10.2/).

Classification – Feature Evaluation

Introduction to WEKA The icon of the Kiwi (see Figure 5.2e) symbolizes the evaluation of the extracted features using the data mining software WEKA. This final step turns the extracted features into a selection of the most appropriate classifiers and the best performing features, and, finally, classification rates.

WEKA is a software tool comprising several modules for the evaluation of different classifiers on the data sets. It consists of several data import and export filters, filters for modifying the data, and a whole lot of classifiers. WEKA is open source software and freely available at http://www.cs.waikato.ac.nz/ml/weka/ [The 10]. The software is completely written in Java® which allows to run it on many platforms. The version applied in this work is 3.6.1.

As WEKA is quite popular, there is a lot of literature available. The most important information for this work was gathered from the WEKA manual [Bouc 08b] which is installed directly with the software. And a very good introduction to data mining itself and the application of WEKA is given in [Witt 05].

The file format of WEKA is the "Attribute Relation File Format" (ARFF). This file format allows to associate attributes with classes, but does not represent – or allows representing – temporal dependencies. Hence, it does not matter in which order the instances appear in the ARFF file. If, however, temporal dependencies are to be considered, then they have to be wrapped in extracted features.

Running WEKA Having run WEKA on a standard PC for almost three months without any result, it was obvious that this procedure would become much too time consuming. This was why the idea to migrate to a computer cluster was born. This computer cluster was located in the High Performance Computing (HPC) department of the Regionale Rechenzentrum Erlangen (RRZE).

As no graphical user interface was available, WEKA Experimenter could not be used. As a workaround the following procedure was established to run WEKA from the command line:

- Use WEKA Experimenter on an office PC to create the experiments, i.e., the compilation of ARFF files and the classifiers to apply.

- Modify the Experimenter XML files to reflect the directory structure of the cluster at RRZE.

- Transfer ARFF and XML files to cluster (using WinSCP, i.e., scp tool for a Windows based PC)

- Start WEKA from command line

One experiment consisted of four ARFF files for one set of features, e.g., the P wave, whereof two files were for the respiratory events and two for the sleep stages. For the Autonomous Model (see /6.3/) there were twelve files because of performing three runs. The feature sets were evaluated individually as the Java virtual machine seemed to have some difficulties keeping up with the memory management.

The last step of starting WEKA was simplified by writing a Linux bash batch file which features:

- Automatic creation of paths to data and XML files according to the directory structure on the cluster

- File names, i.e., anonymous patient names, are stored in an array and can be accessed via an ID sparing the user the effort to type them by hand

5.3. Consistency of the Medical Annotations

	$Kp1$	$Kp2$	bK	nA
a)	5	4	5	86
b)	5	3	22	70

Table 5.2: The results of Figure 5.3 in tabular presentation (in [%])

- Redirection of `stdout` and `stderr` into an appropriately named file which enables to check the protocol for processing errors
- Processes can be pinned to a specific CPU

The batch file is called with:

`runWEKAonRRZEarray TestSetID PatientID FeatureID [CPU-ID]`

In this call `TestSetID` addresses the different test sets which result from different settings in the processing configuration (see /10.2.2/), `PatientID` selects one of the patients, `FeatureID` selects one of the feature sets (see /6.3/ and /6.4/). The last argument, `CPU-ID`, is optional – if supplied, it specifies the ID of the CPU the process shall be started on, if left blank, the process is started on any CPU. The latter argument is intended to spread the different WEKA evaluation processes over the available CPUs in such way that the computational performance is optimized regarding to the hardware of the cluster.

5.3 Consistency of the Medical Annotations

In [Tels 04] and [Dank 01], having evaluated several studies the authors claimed that the interrater variability between two well educated sleep scorers usually does not become better than about 70%. The two involved clinical partners were interested to see how close to this "limit" they would come.

The first approach of judging the consistency of the medical annotations was to plot a pie chart. For this approach all types of SRBD events (see Table 5.1) were grouped in contrast to normal respiration. (Artifacts were excluded from this test.) The periods during which only one clinical partner annotated an event are given by $Kp1$ or $Kp2$, respectively. The periods in which both clinical partners marked a SRBD event are given by bK. The remaining periods which both clinical partner considered healthy are marked with nA. The result is shown in Figure 5.3 as well in Table 5.2.

$$MoC = \frac{p_{K_n} + p_{bK}}{\sum p_K} \qquad (5.1)$$

78   Chapter 5. Acquiring Medical Data

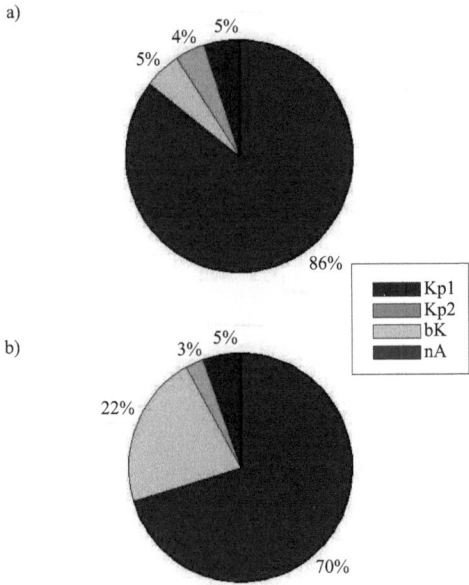

Figure 5.3: Visual representation of the concordance of the annotations of the clinical partners

	$Moc12$	$Moc21$	Moc
a)	0.71	0.64	0.65
b)	0.9	0.83	0.87

Table 5.3: The MoC values for the two examples from Figure 5.3

$p_o\ (\bar{p}_o)$	$\kappa\ (\bar{\kappa})$	$\kappa_{mod}\ (\bar{\kappa}_{mod})$
0.60 - 0.97 (0.79)	0.06 - 0.68 (0.36)	0.40 - 0.76 (0.58)

Table 5.4: The different Kappa coefficients

Assuming that non-annotated, i.e., without any SRBD event, periods are in fact healthy, a measure of concordance MoC for the SRBD annotated periods can be defined as in equation (5.1). In this equation p_{K_n} means the likeliness of one clinical partner annotating an event. Likewise, p_{bK} stands for the likeliness of both clinical partners agreeing on an event and p_K means the likeliness of an event marked by any or both clinical partners. Applying this equation leads to a concordance of the two clinical partners as shown in Table 5.3.

These results can be considered very good. However, the applied MoC is somewhat "special". Thus, to have a more "comparable" view of the degree of concordance, the Kappa κ (see /10.1.1/) and the modified Kappa κ_{mod} (see /10.1.2/) coefficients were computed for the annotations. The coefficients are shown in Table 5.4.

Considering Table 10.2 the overall concordance according to these coefficients must be judged as "moderate". Nevertheless, the achieved interrater concordance exceeds the value of 70% mentioned by [Tels 04].

5.4 Summary and Preview

This Chapter started with an introduction to the BFS project during which most of the data for this work was recorded.

The next Section gave an overview of the data flow chain from the recording of the vital data in the sleep laboratories to the final evaluation of the features which were extracted from the ECG signal. Along with the data flow chain the applied software tools were shortly introduced.

At the end of the Chapter the consistency of the medical annotation of the two clinical partners of the BFS project was evaluated using different approaches. The first one was a visual one in the shape of a pie diagram. The next approach was accomplished by the introduction of the proprietary concordance measure MoC and, finally, the commonly used Kappa coefficients were applied to the annotations.

The next Chapter will introduce the two feature extraction approaches which were developed during this work – the Autonomous Model (see /6.3/) and the morphology based approach (see /6.4/). This Chapter will also provide the linkage between the two Chapters of medical basics and the features which were extracted.

Chapter 6

Proposed Solution for Detecting SRBD Events and Sleep Stages from an ECG Signal

Based upon the medical basics which were introduced in Chapters 2 and 3, this Chapter will present the reasoning for the features extracted and the way this is accomplished.

Two different approaches will be described. Each of them spotlights the heart and its reactions to variations of physiological states from a different perspective. The approaches pursued are based on the fact that the occurrences of SRBD events and sleep stages themselves are represented in the ECG – either by the HR or by its morphology.

Before the actual feature computation, the ECG signal has to be enhanced which is done during the preprocessing step and the distinctive points of the ECG have to be detected. Table 6.1 gives an overview of the four main Sections of this Chapter. Most Sections further split into three Subsections which are a theoretical part which provides the linkage between the medical basics and the features extracted, the implementation, and the results of the intermediate steps when running EVA ml (see /10.2/).

Most of the screen shots have been realized using the file BFS2_01 in the sample range from an offset – due to artifacts at the beginning of the file – of 25000 to the sample at position 50000, i.e., 25000 samples representing approximately 90 seconds, for the morphologic functions. For the HRV evaluation the data was taken from sample 25000 to sample 275000, i.e., 250000 samples representing 15 minutes. During the entire interval the respiratory state is annotated "normal", i.e., healthy.

Processing Step	Page
Preprocessing of the ECG signal	68
Detection of the distinctive ECG points	72
Autonomous Model – Evaluation of the HR and its variation	76
Morphology based features	91

Table 6.1: Overview of the successive processing steps and two feature extraction approaches

In the Figures the values on the coordinate axis representing the amplitude of the ECG wave are given in "units" of AD converter values (ADV), i.e., the digital output representing the analog signal. This "unit" is used as well for the results of the signal processing. Hence, "amplitude" means the digital value.

6.1 Preprocessing of the ECG

In everyday clinical life the quality of the recording is limited by noise and other adverse effects (see /3.1.2/) as the signal amplitude of around $1mV$ is (comparatively) small. The three most important influences on an ECG recording are:

- General noise, e.g., of the measurement equipment
- Influences of the mains supply (50 Hz in Europe)
- Shifts of the DC level caused by movements of the patient or the gradual loss of proper connection of the ECG electrode

The filters designed for EVA ml are FIR (Finite Impulse Response) filters of high order, because this design provides the following advantages:

Linear phase response means that there is no distortion of the signal shape due to frequency dependent delays which is an important prerequisite for the morphology based features.

Small transition bandwidths of approximately 3 Hz, which is a desirable feature of the filters to preserve as much of the ECG frequency spectrum while efficiently suppressing the noisy spectral components.

High attenuation for the noisy components means that the energy in the noisy range of the spectrum is almost completely suppressed.

In the tables describing the properties of the filters "F" stands for "frequency" and "A" stands for "attenuation". "Pass" indicates the frequency up to which the filter retains the spectrum, whereas it suppresses the spectrum in the "stop" range.

6.1. Preprocessing of the ECG

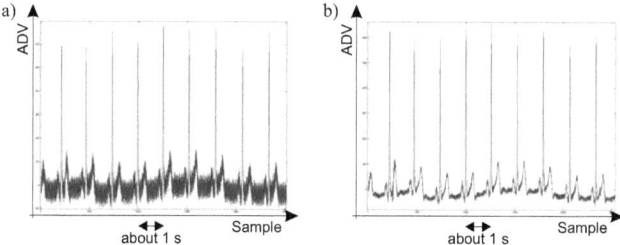

Figure 6.1: Comparison between a) the original ECG and b) the signal cleaned from the mains supply noise by the applied bandstop filter.

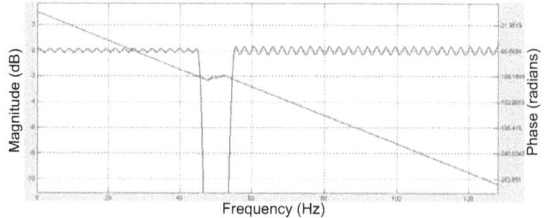

Figure 6.2: Amplitude and phase response of the 50 Hz bandstop filter

6.1.1 Mains Supply

The electromagnetic fields of the mains supply are present "everywhere" and the human body and the measurement wires act as antennas for these fields inducing an electrical voltage.

In Figure 6.1 there is a comparison between the originally recorded ECG signal and the filtered signal. The strong impact on the signal can as well be observed in the spectrum where the mains supply noise results in a pronounced peak (see Figure 6.3).

The type of the filter is a bandstop[1] filter, i.e., it blocks frequencies around its center frequency and lets higher and lower frequencies pass. The amplitude and phase response of the filter are shown in Figure 6.2 and the characteristics are given in Table 6.2.

Figure 6.3 shows the impact of the filter in the frequency domain. In Figure 6.3a there is the spectrum which was generated from a sequence of ECG before the mains supply noise suppression. In blue the original signal and in red the windowed signal (see Figure 6.77) is shown. In Figure 6.3b the same signal sequence is displayed after the invocation of the mains supply filter.

---
[1] Bandstop filters are called "notch filters" as well.

84 Chapter 6. Detecting SRBD Events and Sleep Stages from an ECG Signal

Property	Value
Type	Bandstop
Structure	Direct-Form FIR
Order	198
F_{pass1}	45 Hz
F_{stop1}	48 Hz
F_{stop2}	52 Hz
F_{pass2}	55 Hz
A_{pass1}	0.5 dB
A_{stop}	60 dB
A_{pass2}	1 dB

Table 6.2: Properties of the 50 Hz bandstop filter: the very narrow transition range enables efficient filtering of the mains supply influences, while keeping as much of the morphological information as possible.

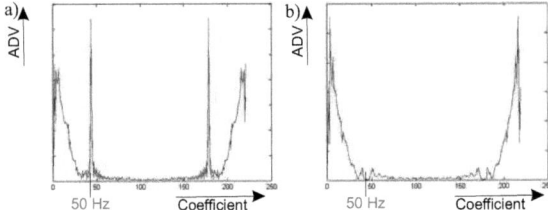

Figure 6.3: Comparison of the impact of the mains supply filter in the frequency domain: in a) the original signal and in b) the signal after the bandstop filter was applied (The slight shift of the 50 Hz marker against the coefficient 50 on the abscissa results from the fact that the signal was sampled with 256 Hz, but the DFT was performed on a window length of 221 samples, which means that one coefficient represents about 1.16 Hz).

6.1. Preprocessing of the ECG 85

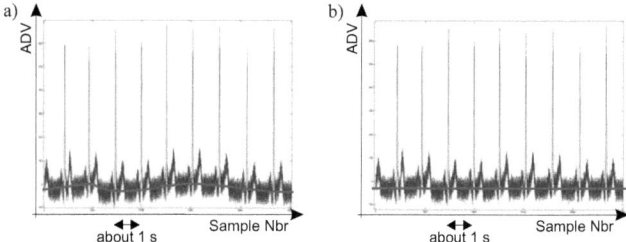

Figure 6.4: Compensation of DC-shifts by a highpass filter: The effect can be observed by looking at the red lines which (approximately) mark the iso-electrical potential.

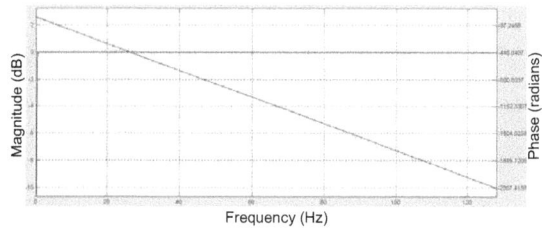

Figure 6.5: Amplitude and phase response of the highpass filter compensating DC-shifts

6.1.2 DC-Shifts

The DC-shifts are caused, for example, by movements of the patient or electrode displacements entailing a change in the impedance between the electrode and the patient's skin. Compensating the DC-shifts is of high importance for the morphological features, because DC-shifts outrange the ECG amplitude by far, i.e., several 100 mV of DC-shift compared to about 1 mV of ECG signal.

As DC-shifts can be considered signals with a frequency of (about) 0 Hz, they are canceled by applying a highpass filter, i.e., a filter letting high frequencies pass and blocking low frequencies. The comparison of the original and the filtered signal is given in Figure 6.4. The filter's amplitude and phase response are depicted in Figure 6.5. The characteristics of the filter are given in Table 6.3.

6.1.3 General Noise

Under the terminus "general noise" all the remaining adverse impacts on the measurement are summarized. It includes electromagnetic influences as well as the

86   Chapter 6. Detecting SRBD Events and Sleep Stages from an ECG Signal

Property	Value
Type	Highpass
Structure	Direct-Form FIR
Order	1408
F_{stop}	0.001 Hz
F_{pass}	0.5 Hz
A_{stop}	80 dB
A_{pass}	1 dB

Table 6.3: Properties of the applied high pass filter

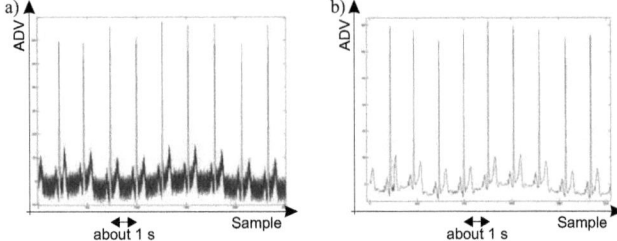

Figure 6.6: Comparison of the ECG signal before and after the lowpass filtering

shortcomings of the technical equipment. Technically, this filter is a lowpass filter, i.e., it suppresses frequencies higher than its cut-off frequency F_{stop}.

Figure 6.6 shows the original signal on the left side, whereas the lowpass filtered signal is on the right. Figure 6.7 shows the amplitude (blue) and the phase response (green) of the designed filter. The characteristics of the filter are given in Table 6.4.

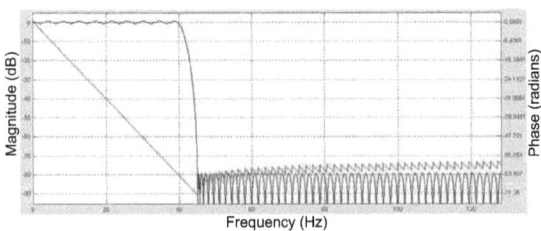

Figure 6.7: Amplitude and phase response of the applied low pass filter

6.1. Preprocessing of the ECG

Property	Value
Type	Lowpass
Structure	Direct-Form FIR
Order	130
F_{pass}	40 Hz
F_{stop}	45 Hz
A_{pass}	1 dB
A_{stop}	80 dB

Table 6.4: Properties of the applied low pass filter

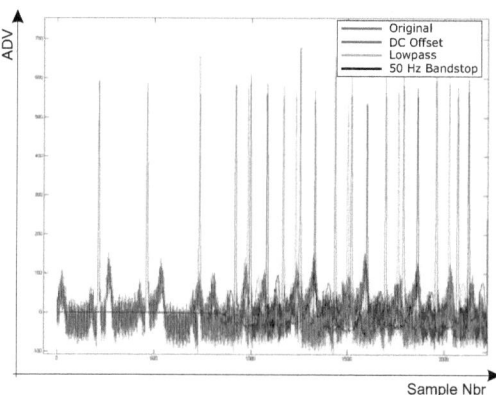

Figure 6.8: Original ECG signal (blue) and the delayed ECG signals after the application of the filters: As the DC-shifts filter is the first one to be applied and the one of the highest order, the delay is most obvious here (red).

6.1.4 Compensating Filter Delays

An additional aspect to consider is that the application of any of the filters leads to a delay of the filtered signal. For FIR filters this delay equals half the order of the filter as can be seen in Figure 6.8 where the filters have been applied successively.

This delay leads to a displacement of the ECG with respect to the SRBD annotations and the hypnogram. This displacement reaches its maximum of 868 samples – approximately 3.5 s – when all the filters are activated. This may not be important for an evaluation period of 30 seconds, but it may be relevant for the beat-to-beat evaluation.

To compensate for the filter delays and, accordingly, resynchronize the annotations, the number of samples given by half the filter order are cut from the beginning of the ECG recording.

88 Chapter 6. Detecting SRBD Events and Sleep Stages from an ECG Signal

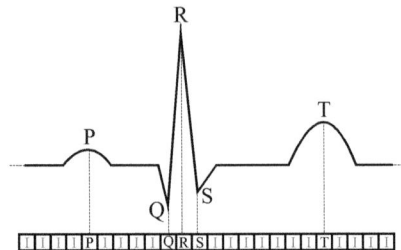

Figure 6.9: Principle of labeling the distinctive points in the ECG: this is a stylized view, as in the real data there is an annotation entry for each ECG sample. Hence, the resolution of the annotation track is much higher than in this Figure, but this reduction improves clarity.

6.2 ECG Distinctive Point Detection

The first step in each of the two different approaches is the labeling of the distinctive ECG points (see /3.1.1/). The only difference is that for the HR evaluation just the R-peaks are extracted, whereas for the morphologic approach all distinctive points are extracted.

6.2.1 Labeling the Distinctive Points in the ECG

In Figure 6.9 there is an illustration of the principle of labeling the distinctive ECG points. In the upper pane there is a standard ECG wave and in the lower pane there is a representation[2] of the data vector containing the distinctive point labels.

The data vector is allocated with the same length the ECG vector. During initialization each element is set to "I" standing for "intermediate point", a point between the distinctive points.

The first distinctive points labeled are the R-peaks as these are most dominant. Each found R-peak is labeled with an "R" in the data vector. The remaining points are all found according to the same principle: compute borders within which the distinctive point of interest has to be in a healthy heart beat and search the maximum (P-wave, T-wave) or minimum (Q-peak, S-peak), respectively. Each found maximum or minimum is labeled with the corresponding letter, e.g., "P", "Q", and so on.

The search is performed from "close to the R-peak to far from the R-peak" to adjust the search borders to the current heart rate, i.e., the search order is:

---

[2]This representation is not to the scale as there are about 256 samples for each heart beat

6.2. ECG Distinctive Point Detection

$$R \longrightarrow Q \longrightarrow S \longrightarrow P \longrightarrow T$$

After the labeling the data vector looks something like in Figure 6.9.

6.2.2 R-Peak Detection

The algorithm used for the R-peak detection is based on the algorithm described in [Fuhr 04] which itself is based on [Lee 02]. The algorithm has been modified for the usage with EVA ml. The main difference is that the version for EVA ml does not operate on the complete ECG recording but on intervals whose length in seconds is specified by the parameter `Evaluation Period` on EVA ml's GUI (see Figure 10.1). This yields two advantages: First, the algorithm is much – approximately ten times – faster which seems to be due to the memory management of Matlab (see p. 82). Second, the splitting of the records allows implementing a progress indicator which is a quite comforting feature as the R-peak detection takes about one hour for an overnight recording.

6.2.3 Detection of the Remaining Distinctive ECG Points

After the detection of the R-peaks the boundaries of each ECG wave are well defined which enables detecting the remaining distinctive ECG points by means of the following principle:

- Take the position of the corresponding R-peak
- Compute the distance to the previous or following R-peak, respectively
- Compute lower and upper boundaries for the range within which the point of interest is expected to be located.
- For the distinctive points "far from" the R-peak, i.e., P and T, find intermediate points, i.e., Q and S, according to search order
- Find maximum (P, T) or minimum (Q, S) within boundaries, respectively
- Label point accordingly

Table 6.5 gives an overview over the boundaries that are applied for each distinctive point. Each label, for example "R", stands for the position (on the time, i.e., sample, scale) of the point, and RR means the length of the current RR interval.

Figure 6.10 shows the results of the detection of the distinctive ECG points.

Chapter 6. Detecting SRBD Events and Sleep Stages from an ECG Signal

Distinctive Point	Begin	End
Q	R - $\frac{1}{8}$RR	R
S	R	R + $\frac{1}{6}$RR
P	R - $\frac{1}{4}$RR	Q
T	S	R + $\frac{1}{2}$RR

Table 6.5: Distinctive ECG points and their corresponding search boundaries

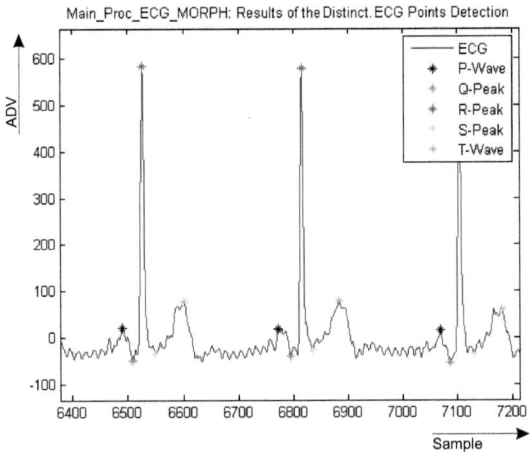

Figure 6.10: Results of the ECG distinctive points detection

6.3 Autonomous Model

The model which is described in this Section is based on the physiological fact that the HRV, i.e., the change of the heart rate, is controlled by the balance of sympathetic and parasympathetic activity. Both, the SNS and the PNS, are modeled as generators which have their own properties and contribute to the HRV (see /3.2/ and /3.3.1/). As the sympathetic and the parasympathetic nervous system constitute the autonomous system, the model presented here is called the *Autonomous Model*, *AM*.

6.3.1 Technical Description of the Model

This Section examines the autonomous model from an electrical engineering point of view. It start with the "schematic" of the model which is shown in Figure 6.11a. It consists of the main voltage controlled oscillator (VCO[3]). This oscillator is to represent the heart as indicated by the pictogram of the heart. It produces the ECG waves (not shown) at a frequency of f_{HR} (see Figure 6.11b), the heart rate. The input of the VCO comprises the three (analogue) voltages $u_{1...3}$ which are produced by three signal generators named G_{Resp}, G_{Symp}, and G_{Noise}, respectively.

Generator G_{Resp} outputs a "sine" wave, generator G_{Symp} emits rectangular bursts sporadically at times t_{Ev}, and the last generator G_{Noise} produces *Noise* which is to be read "a wave form showing no regularities".

The output frequency of the VCO equals:

$$f_{HR}(t) = f_0 + \frac{df_{HR}}{du_1} \cdot u_1(t) + \frac{df_{HR}}{du_2} \cdot u_2(t) + \frac{df_{HR}}{du_3} \cdot u_3(t) \quad (6.1)$$

In equation (6.1) f_0 is the fundamental frequency, i.e., the output frequency of the VCO without any input voltage. $\frac{df_{HR}}{du_1}$, $\frac{df_{HR}}{du_2}$, and $\frac{df_{HR}}{du_3}$ give the changes of f_{HR} depending on changes of u_1, u_2, and u_3, respectively – it's the sensitivity of f_{HR} to changes of the input voltages at the respective inputs or – in more technical nomenclature – the control ratio.

Assuming that $\frac{df_{HR}}{du_1} = \frac{df_{HR}}{du_2} = \frac{df_{HR}}{du_3} = \frac{df_{HR}}{du}$ equation (6.1) can be rewritten into equation (6.2) where the "sum of influences" is symbolized by the Σ symbol.

$$f_{HR}(t) = f_0 + \frac{df_{HR}}{du} \sum_{n=1}^{3} u_n(t) \quad (6.2)$$

---

[3] A VCO is a frequency generator whose output frequency is controlled by one (or the sum of more) input voltages. Accordingly, it produces a frequency modulated signal.

92   Chapter 6. Detecting SRBD Events and Sleep Stages from an ECG Signal

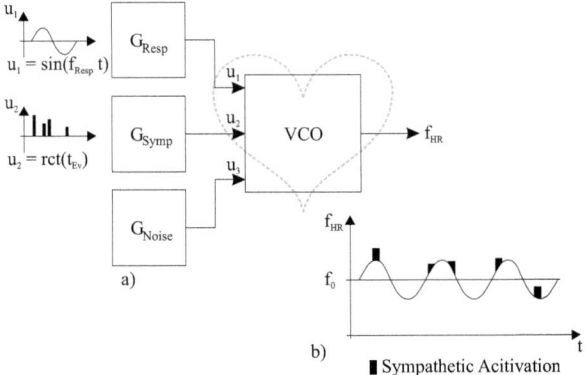

Figure 6.11: In a) there is the Autonomous Model from an electrical engineering point of view. It consists of a VCO which generates the HR according to the different influences at its inputs. These influences derive from the ANS (see text). In b) there is a (stylized) graph of the produced output **frequency** according to the different influences.

Given the (stylized) output voltages of the generators G_{Resp}, G_{Symp}, G_{Noise} (see Figure 6.11a), and equation (6.1) a curve of f_{HR} (stylized as well) is shown in Figure 6.11b: the output frequency f_{HR} is centered around the fundamental frequency f_0 and the influence of generator G_{Resp} leads to a sine like swing of the output frequency around f_0. The rectangular bursts of generator G_{Symp} result in superimposing bursts of f_{HR}. The influence of the last generator G_{Noise} is not shown in Figure 6.11b – the superimposed noise simply leads to a "blurring" of the curve of f_{HR}, i.e., it introduces a jitter of f_{HR}.

6.3.2 Model and Physiology (Hypothesis)

Even though the names of the generators in Figure 6.11a already hint on their relation to the physiology of the heart rate regulation, it will be explained in more detail.

The fundamental frequency f_0 of the VCO relates to the heart rate at rest – without any influences from the inside or outside. Of course, it is not possible to determine this frequency, because it is not feasible to block all influences. Hence, as a "workaround", this frequency is approximated by the mean of the heart rate over a long period at rest, i.e., over the night.

6.3. Autonomous Model

The generator G_{Resp} produces the heart rate fluctuations which are caused by the sinus arrhythmia (see /3.3.1/). These are fluctuations of the heart rate caused by respiration. They are considered to be under the control of the PNS, which is thought to have a response delay of 4 - 8 seconds.

The generator G_{Symp} stands for the influences of the SNS. This is the part of the autonomous system which is (said to be) activated by an arousal or during a transition between sleep stages. The sympathetic nervous system is considered to have a response delay of 20 - 40 seconds.

Apart from the influences discussed so far there are of course many more, which do not have a special meaning in the scope of this model or which are simply much too complex. That's why they are named "Noise" and summarized in the last generator G_{Noise}. One of these influences is for example the REM sleep stage with its massive heart rate fluctuations. Inversely, a turbulent f_{HR} may hint on the REM sleep stage.

Arousals are known to be short bursts of sympathetic activity which happen to restore the wake state respiration. One result is a short time rise of the heart rate. Accordingly, the bursts of f_{HR} shown in Figure 6.11b might relate to events like apnea, hypopnea, and/or sleep stage changes, respectively.

Of course, there are other effects which are known to have impact on the heart rate. These will be discussed here shortly. Arrhythmia leads to ectopic bursts, i.e., short time disturbances of the RR-peak sequence. Therefore, in principle it should be noticed as an output of generator G_{Symp}, i.e., interpreted as an apnea event. First, this would be a misinterpretation as the occurrence of an ectopic heart beat does not necessarily mean there is an apnea. Second, nevertheless, arrhythmia is known to happen under apnea condition sometimes which is especially true for CSAS /2.5.4/. Therefore, in otherwise healthy subjects – as far as the cardiovascular system is considered – ectopic heart beats might well hint on an apnea event or help to distinguish CSA from OSA. Third, during the processing of the AM there is quite a lot of low pass filtering – in the sense of suppressing such "noises".

The sleep apnea induced hypoxemia (see /3.3.1/ and Figure 3.11) should be noticeable in an increased activity of generator G_{Resp} in the phase of decreasing HR, followed by an increase in the activity of generator G_{Symp} during the compensation phase.

Figure 6.12 is to illustrate some reasoning about the short time dynamics of the HR. A stable condition of the body relates to an almost constant HR. Considering the spectrum of the HR, a constant HR results in a sharp, i.e., narrow, peak. This

94   Chapter 6. Detecting SRBD Events and Sleep Stages from an ECG Signal

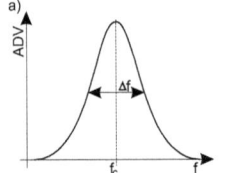 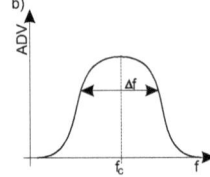

Figure 6.12: This Figure serves as an illustration how to derive the stability of the body state from the shape of envelop curve covering the frequencies belonging to one of the generators. In a) the spectrum resembles a narrow peak which means the frequency of the generator is quite stable, i.e., there are no fluctuations due to transitions of the body state. Vice versa, in b) the peak resembles a wide "bell shape" which means that the frequencies of this one generator are spread in the spectrum. Assumingly, this high variability around the center frequency is caused by fluctuations of the body state.

can be seen in Figure 6.12a: a high peak due to condensed energy with a small Δf around the center frequency f_c of the respective oscillator.

Vice versa, fluctuations of the HR hint on instabilities in the regulation of the HR, thus, indicating transitions of the body condition. Again, considering the spectrum, fluctuations of the HR result in a soft and wide bell shaped curve. This is shown in Figure 6.12b: a less high peak due to "blurred energy" with a high Δf.

All three introduced "intuitive" values describing the shape, i.e., amplitude and Δf, and position, i.e., f_c, of the "body state stability curve" will be given a more mathematical character in later Sections.

6.3.3 Implementation of the Autonomous Model

To extract the information about changes in the subject's physiological state, EVA ml has to "reverse-process" the model, i.e., to compute the properties of the generators from the HRV. Figure 6.13 illustrates the required steps in a flow chart.

Each of the steps depicted in the flow chart will now be explained in more detail.

Compute HR and Detect Anomalies

In the first step EVA ml extracts the positions of the R-peaks along the time axis and computes the HR therewith (see Figure 6.13a) according to equation (6.9). Subsequently, the computed HR is put to tests for bradycardia and tachycardia (see /3.2/) as well as for extensive, i.e., physiologically unlikely, fluctuations of the heart rate.

6.3. Autonomous Model

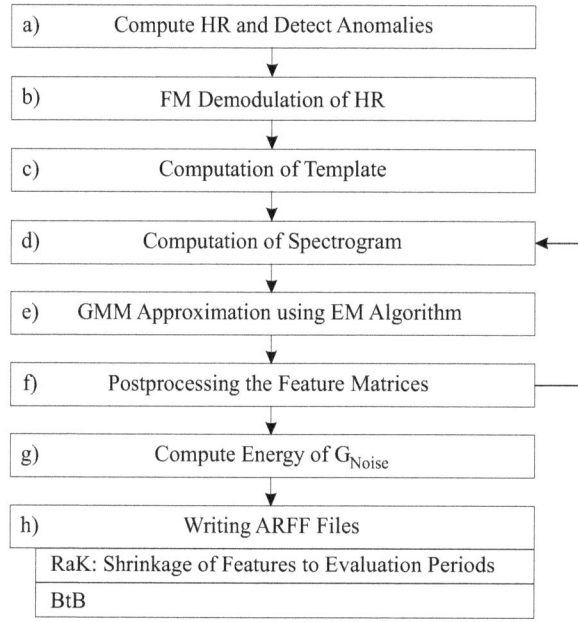

Figure 6.13: Flow Chart of EVA ml processing the Autonomous Model

96   Chapter 6. Detecting SRBD Events and Sleep Stages from an ECG Signal

In the case of very low or high HR, respectively, EVA ml simply issues a note and the index of the corresponding R-peak, at whose position the event was detected[4]. In the case of high fluctuations EVA ml additionally replaces the "dubious" value with the mean of the surrounding values, i.e., $m_c(HR, 5)$ (see equation (10.9b)).

FM Demodulation of HR

The next step in the "reverse modeling" is the FM demodulation (see Figure 6.13b) which undoes the influence of the VCO (see /6.3.1/) and delivers the "sum of all influences" (see equation (6.2)) of the generators representing the autonomous system.

Before the actual FM demodulation of the HR series, this vector is resynchronized to the ECG signal, i.e., its former length is restored. This is required due to the fact that the vector containing the HR is derived from the vector of R-peak positions, accordingly, it has the same length like the number of R-peaks in the recording. The resizing of the vector is done in the following steps:

- A vector of the same length like the number of ECG samples is allocated.
- The positions of the R-peaks are reconstructed.
- The samples between two R-peaks are filled with the repeated HR value from the beginning of the interval.

This procedure results in a step curve which is shown in Figure 6.14.

The FM demodulation requires two preconditions: First, the input signal must be differentiable, and second, the fundamental frequency of the VCO. The first requirement is fulfilled by smoothing the step curve from the previous processing step in an AM demodulation derived processing[5], i.e., an envelope function of the HR series is computed. The result is shown in Figure 6.15 in the upper panel in a zoomed view. The blue signal is the step curve and the red one the envelop signal.

For the second requirement, as the actual base frequency f_0 of the body is not accessible, it is computed as the mean $m(HR)$ of the HR over the complete night.

During the evaluation of the complete overnight recordings the limitations of Matlab's memory management became obvious: Matlab aborted the processing issuing an `Out-of-Memory` warning. To overcome this limitation the FM demodulation of the HR series is separated into chunks of data. As the FM demodulation

---

[4] This feature was implemented mainly for debugging purposes, i.e., to verify whether the R-peak detection worked properly.

[5] AM demodulation is performed by means of the function `smoothHRSeriesforFM()` (essentially the same as `BreathEnvelopeADM()` in /10.3/)

6.3. Autonomous Model

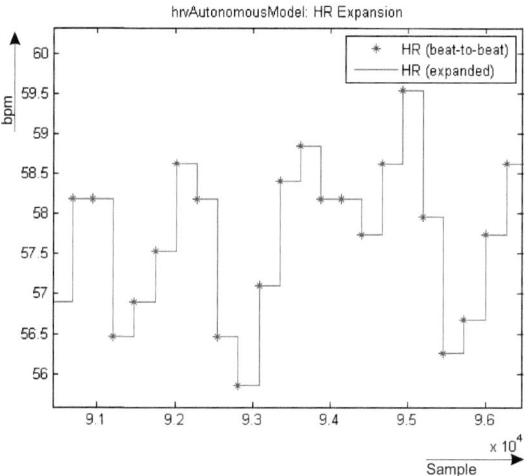

Figure 6.14: Expanded HR: The blue asterisks denote the HR series (readjusted to the positions of their corresponding R-peaks) and the red step curve shows the expanded HR series.

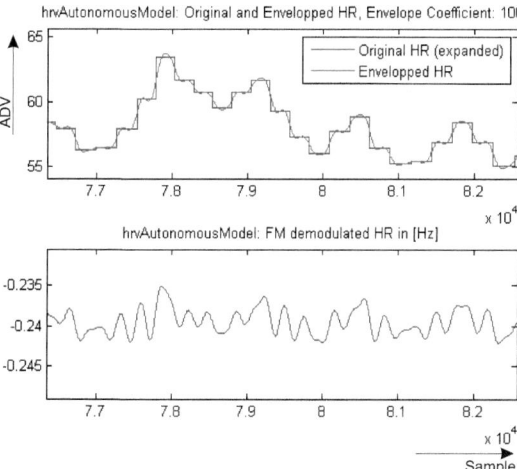

Figure 6.15: FM demodulation of the HR series: In the upper panel, there is the step curve of the HR series (from the previous Figure) in blue and the smoothed envelope curve in red. In the lower panel, there is the FM demodulated signal whose fundamental frequency was estimated by the mean of HR over the complete night.

98   Chapter 6. Detecting SRBD Events and Sleep Stages from an ECG Signal

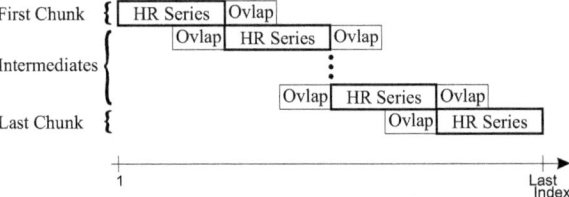

Figure 6.16: Computing the FM demodulated signal from HR series chunks

functions needs "some time", i.e., samples, to engage into the HR series, the actually evaluated data is extended with additional data on either side. The principle is shown in Figure 6.16. The center part named "HR Series" is the actually processed data. The additional data at either side is named "Ovlap". The first and the last chunk of data differ from this principle as there is no data which could be used for the overlap.

As the first and the last chunk of data showed some extra (engagement process related) noise compared to the FM demodulation "in one whole", an additional method was evaluated. It consisted of extending the first and the last chunk with zeros to have the actual HR series situated "protected in their mids". Figure 6.17 shows the results of a comparison of the three different FM demodulation methods. The blue curve is the result of the FM demodulation in "one whole", the red one according to the principle of overlapping as in Figure 6.16, and the green the one with the zero-padding at either end. It can be seen that the red curve swings around the blue one which accounts for introduced high frequency noise. The green curve not only shows higher noise amplitudes, but it is not even centered around the blue one. Accordingly, the method producing the red curve was chosen.

The values for the chunk length of the HR series and the degree of overlap were found heuristically: the length of the HR series is a compromise between the fact that the first and the last chunk of data is polluted with high frequency noise, i.e., the length should be small, and the processing speed, i.e., the length should be as big as possible. A value of 50000 samples showed good results. For the value of the overlap length the compromise is between a perfect engagement of the demodulation function, i.e., the length should be big, and the processing speed, i.e., the overlap should be as small as possible. Good results were produced setting this value to 15000 samples. Table 6.6 finally shows the achieved SNR values for the chosen FM demodulation method.

6.3. Autonomous Model

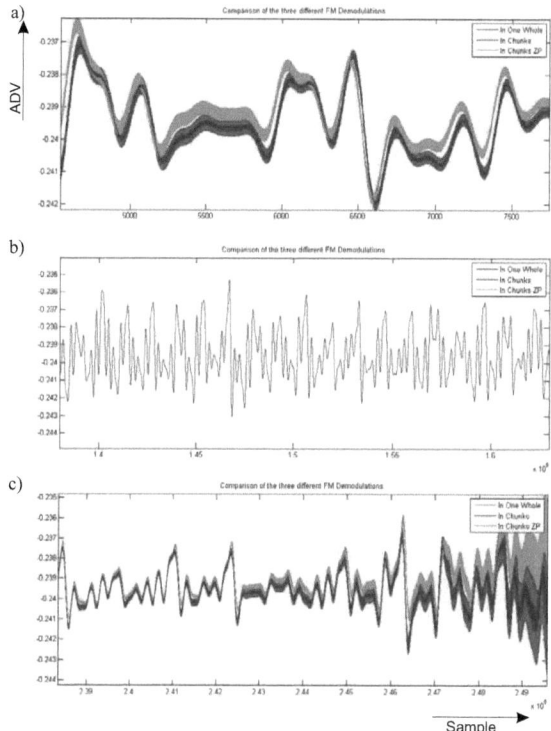

Figure 6.17: Comparison of different methods of split FM demodulation: in blue the FM demodulation "in one whole", in red FM demodulation in chunks, and in green the chunks extended with zero-padding.

Chunk	Beginning	Intermediate	End
Complete	21.1 dB	87.5 dB	25.8 dB
1000 samples missing	60.3 dB	87.5 dB	62.8 dB

Table 6.6: SNR values for the 'chunk-wise' FM demodulation: "Complete" means the *complete* first and the last chunk was evaluated, respectively. "1000 samples missing" means that the data considered for the SNR evaluation started at the 1000th sample or ended at the 1000th before the end of the recording. From the SNR values it can be clearly seen that the noise level decays rapidly along the samples. The achieved SNR values – especially for the intermediate chunks – can be considered very good. Moreover, the (low pass) filtering in the processing stages to come will make sure that this noise does not influence the evaluation of the HR series.

Computation of Template

In order to separate the influences of the generators from one another, EVA ml computes a template in the third step (see Figure 6.13c). This template contains the maxima (in frequency of occurrence) of the spectrogram where the different generators are represented as a series of peaks or "bells", respectively (see Figure 6.12). This spectrogram is required to calculate a template which is used during the feature computation to track the different spectral maxima. Each of these maxima belongs to a generator of the autonomous model (see Figure 6.11) and reflects its properties (sympathetic or parasympathetic activity, degree of influence, stableness, and so on).

The first step for the creation of the template is the computation of a spectrogram[6]. For the creation of the spectrogram the FM demodulated signal is split into pieces of a length defaulting to 24000 (given by the parameter lenTemplate). Hence, the matrix which is returned features the dimension 12000 by 10: the first figure is the number of DFT coefficients purged from the redundant ones and the second figure is the number of pieces which can be cut from the ECG signal (the data for creating the Figures of the AM consists of 250000 samples, see p. 68).

In the following step the computed spectrogram is "smoothed", i.e., lowpass filtered, by grouping a number of spectra along the time axis and computing the mean $m(Coef_f)$, i.e., the spectral coefficients belonging to the same frequency. The parameter nbrSubSections defines how many subsections, i.e., groups of spectra, shall be created from this spectrogram. As the default value of 30 for nbrSubSections is far to large for the test ensemble (there are only ten spectra in the spectrogram), EVA ml automatically corrects this value in such a way that there are at least two spectra combined for the mean $m(Coef_f)$.

The previous step is done to subdue the influence of noise and outliers. Subsequently, these spectra are processed by a Gaussian filter (whose kernel length is set by the parameter coefGaussianFilter, best results with values 4 & 5, default 5). The results so far are shown in Figure 6.18 for *one* of the subsections. The blue curve is the spectrum before and the red one after the Gaussian filtering.

For each of these filtered subsections the maxima are detected as these most likely belong to the dominant generators. This is done in two steps which are illustrated in Figure 6.19: In the first step the possible, i.e., local, maxima are detected by evaluating the first derivative. The positions of the possible maxima are marked with red asterisks. In the second step the global maxima are filtered

---

[6] A spectrogram is the sequence of spectra for subsequent time windows. It is a 3D plot with the axes time, frequency, and amplitude (of frequency components)

6.3. Autonomous Model

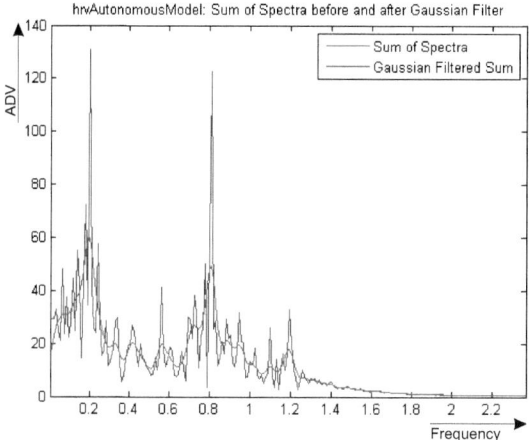

Figure 6.18: Spectra before and after Gaussian filtering

out by applying two criteria to each possible maximum: within a neighborhood of five (default) samples the value must be 0.002 (default) higher than any other. If a possible maximum satisfies these criteria, it is considered a global maximum. The filtered maxima are marked with green asterisks in Figure 6.19. The positions of the detected maxima are remembered for further processing.

The next step is to create a histogram from the previously computed maxima positions, i.e., a numerical pattern which matches their positions and distributions. To do so, all the computed maxima positions are sorted in ascending order. Subsequently, the histogram of the sorted maxima positions is created which serves to group (position) and count (distribution) the maxima positions (from the subsections of the spectrogram). Afterwards, the histogram is normalized and a Gaussian filter is applied. The result of the operations so far is shown in Figure 6.20a. The blue curve represents the histogram and the red one the Gaussian filtered one. The same maxima detection algorithm as explained by means of Figure 6.19 is called to derive the maxima of the histogram which is illustrated in Figure 6.20b. The detected maxima of this histogram are the positions within the spectrogram where most of the coefficients – with the highest amplitudes in their respective subsection – are located, i.e., these frequencies are dominant in the subspectrograms.

For the actual generation of the AM based features a higher temporal resolution is chosen to increase the sensitivity to physiological dynamics. The slice of data extracted from the ECG signal for the generation of a new spectrogram is determined by the parameter lenChHR defaulting to 4000. This increases the temporal resolution

102 Chapter 6. Detecting SRBD Events and Sleep Stages from an ECG Signal

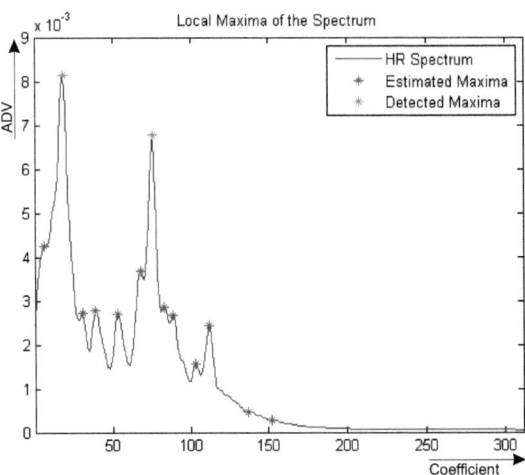

Figure 6.19: Local maxima for the template

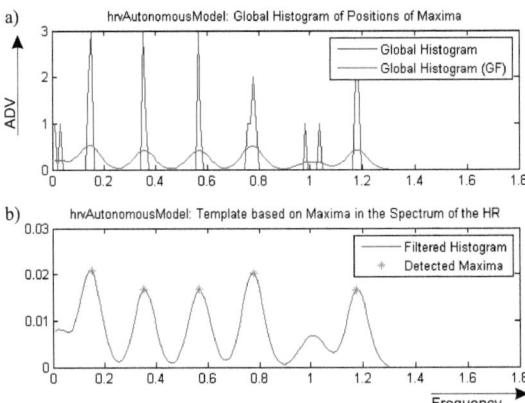

Figure 6.20: Global histogram of maxima for all periods and the template

6.3. Autonomous Model

by a factor of six. The returned spectrogram features a dimension of 2000 by 62. The later number is the number of spectra within the spectrogram and for each of these spectra EVA ml derives the features of the autonomous model. Accordingly, there are 62 evaluation periods.

As the procedure of increasing the temporal resolution effects the spectral resolution as well, the detected maxima positions of the template have to be (linearly) "stretched" to the new spectral position (one sixth). This is performed in the final postprocessing step of the template generation.

Computation of the Spectrogram

After these preliminary steps, in the fourth step EVA ml computes the spectrogram which is used for extracting the features (see Figure 6.13d). This step resembles the last two steps, but with a much shorter, i.e., one sixth (in the default setting), window length to increase the temporal resolution, thus, making EVA ml more responsive to sudden changes of the bodily states.

At a sampling frequency of 256 Hz the temporal resolution is around 15 seconds for a DFT length of 4000 samples which is half the standard evaluation period of 30 seconds (see /2.8.1/). But before the processing nbrSpecsToGroup (default 5) spectra are summed up and Gaussian filtered (see Figure 6.18 and the corresponding explanation) to suppress outliers which reduces the temporal resolution to around $1\frac{1}{4}$ minutes. Hence, EVA ml computes features for around every two standard evaluation periods.

Prior to calling the EM algorithm, the number of Gaussian curves to use for the GMM is heuristically estimated by considering the number of maxima in the spectrum. On the test data the estimated number of Gaussian curves is five.

After all these initializing steps EVA ml enters the main feature extraction loop. At its beginning the spectrum is preprocessed analog to the creation of the template, i.e., Gaussian filtering and normalizing. Subsequently, to extract the features from the spectra, each spectrum is approximated applying a Gaussian Mixture Model (GMM, see /10.4/). This means that the spectrum for each evaluation period is reconstructed by adjusting the means, sigmas, weights of "some" Gaussian distributions. These parameters describing the GMM are the features EVA ml produces as each maximum represents a generator and its properties.

GMM Approximation using EM Algorithm

In the fifth step EVA ml approximates each spectrum (see Figure 6.13e), i.e., a "slice" of the spectrogram, for each evaluation period by a GMM. This step reduces

104   Chapter 6. Detecting SRBD Events and Sleep Stages from an ECG Signal

the numerous coefficient values of the spectrum to just a few parameters which are easier for the classifier to process. These parameters are the mean, the variance, and the weight of each Gaussian distribution contributing to the approximation of the spectrogram currently considered. For the approximation of the spectrograms by means of a GMM, the Expectation-Maximization (EM, see [Schu 95]) algorithm is applied.

The algorithm which is used in this work was implemented by Joni Kamarainen and Pekka Paalanen from the Lappeenranta University of Technology (see [Kama 07]). For the initialization of the EM algorithm two initialization methods are available (see [Witt 05]):

c-means clustering is the classical approach: a number of "c" random centers is chosen as initial starting points.

maximum likelihood is a method for estimating probability distributions based on a relatively small number of samples.

The results of this work are based on the "c-means" initialization. The EM algorithm is set to create five Gaussian curves for the approximation of each spectrum. However, in a subsequent step the components of the Gaussian approximation are assessed considering their contribution to the approximation. Components are considered "needless" – and, hence, deleted from the GMM approximation – if they fulfill any of the following criteria:

- The weight of the component is too small, i.e., the overall contribution of this component is only limited.

- The component is not "pronounced", i.e., figuratively spoken, the top of the component is flat. Put another way, the component may be considered "blurred", i.e., not attributable to a certain generator. This property is "measured" by its weight-to-sigma ratio.

- The peak of the component is too close to a more pronounced peak of another component.

- The complete GMM approximation of the current spectrum is abandoned, if the approximation error exceeds a given threshold.

A showcase result for the EM algorithm is shown in Figure 6.21. The Figure focuses on the first coefficients as the remaining ones are negligible. The blue curve

6.3. Autonomous Model

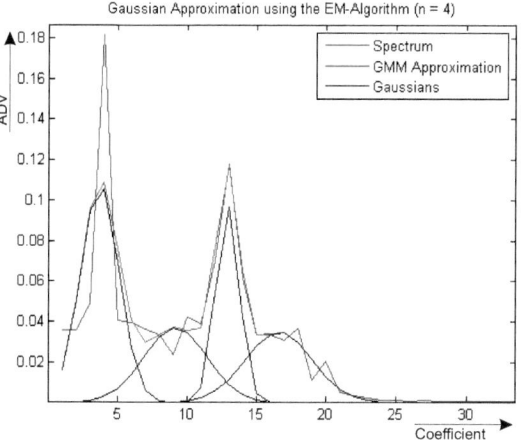

Figure 6.21: Approximation of the spectra by means of the EM algorithm: The blue curve is the original spectrum. The GMM approximation is shown in red whose individual GMM components – four in this case – are plotted in black.

is the spectrum to be approximated. The red curve is the resulting GMM approximation which consists of the black Gaussian bell-shaped curves. The parameters defining these Gaussian bell-shaped curves, i.e., weight, mean μ, sigma σ, and the amplitude of the spectrum at the positions of the μs are the features which are extracted for each evaluation period. Sometimes, as in Figure 6.21, narrow peaks are not reproduced properly which affects the variance of the Gaussian curve, while the μ values are correct. Considering the model, this approximation error results in a false assessment of the stableness of a generator while its center frequency is correctly detected. This behavior may show some effect in sleep stages which are characterized by constant HRs, e.g., the deep sleep stages. Recalling that even during these sleep stages the HR is affected by the SA (see /3.3.1/), the overall effect should be negligible.

In the next step the different μ values are assigned to the their corresponding maxima of the template. This matching is based on the distances of the μ values of the current approximation and the distances of the maxima of the template. Subsequently, the GMM parameters are stored as the properties of the generators for the current evaluation period. In addition to the GMM parameters, the amplitudes of the current spectrum at the frequencies indicated by the μ values are stored as an additional indicator for the "importance" of each generator.

106   Chapter 6. Detecting SRBD Events and Sleep Stages from an ECG Signal

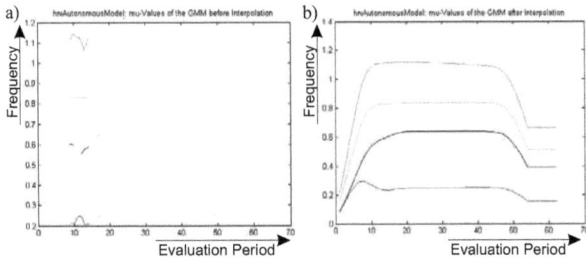

Figure 6.22: On the left side this Figure shows the μ (mu) values after all evaluation periods have been processed. Each curve belongs to a different Gaussian distribution, i.e., four curves mean that the approximation of the spectra was computed with four Gaussian distribution. The missing values, i.e., the gaps between the curves, belong to evaluation periods where the EM algorithm failed to find proper GMM parameters. On the right side the same curves are shown after the missing values have been interpolated.

At the end of the computations for the current evaluation period the template is adjusted to keep track of the changes of the GMM μ values. This is accomplished by computing a weighted mean between the value of the template μ_t and the current GMM value μ_c (see equation (10.9b)) where the template value and the GMM value have a ratio of 40 : 60 (see equation (6.3)). This is performed for each maximum of the template.

$$\mu_n = 0.4 \cdot \mu_t + 0.6 \cdot \mu_c \qquad (6.3)$$

Postprocessing the Feature Matrices

As the EM algorithm sometimes fails to produce a satisfying approximation, in the seventh step EVA ml performs a postprocessing of the GMM parameters (see Figure 6.13f). During this process the missing values are interpolated linearly.

After the main processing loop the values for abandoned GMM parameters are filled in. Figures 6.22a & b show as an example one of the parameters of the GMM – the means of the Gaussian distributions – over all evaluation periods where Figure 6.22a is before and Figure 6.22b after the interpolation of the abandoned values of the previous step. Figure 6.22a clearly shows that the EM algorithm quite often fails to produce a successful GMM (in the data used to plot the Figures): all the spaces in the four curves belong to abandoned values. The four curves – for the means – in each of the Figures belong to the different Gaussian distributions the GMM is composed of.

6.3. Autonomous Model

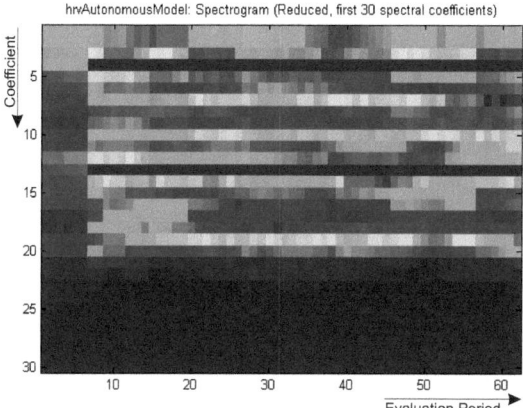

Figure 6.23: Spectrogram zoomed to reveal only the first 30 coefficients as the remaining coefficients are negligible.

Figure 6.23 shows the spectrogram over all the evaluation periods. The horizontal "lines" can be seen as belonging to the maxima of the template, i.e., the different generators of the autonomous nervous system.

Compute Energy of G_{Noise}

In the eighth step EVA ml computes the energy of the generator G_{Noise} (see Figure 6.13g). This is done by extinguishing the spectral ranges of the other generators from the spectrum and subsequently summing up the remaining spectral components. This reflects the idea that the generator G_{Noise} sums up all the influences which could not be assigned to one of the generators representing the activity of the ANS. These frequency ranges gain energy during fluctuations of the ANS generators, i.e., the higher the energy of the generator G_{Noise}, the higher the likeliness that the subject's body is in an unstable state due to a SRBD event or a change of the sleep stage.

Figure 6.24 shows the principle: the blue curves are the spectra of the different evaluation periods. The maxima of the template, i.e., the well assigned generators, are indicated by the red vertical lines. In the first step ranges around the maxima are deleted, i.e., their amplitudes are set to zero. In the second step the remainders of each spectrum are summed up to deliver a measure for the energy of the noise generator. The width of the ranges around the maxima which are considered "well assignable" can be adjusted by the parameter `specRangeToDel` which defaults to 10

108   Chapter 6. Detecting SRBD Events and Sleep Stages from an ECG Signal

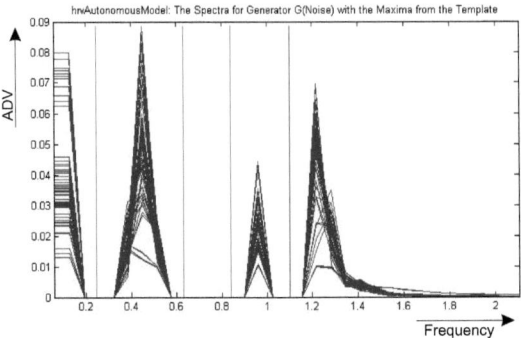

Figure 6.24: Spectrum with template and the deleted ranges for the generator G_{Noise}

coefficients (approximately 0.64 Hz) to either side. Likewise, the frequency range higher than twice the frequency of the highest maximum is deleted.

Figure 6.25 finally shows the energy of the noise generator over the evaluation periods. Like in some other features which EVA ml computes as "energy" this feature is actually the sum over the amplitudes of the spectrum which means it is rather an amplitude than an energy. This is done to keep the values in practical, i.e., processable, range.

Writing ARFF Files

In the final step EVA ml writes the computed model properties to ARFF files (see Figure 6.13h). Depending on the processing options chosen (see /10.2/), files for "all features" and/or "each feature group" are written, respectively (see p. 201).

6.4 Morphological Features

The features of the morphological approach are based on Chapters /3.4/ and /3.5/. The first one explains the correlation between the changes of the ECG shape and the load condition. The second one introduces the ischemia driven morphological changes.

In Table 6.7, there is an overview over the morphological functions and the number of parameters extracted (using the standard processing configuration file initial.epc, see /10.2.2/).

6.4. Morphological Features

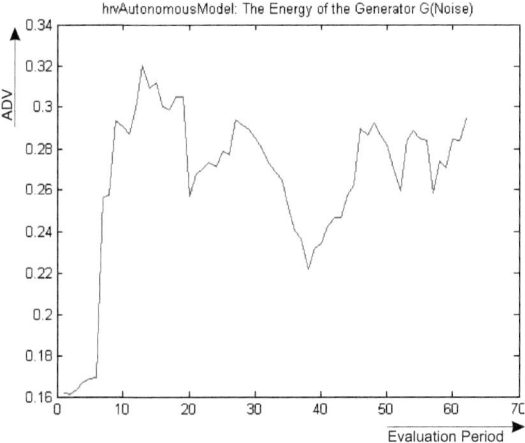

Figure 6.25: Energy of the generator G_{Noise}

Function	Local Parameters	Global Parameters
morphPWave()	5	14
morphRPeak()	9	22
morphSTSegment()	16	32
morphTWave()	13	26
morphTiming()	9	20
morphShape_Dev()	4	12
morphShape_CA()	47	94
morphShape_Spec()	120	240
morphShape_SpecDiff()	80	160

Table 6.7: The processing functions and the number of extracted local and global parameters, respectively

110   Chapter 6. Detecting SRBD Events and Sleep Stages from an ECG Signal

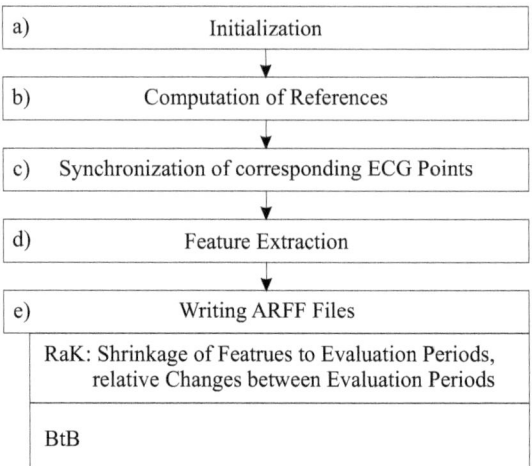

Figure 6.26: Overall flow chart of the morphological functions

6.4.1 Common Features of the Morphological Functions

This introductory Section gives a short overview of the processing steps which are generally speaking identical to all morphological functions. These steps are discussed along the flow chart given in Figure 6.26.

EVA ml starts processing the morphological functions with the initialization (see Figure 6.26a). At the beginning of this step variables are initialized along with the verification of some function specific prerequisites, e.g., whether preprocessing was applied to the ECG signal. Subsequently, the distinctive ECG points (P, Q, R, ...), which are required for the current function, are retrieved from the data vector which was created by labelECGPoints() (see /6.2/).

Afterwards, EVA ml computes required reference signals (see Figure 6.26b). Three types of reference values are computed: the first one is the "overall mean", i.e., $m(...)$ (see equation (10.9a)), of the amplitude of a distinctive point, e.g., the P-wave. This is considered the default value of the amplitude of a distinctive ECG point for the specific subject. The next reference value is the floating mean and exists in two characteristics: a) the window of the floating mean is centered around the current value, i.e., its past and future (values) are considered, i.e., $m_c(..., flmenLen)$ (see equation (10.9b)), and b) the window is delayed, i.e., it lies completely in the past of the values, i.e., $m_d(..., flmenLen)$ (see equation (10.9c)). Even though both values only differ in a time shift, they describe a different chronological development: In the first case the value of interest is considered in its proximity and

6.4. Morphological Features

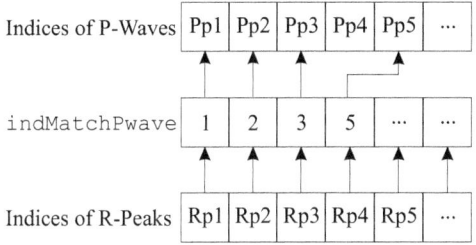

Figure 6.27: Mechanism of synchronizing the corresponding ECG points as detected by labelECGPoints()

in the latter case the value of interest is considered in the way it is different from its predecessors. The number of predecessors and/or successors, i.e., the length of the window, is set by the parameter flmenLen in the processing configuration (see /10.2.2/). The floating means take into consideration the dynamics of a parameter over the night and during load changing events, e.g., SRBD events and changes of sleep stages. Thus, they allow deciding, whether there was a significant change, i.e., a possible event, during the last few heart beats.

Next, to compensate false detections of the distinctive points, EVA ml synchronizes the distinctive ECG points (see Figure 6.26c). Thus, EVA ml makes sure that the required subset of distinctive points belongs to a *single* ECG wave, i.e., they appear in the proper temporal order and follow the physiological restraints. The mechanism to achieve this is shown in Figure 6.27.

This mechanism is now explained for the synchronization of the P- and R-points: Having extracted the distinctive ECG points positions of the labelECGPoints() vector, EVA ml keeps these positions in two data arrays "Indices of R-Peaks" and "Indices of P-Waves", i.e., Rp1 is the position (index) of the first R-peak in the ECG recording and so on and the same applies for the P-waves. During the synchronization EVA ml creates a third data vector, e.g., indMatchPwave. This vector contains the *ind*ices of the *Match*ing *P-wave*s which are used for indirection. For example, in Figure 6.27 the first three P-waves directly match the R-peaks of the same index resulting in the indirection vector showing the values 1, 2, 3. But the fourth R-peak matches the fifth P-wave indicated by the value 5 in the indirection vector when there should have been 4. The matches are found by searching for the P-wave "closest in front of" the current R-peak. The likewise principle is applied for the other distinctive ECG points.

Subsequently, the consistency of the labeled ECG points is verified. This is done in two ways: the first test checks, whether the derivation of indMatchPwave is constantly the value 1. This is only true, if no adjustment has had to be done and the values in indmatchPwave run from 1 to the total of P-waves in the recording. The second test applies physiological restraints, i.e., it checks whether the distance between the P-wave and the R-peak remains "approximately constant" which is within a window of 30%. This is enough to allow all physiological variations, but reliably catches false distinctive ECG points detections[7].

The next processing step of EVA ml is the feature extraction (see Figure 6.26d). It is performed by nine individually called functions (see Figure 10.2) which are listed in Table 6.7. Each of them deals with a distinctive ECG point or the ECG shape as a whole. Accordingly, they are called morphPWave(), morphQPeak(), and so on, or morphShape_Dev() and so on. A more detailed description of these functions is provided in the following Sections.

The final processing step is the writing of the ARFF files (see Figure 6.26e). During this step the computed features are written to two different ARFF files: one on a beat-by-beat basis and the other on a evaluation period basis (see /10.2.3/). The latter is mainly done by means of computing the mean and the standard deviation of the feature values which fall within one evaluation period.

6.4.2 P-Wave

The P-wave results from the contraction of the atria. It is shown in Figure 6.28. This Section will explain which features are extracted and why, i.e., the physiological changes accompanying a respiratory event and their impact on the morphology of the P-wave. The features of the P-wave are computed in the function morphPWave().

The obstruction of the airways (during an apnea) leads to an increase of blood pressure in the pulmonary circulation which almost instantly provokes the symptoms of a "P pulmonal" (see /3.4.1/) or a "P dextroatrial" as they are the markers for an increase in pressure and/or volume load. Both cause a high P-wave. However, the provoked increase usually remains less than 10%, which makes the effect hard to detect.

Figure 6.29 shows the results of the reference computation (see Figure 6.26b) of morphPWave(). The Figure shows the corresponding values over the complete interval of 90 heart beats.

The red curve shows the progression of the floating mean of the P-wave amplitudes over a centered interval of flmnLen (set in the processing configuration)

---

[7] If either test should fail, EVA ml dumps the positions where resynchronization was necessary to the Matlab console. This allows to check (manually), whether the reason for the resynchronization is due to an error of labelECGPoints() or an anomaly in the ECG recording.

6.4. Morphological Features

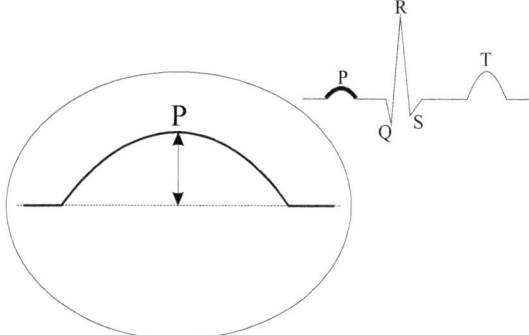

Figure 6.28: The P-wave highlighted in the ECG wave and an adumbration of some P-wave features

values. The default value of five is chosen to retain the trend of the P-wave amplitudes. Thus, it emphasized the local dynamics, because the short time reference suppresses long time drifts during the night.

To evaluate the dynamics of the P-wave amplitude, the following features are extracted for each P-wave and written to the "each feature group" ARRF file:

P-Wave amplitude relative to reference The amplitude of the current P-wave is computed to the reference $m(P)$ for the P-wave.

P-Wave amplitude relative to the floating mean The amplitude of the current P-wave is computed to the floating mean $m_d(P, \text{flmnLen})$ values of the P-wave amplitude. The value flmnLen is set in the processing configuration file and defaults to 5.

Floating mean relative to the reference The floating mean $m_d(P, \text{flmnLen})$ is related to, i.e., divided by, the overall reference of the recording.

Periods of increasing load After the obstruction of the airways the load of the heart increases over time until an arousal wakes the patient. This increase is captured by this feature: it counts the number of subsequent heart beats with increasing or decreasing amplitudes, respectively. Accordingly, the values of this feature are natural numbers (1, 2, 3, ...) with positive sign for increasing and negative sign for decreasing load.

Figure 6.30 shows as the blue curve the P-wave amplitudes (as in Figure 6.29). The red curve represents the "periods of increasing load". Accordingly, the value of

114   Chapter 6. Detecting SRBD Events and Sleep Stages from an ECG Signal

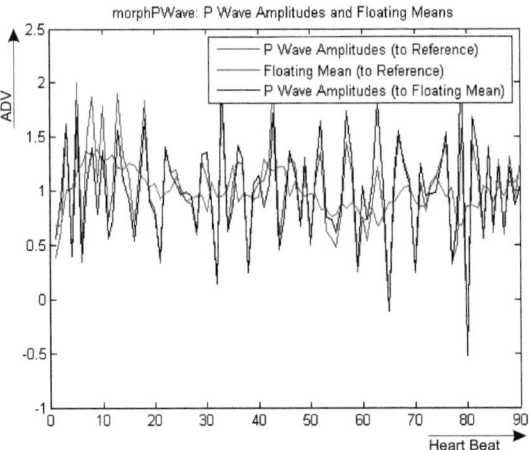

Figure 6.29: Dynamics of three P-wave features over the extracted interval: the P-wave amplitude in relation to the reference in blue, the floating mean over the two surrounding values in relation to the reference, and the P-wave amplitudes in relation to the floating mean.

the red curve is higher, when the amplitudes of subsequent P-waves rise, and vice versa.

Relation between P-wave and R-peak amplitude   The amplitude of the P-wave is compared to the amplitude of the corresponding R-peak. This feature is included as sympathicotonia and parasympathicotonia may have a higher impact on the R-peak amplitude than on the P-wave amplitude.

Usually, for each beat-to-beat (BtB) feature there are two corresponding RaK[8] features which are created by computing the mean $m(feature)$ and the standard deviation of all feature values within one evaluation period. The following features are exclusive to the RaK features or were computed differently:

Periods of increasing load (RaK)   This feature is analogue to the BtB feature that describes the length – in heart beats – of periods of increasing or decreasing cardiac load. But for this feature the adaption to the RaK interval is accomplished by the functions max() or min() (for the decreasing periods because of the negative sign), respectively, which return the longest increasing or longest decreasing during this interval.

---
[8]The abbreviation "RaK" was chosen to recall that the standard evaluation period of 30 seconds was suggest by *R*echtschaffen and *K*ales.

6.4. Morphological Features

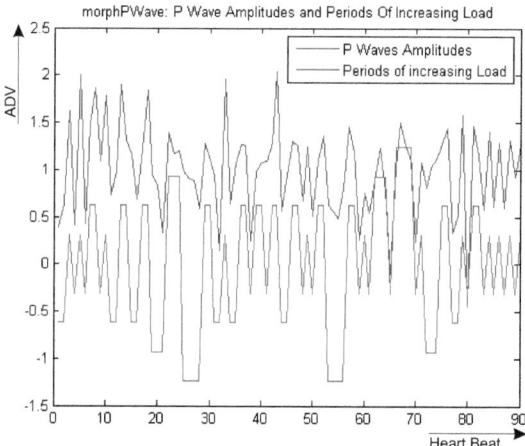

Figure 6.30: Amplitudes of the P-waves and the values of the feature "periods of increasing load" over the complete interval. Note that the red curve is rescaled to match the amplitude of the P-waves (only for plotting purposes) which means that it does not show absolute values, but only trends.

P-wave amplitude relative to R-peak amplitude The same feature as the BtB one. In addition to the standard mean and standard deviation approach, max() and min() are evaluated.

Subsequent means of P-wave amplitudes This feature accounts for dynamics in *subsequent evaluation periods*: it takes the amplitude means of two subsequent evaluation periods and computes their difference and standard deviation.

6.4.3 R-Peak

The R-peak is the electrical representation of the contraction of the ventricles. It is shown in Figure 6.31 along with some of the extracted features. The (morphological) features of the R-peak are computed in the function morphRPeak().

The activation of the SNS due to an SRBD event entails a rise of the blood pressure. Hence, the heart has to work harder. morphRPeak() implements different features which reflect this increased load condition.

The features which are extracted on a BtB basis are the following:

Absolute amplitude of the R-peak relative to the reference This feature tracks the absolute amplitude A_{abs} of the R-peak relative to the subject's standard

116 Chapter 6. Detecting SRBD Events and Sleep Stages from an ECG Signal

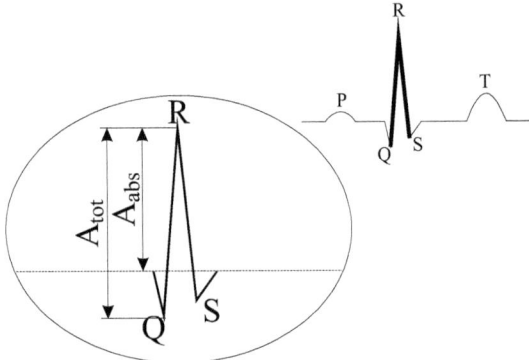

Figure 6.31: Some features of the R-peak

amplitude, i.e., $m(R)$ (see equation (10.9b)). The R-peak is expected to increase under load conditions, e.g., after an arousal (see /3.4.2/).

Absolute amplitude of the R-peak to the floating mean This feature puts the current R-peak amplitude in relation to the surrounding R-peak amplitudes, i.e., $m_c(R, \texttt{flmnLen})$ (see equation (10.9b)). Hence, it characterizes the short time dynamics.

Figure 6.32 shows the amplitudes of the R-peaks of the interval in relation to the reference $m(R)$ (blue) or the floating mean $m_c(R, \texttt{flmnLen})$.

The effect of emphasizing local dynamics is more pronounced in Figure 6.32 than in Figure 6.29: while the amplitudes of the R-peaks decrease between R-peak 0 - 30, the floating mean related values drop even further, and while the R-peak amplitude rises between R-peak 50 - 70, the floating mean related values rise more significantly.

Floating mean of the R-peak amplitude to the reference The floating mean $m_c(R, \texttt{flmnLen})$ compared to the subject's standard amplitude $m(R)$. Thinking of $m_c(R, \texttt{flmnLen})$ as a low pass filtered signal, this feature describes the current trend of the R-peak amplitude while suppressing outliers.

Total amplitude of the R-peak The total amplitude A_{tot} is measured from the base point of the Q- to the crest of the R-peak[9]. This feature – in conjunction with the following – is intended to indicate the performance of the cardiac conduction system which itself is under the influence of the ANS.

---
[9] The delay between the Q- and the R-peak is given by the speed at which excitation propagates along the conduction system – it will, therefore, be a feature of morphTiming()

6.4. Morphological Features

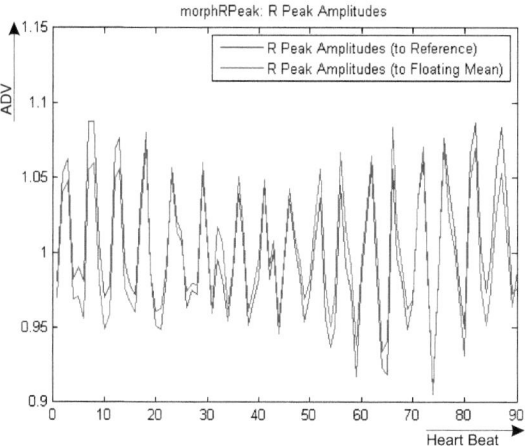

Figure 6.32: Amplitudes of the R-peaks in relation to the overnight and the floating mean reference, respectively

Steepness of the QR-ascent This features is the linear slope which results from the total amplitude A_{tot} and the required rise time. Accordingly, this feature is a combination of the amount of muscle strands responding and their response time.

Figure 6.33 shows parameters that relate to the steepness of the Q-R-segment and the periods of increasing load. The blue curve is the amplitude of the R-peak starting from the base of the Q-peak. The red curve displays the computed steepness which is computed from the QR-amplitude and the delay between the Q- and the R-peak. As the two curves show different dynamics at several points, it seems quite obvious that the dynamics of the delay play an important role – but they are not evaluated here, but in morphTiming().

Periods of increasing cardiac load The green curve at the "bottom" of Figure 6.33 is the already known "periods of increasing load" parameter (for an explanation see /6.4.2/).

Periods of increasing cardiac load relative to delayed floating mean This feature is essentially the same as the previous one, but reflects a different timing.

Difference of R-peak amplitude and delayed floating mean This feature is computed as the absolute increase of the R-peak amplitude against the mean of the "short past". It is intended to denote the acute increase of cardiac load.

118   Chapter 6. Detecting SRBD Events and Sleep Stages from an ECG Signal

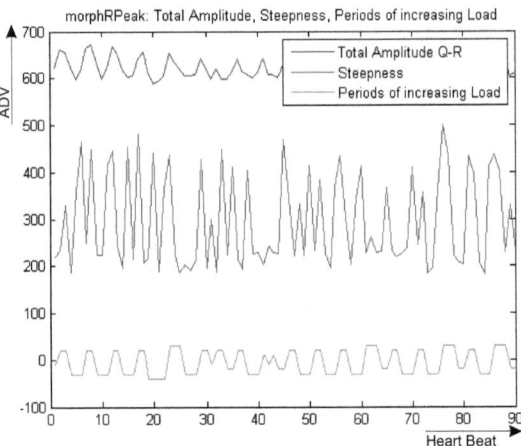

Figure 6.33: Total amplitudes A_{tot} and steepness of QR-segments

Relation of amplitudes of R-peak and corresponding P-wave This feature is mathematically the reciprocal of the value computed in `morphPWave()`. It is included in `morphRPeak()` mainly to make this feature available in the BtB ARFF file.

Most of the RaK features of `morphRPeak()` are derived from the corresponding BtB features by mapping them to the evaluation periods using mean and standard deviation. But there are two additional features, each in two characteristics as mean and standard deviation:

Difference between R-peak amplitudes This feature computes the difference of R-peak amplitudes between the current evaluation period and the previous one.

Relation of R-peak amplitudes This feature is very much like the previous one, but computes the relation between evaluation periods.

6.4.4 ST-Segment

The ST-segment (in conjunction with the T-wave, see /3.5.3/) plays an important role for the detection of fluctuations in PNS activity as well as critical load conditions. The ST-segment is displayed in Figure 6.34. The features of the ST-segment are computed in the function `morphSTSegment()`.

6.4. Morphological Features

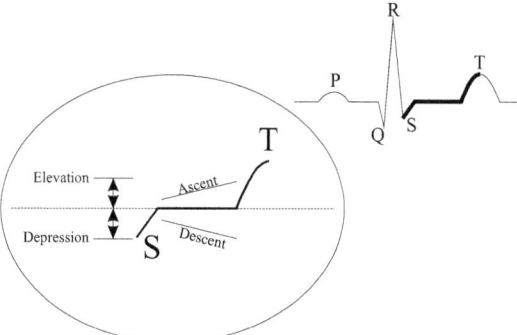

Figure 6.34: Some features of the ST-segment

Summarizing the Section on the ST-segment in the medical basics, it can be stated that the important ST-segment features are the degrees of ascent or descent and the degrees of elevation or depression.

Extracting the ST-Segment

Figure 6.35 shows some intermediate values computed during the initial processing of the ST-segment features. The green curves represent the amplitudes of the S-peaks – the continuous one the current amplitude and the dotted one the floating mean $m_c(S, \texttt{flmnLen})$. The two red curves are the corresponding curves for the T-wave amplitudes.

To compute the features based on the ST-segment, the first step is to extract the ST-segment. For the extraction of the ST-segment constant offsets to either limiter, i.e., the S-peak and the T-wave, respectively, are used. These offsets were derived heuristically: the ST-segment was found to start at 1.5% of the RR interval after the S-peak and end at 2.5% of the RR interval in front of the T-wave.

Degree of Ascent or Descent

As the horizontal gradient of the ST-segment is of great importance, the ascending or descending character is computed in different ways.

The first approach is a polynomial approximation of the extracted ST-segment. The number of coefficients is given by `nbrPolySteepCoefs` whose value is set in the processing configuration and defaults to 2. The actual number of returned coefficients is one more which results from the called function. From this feature two different versions exist: The one that approximates the ST-segment directly and the

120   Chapter 6. Detecting SRBD Events and Sleep Stages from an ECG Signal

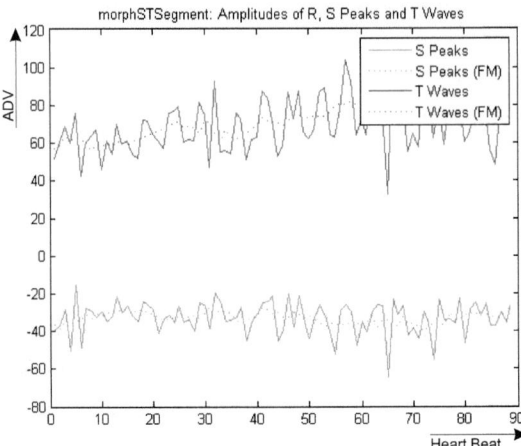

Figure 6.35: Amplitudes and floating means $m_c(.,\texttt{flmnLen})$ of the S-peaks and T-waves

other that approximates the ST-segment in relation to the scaling amplitude from $m(S)$ to $m(T)$.

The second approach is simply the linear approximation of the gradient between S-peak and T-wave. This feature considers only the start and end point for the computation of the sloop. (The previous features would approximate the sloop by a regression line, if `nbrPolySteepCoefs` was set to 1.) Again, from this feature, there are the two versions as described in the previous paragraph.

The results of the linear and regression based approximation of the ST-segment are shown in Figure 6.36. The blue curve is the original ECG signal, upon which the S-peak is marked in yellow and the T-wave in black as small circles. The red curve is the extracted ST-segment, i.e., the ECG curve between the S-peak and T-wave without the fringes whose widths were computed as a fixed percentage of the RR-interval at either end.

The green curve in Figure 6.36 is the regression approximated ST-segment. As the parameter `nbrPolySteepCoefs` is set to 2 in the processing configuration, resulting in a second order polynomial, its shape resembles a parable. The black curve is the linear interpolation of the extracted ST-segment.

The third approach is the stepwise linear approximation of the ST-segment. This delivers a "low-resolution" gradient, i.e., the derivation, of the ST-segment. The number of nodes is given by `nbrGradSmpls` whose value defaults to 5. Between these nodes the gradients of the segments are computed. Subsequently, the number of

6.4. Morphological Features

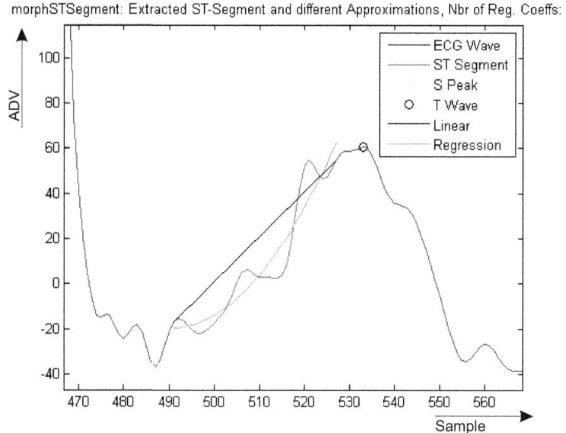

Figure 6.36: Extracted ST-segment and its linear approximation

gradients whose value is lower than a threshold given by gradHorizThresh (default 1) is counted and set into relation to the number of nodes (see equation (6.4)). Accordingly, the higher this value, the higher the measure of "horizontality" and/or "descentality[10]" of the current segment. This procedure catches horizontal as well as descending segments as both are indicators for an unusual cardiac load and/or condition.

$$\%AscendingGrads = \frac{|Grad < \texttt{gradHorizThresh}|}{\texttt{nbrGradSmpls}} \qquad (6.4)$$

Figure 6.37 shows the result of the successive gradient approximation of the extracted ST-segment as the green curve. The remaining features are the same ones as in Figure 6.36.

Elevation and Depression

The elevation and the depression of the ST-segment are essentially the same value – except for the sign. To gain additional information both features are computed differently by EVA ml: The elevation is computed simply as the mean $m(ST)$ of the extracted ST-segment. This method was chosen as many of the available recordings did not show a distinct horizontal segment.

The depression is computed as the difference to a reference point. The reference point is calculated as the mean $m(\tilde{P}\tilde{Q})$ of the segment between P-wave and Q-peak

---

[10] Made-up word to mimic the appearance of "horizontality".

122   Chapter 6. Detecting SRBD Events and Sleep Stages from an ECG Signal

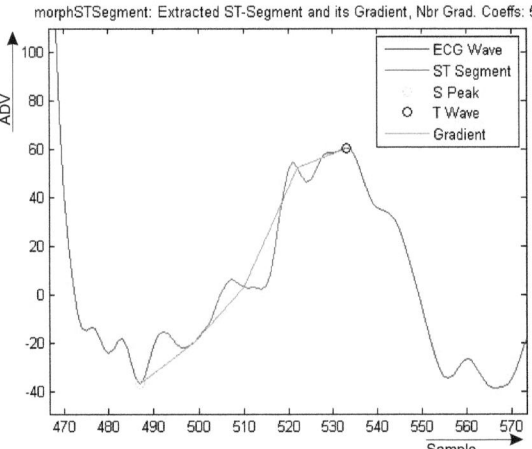

Figure 6.37: Extracted ST-segment and its gradient approximation

(none of them included). The extracted PQ-segment starts at 2% of the RR-interval after the P-wave and ends at 2% of the RR-interval in front of the Q-peak.

Figure 6.38 shows the result of the computation of the PQ-level which is used to detect ST-segment depressions (see p. 44). Just like in the previous Figures the blue curve represents the ECG signal, upon which the P-wave is marked black and the Q-peak yellow. The red curve is the extracted $\tilde{P}\tilde{Q}$-segment and the PQ-level indicated by the green horizontal line is computed as the mean $m(\tilde{P}\tilde{Q})$.

Along with the features introduced so far, the following feature is included in the ARFF file.

Absolute amplitude of ST-segment The amplitude of the ST-segment is set in relation to the amplitude of the floating means $m_c(S, \texttt{flmnLen})$ and $m_c(T, \texttt{flmnLen})$. This feature represents a measure for the dynamics of the complete segment.

The number of BtB features depends on the settings in the processing configuration and is given by equation (6.5).

$$n_{ST-Segment} = 2 \cdot (n_{nbrPolySteepCoefs} + 1) + (n_{nbrGradSmpls} - 1) + 6 \qquad (6.5)$$

The RaK features of morphSTSegment() are derived from the corresponding BtB features by mapping them to the evaluation periods by means of computing their

6.4. Morphological Features

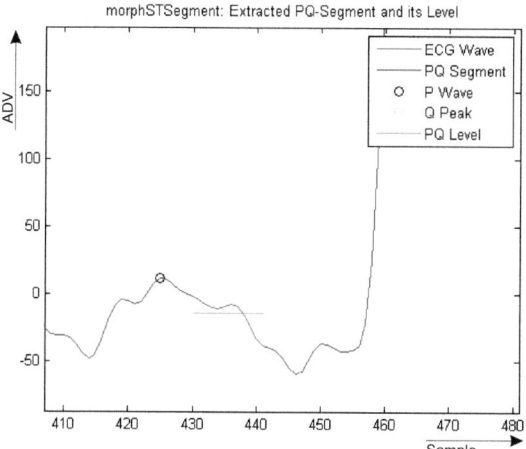

Figure 6.38: Extracted $\tilde{P}\tilde{Q}$-segment (red) and the iso-electric potential (green) which is computed from this segment. It is used to calculate the degree of ST-depression.

means or standard deviations. The number of RaK features can be computed by equation (6.6).

$$n_{ST-Segment} = 4 \cdot (n_{nbrPolySteepCoefs} + 1) + 2 \cdot (n_{nbrGradSmpls} - 1) + 12 \quad (6.6)$$

6.4.5 T-Wave

The T-wave is closely linked to the ST-segment which is why some of the reasoning given here may well sound familiar. According to its relation to the ST-segment, the T-wave can be evaluated to detect abnormal conditions of the heart. The T-wave and some of the extracted features are shown in Figure 6.39. The features of the T-wave are computed in the function morphTWave().

The correlation between the behavior of the T-wave and changing load conditions is explained in /3.5.4/. Hence, as the T-wave greatly reacts to different load and oxygen supply conditions, the first parameters extracted directly rely on this behavior. The overall dynamics of the T-wave is considered by evaluating its amplitude against the overnight reference $m(T)$ as relation and as difference. The latter is expected to show a higher "event resolution", i.e., to exhibit larger value swings during an SRBD event.

124   Chapter 6. Detecting SRBD Events and Sleep Stages from an ECG Signal

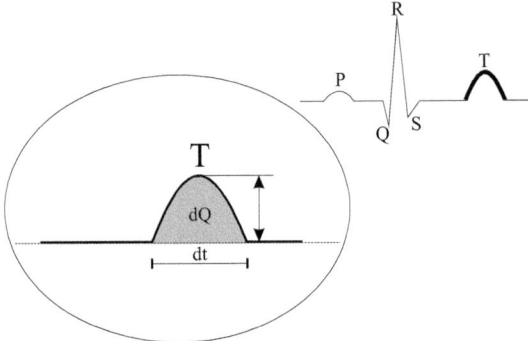

Figure 6.39: Some features of the T-wave as well as the funny current I_f

Figure 6.40 shows some reference values which are computed in an early stage of morphTWave(). The blue curve depicts the amplitudes of the T-waves in the interval. The green and the red curves are the floating means $m_c(T, \texttt{flmnLen})$ and $m_d(T, \texttt{flmnLen})$, respecitvely. The black horizontal line is the value of the overnight reference value $m(T)$.

The next two features examine the short time dynamics which is done by comparing the current T-wave amplitude to the floating means $m_c(T, \texttt{flmnLen})$ and $m_d(T, \texttt{flmnLen})$. The current T-wave is evaluated against both floating means as relation and as difference. Figure 6.41 shows these features based on the computed references. Figure 6.41a shows the amplitudes of the T-waves relative to the different references: the blue curve reflects the amplitude relative to the overnight reference, the green and the red curve represent the amplitude in relation to the two different floating means. The features based on the *differences* (see Figure 6.41b) appear to be quite promising as they directly consider the dynamics of the T-wave (see /3.5.4/).

The next features directly focus on the dynamics and the negativeness of the T-wave amplitude and express it with different properties. They are summarized in Figure 6.42.

Negativeness of T-wave The first of these feature (not shown in Figure 6.42) is a measure for the "negativeness of the T-wave". A decreasing T-wave accompanies phases of bad oxygen supply as expected to be induced by disturbed respiration. This feature indicates the "negativeness of the T-wave" by just letting pass the negative values and setting the positive values to zero.

6.4. Morphological Features

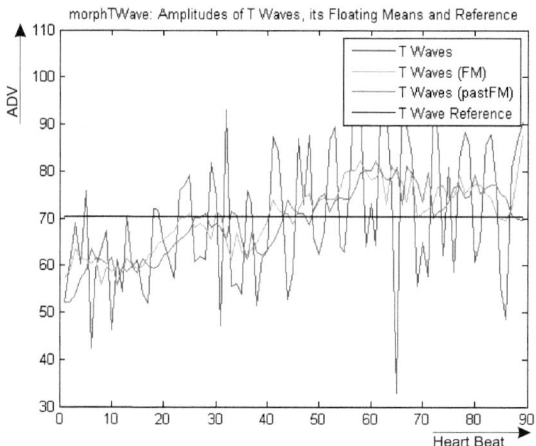

Figure 6.40: Amplitudes of T-waves and the derived references: two different types of floating means concerning their timing and the overnight reference

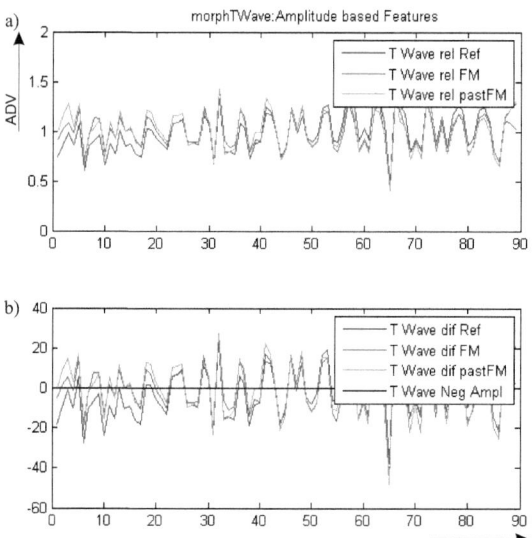

Figure 6.41: Amplitudes of the T-wave in relation to the different references: in the upper panel the amplitude is relative to the references and in the lower panel the reference were subtracted from the amplitudes.

Periods of decreasing T-wave The next feature is less "sharp" than the previous one. It computes the number of subsequent heart beats with decreasing T-wave amplitudes. It is derived from the (negative) first derivation. In this approach the absolute amplitude of the T-wave may still be positive, while the decaying trend is caught. This is similiar to the "periods of increasing load" feature, however, in this case the important trend is the decrease of the amplitude (see /3.5/). The results of this feature are shown as the blue curve in Figure 6.42.

Accumulated negative trend Whereas the previous feature only considers qualitative aspects, i.e., whether the amplitude drops or rises, this features adds the quantitative aspect: it computes the accumulated negative trend of the last nbrPastGrad (value is set in the processing configuration and defaults to 5) T-waves. It does so by taking the differentiated T-wave amplitudes curve and summing up only the negative values. The accumulated negative trend is depicted in the red curve of Figure 6.42.

Prevailing trend of the T-wave The next feature is a measure for the prevailing trend of the T-wave amplitude within the last nbrPastGrad T-waves. It counts the transitions from one T-wave to the next one with dropping amplitude and relates this count to the length of the evaluation period given by (nbrPastGrad - 1). The result is shown in Figure 6.42 as the green curve. It reflects the percentage of decreasing amplitudes within an observation interval, e.g., if the length of the evaluated interval is five beats and within this interval three amplitudes (not necessarily subsequent) show a decrease, then the value for this interval is 60%, i.e., $\frac{3}{5}$ (for analogon see equation (6.4)).

The T-wave amplitude strongly depends on the oxygen supply and the ANS activity. Therefore, the duration and the integral over the amplitudes of the T-wave should be an indicator for the subject's current condition. From these parameters a third one is computable as the quotient of the both. The quotient serves for two reasons: First, the proper detection of the onset and offset of the wave might sometimes be faulty, but as both – numerator and denominator – depend on the detected width, the error is somewhat compensated. And second, the quotient may be considered as a representation of the "funny current" (see /3.3.1/ and Figure 3.10) which itself is an indicator of the activity of the SNS. This is analogue to equation (6.7) which defines the relation between charge Q and current i. In this analogon Q represents the "charge" of the heart muscle which needs to be reloaded during the repolarization, time t is the duration of the T-wave, and the current i stands for the funny current. (This is of course a very simple analogon as the funny current

6.4. Morphological Features

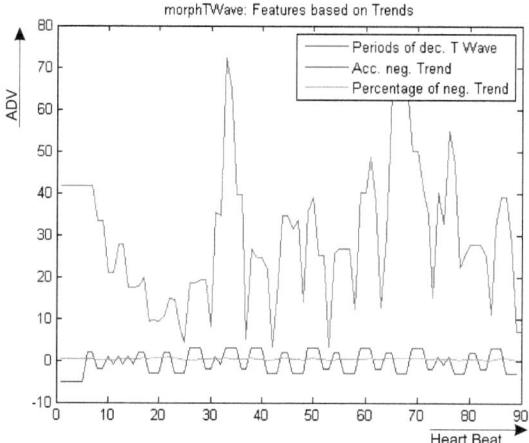

Figure 6.42: Trends of the T-wave amplitude which reflect changes of the ANS and/or the oxygen supply.

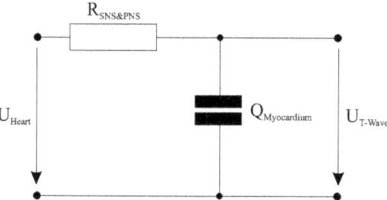

Figure 6.43: Simple model for the funny current I_f and the measured amplitude of the T-wave.

depends on the activity of the autonomous system as well – which introduces a kind of "resistor", see Figure 6.43.)

$$i = \frac{dQ}{dt} \qquad (6.7)$$

In the next two successive steps the duration of the T-wave is computed: First, an interval around the T-wave peak is set by ± 10% of the RR interval. Next, the deviation is computed for the extracted interval. To find the onset point of the T-wave the computed deviation is compared to a threshold which is computed from the value of thresTwaveRise (defaulting to 4) and the amplitude of the current T-wave. The likewise procedure is performed with the parameter thresTwaveDrop whose default value is 7 to find the offset (end) of the T-wave. In case the deviation approach does not yield reasonable results, i.e., the resulting T-wave would be too

128   Chapter 6. Detecting SRBD Events and Sleep Stages from an ECG Signal

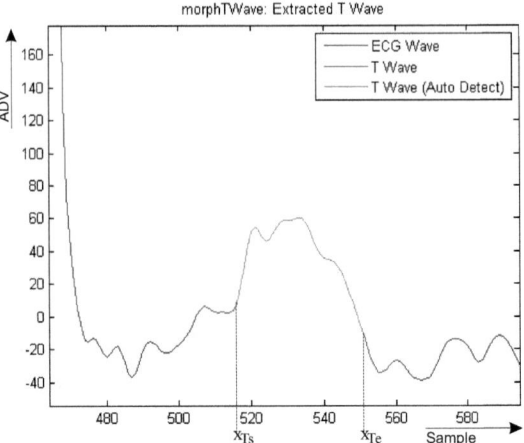

Figure 6.44: Result of an automatically detected T-wave as an intermediate step of computing the repolarization features

small or too wide, the limiters are set to ± 5% of the RR interval around the T-wave peak.

The result of the automatic T-wave detection is illustrated in Figure 6.44. The blue curve is the recorded ECG wave. The red curve is the extracted T-wave based on the fixed percentage of the RR-interval from either side. Finally, the green curve is the estimated T-wave based on thresholds for the ascent and descent, respectively, whose start and end positions are marked with x_{Ts} and x_{Te}. In case the threshold based estimation should fail which is detected, if the computed boundaries of the T-wave are too narrow or too wide, morphTWave() uses the boundaries indicated by the red curve. From the computed T-wave the features of the repolarization – see next Figure – are derived.

Subsequently, the time is computed as the difference between onset x_{Ts} and offset x_{Te} of the detected T-wave according to equation (6.8a) with f_s being the sampling frequency of the ECG signal. The integral, i.e., the "charge", is calculated as the sum of the ECG wave amplitudes within the detected range according to equation (6.8b).

6.4. Morphological Features

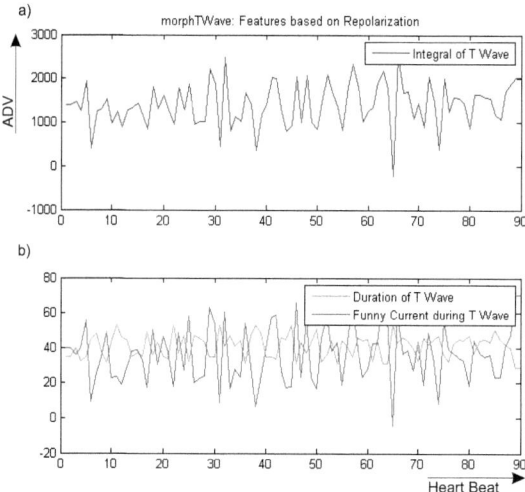

Figure 6.45: Features to describe the repolarization period

Finally, the "funny current" is derived from their quotient according to equation (6.7) (see Figure 6.39).

$$t = \frac{1}{f_s} \cdot (x_{Te} - x_{Ts}) \tag{6.8a}$$

$$Q = \sum_{n=x_{Ts}}^{x_{Te}} T(n) = \sum_{n=x_{Ts}}^{x_{Te}} ECG(n) \tag{6.8b}$$

The features reflecting the repolarization period of the heart are shown in Figure 6.45. In the upper panel there is the integral of the T-wave which represents the "charge" which has to be loaded during the repolarization process. In the lower panel two curves are given: the green one shows the duration of the T-wave and the red one the "funny current" (see /3.3.1/ and /6.4.5/) which is an indicator of the activity of the ANS.

All of the described features are written to the ARFF files. The RaK features are generated by mapping the beat-to-beat features to the 30 second evaluation period by computing the means and standard deviations of the feature's values within one evaluation period.

130   Chapter 6. Detecting SRBD Events and Sleep Stages from an ECG Signal

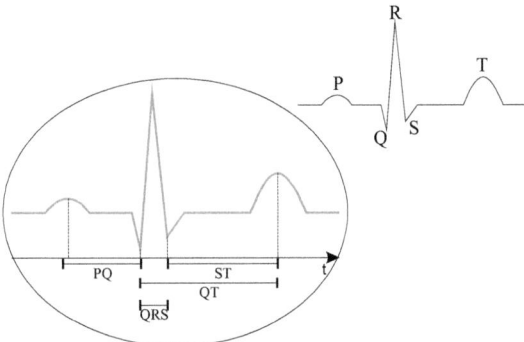

Figure 6.46: Some features based on the timing of the ECG, i.e., the relative dislocations of the distinctive points of the ECG (due to influences of the cardiac conduction system and the ANS)

6.4.6 Timing

The timing of the heart should be affected by different levels of autonomous activity as both the cardiac conduction system and the control of the muscle are driven by physiological processes which are directly affected by the ANS.

Parasympathicotonia – high PNS activity – provokes a prolonged PQ-time while reducing the QT-time. The same holds true for ischemia. The problem is that the QT-time depends on the current heart rate, i.e., it becomes shorter with tachycardia and longer with bradycardia (see Figure 3.12). Therefore, for diagnosing possible heart diseases the measured value would have to be compared to the "frequency corresponding norm value". But in the context of this work this might not be necessary as an increasing heart rate itself is an indicator for an activation of the SNS, thus, an indicator for the events EVA ml aims at detecting. Even though EVA ml does not consider the equation (3.1), the heart rate and its floating mean are computed for reference purposes.

The timing features are computed as differences between the distinctive ECG points. By taking into account the sampling rate of the ECG signal, the "differences in samples" are converted into "durations in seconds". The computed references are the absolute HR $m(HR)$ and the floating mean $m_c(HR, \texttt{flmnLen})$ of the HR. The HR is computed according to equation (6.9).

$$HR = 60 \cdot \frac{f_s}{diff(RR)}, \text{ in [bpm]} \qquad (6.9)$$

6.4. Morphological Features

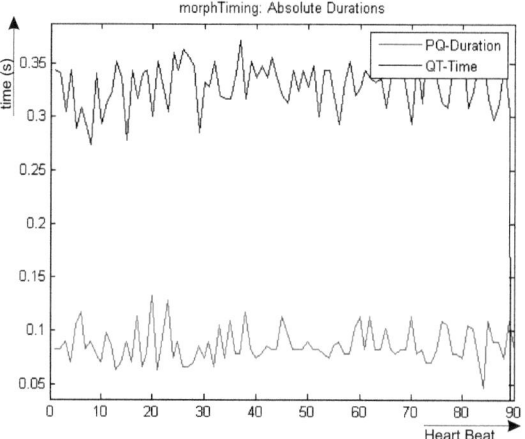

Figure 6.47: Absolute durations of the PQ- and the QT-timing

The timing features are computed in the function morphTiming(). These features relate to variations of the relative timing of the different ECG distinctive points to one another and not to variations in the heart rate (These features are considered by the AM, see /6.3/). Some of the features computed by morphTiming() are displayed in Figure 6.46. morphTiming() extracts the following features:

PQ-time The PQ-time is the AV-delay, i.e., the duration it takes the conduction system to pass the excitation from the atria to the ventricles. As the AV-node is sensitive to SRBD events (at least in the shape of the AV-blocks), variations in the conduction delay may relate to them. This feature is computed in seconds by taking into consideration the sampling frequency f_s of the ECG signal (see /3.3.2/).

PQ-time relative to floating mean of the HR To consider relative changes of the PQ-time to the absolute timing of an ECG wave which is governed by the HR, this feature is computed from the previous one by referring it to $m_c(HR, \texttt{flmnLen})$ according to equation (6.10).

$$PQ_{relHR} = \frac{PQ - time}{m_c(HR, \texttt{flmnLen})} \qquad (6.10)$$

Two features of morphTiming() are shown in Figure 6.47: The PQ-time (blue) which is mainly the delay of the AV-node and the QT-time (black) which is dominated by the repolarization time. From looking at the black curve the QT-time is

132   Chapter 6. Detecting SRBD Events and Sleep Stages from an ECG Signal

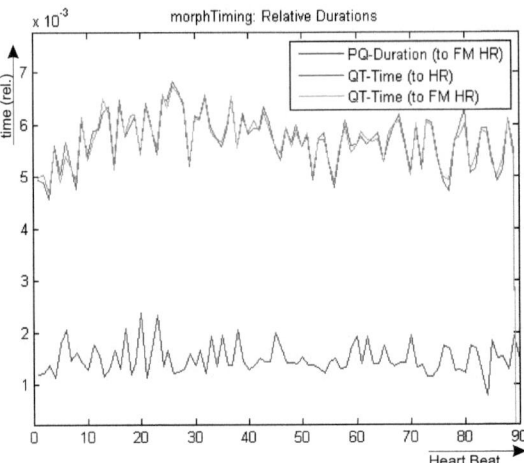

Figure 6.48: Timing of the distinctive P-Q-T-points in relation to the current HR or its floating mean, respectively (see equation (6.10) for principle)

read off as 0.34 s which matches the upper limit of Figure 3.12 considering the HR of 58 bpm.

QRS-time   The QRS-time is the duration it takes the cardiac conduction system to fully propagate the excitation along the ventricles.

QRS-time relative to floating mean of the HR   This feature is similar to the previous one but with respect to $m_c(HR, \mathtt{flmnLen})$ (see analog equation (6.10)).

As the absolute HR changes, the timing parameters of the heart, i.e., their relation to one another, do so as well. To compensate for this effect[11], the timing parameters are put in relation to the current HR and its floating mean. The results of this compensation are depicted in Figure 6.48. The blue curve is the PQ-Duration in relation to the floating mean of the HR. The QT-time is related to both the current HR and its floating mean with the results shown in the red and green curves.

QT-time   The QT-time describes the timing of the working cycle of the ventricle and the repolarization of the myocardium. It depends on the ANS activity level.

---

[11]This compensation is not truly physiological (see e.g., Figure 3.12), but is sufficient for the purpose of this work.

6.4. Morphological Features

QT-time relative to current HR As the QT-time seems to be one of the most important features for analyzing the ECG, a total of three features is derived from it: the absolute QT-time (previous), the QT-time in relation to the current HR (this feature), and the QT-time in relation to $m_c(HR, \texttt{flmnLen})$ (next ,feature) (see analog equation (6.10)).

QT-time relative to the floating mean of the HR As already mentioned this feature relates the QT-time to $m_c(HR, \texttt{flmnLen})$ to compensate influences of short time HR fluctuations (see analog equation (6.10)).

ST-time The ST-time is the duration of the repolarization. As the repolarization is sensitive to the activity level of the ANS, this feature should show dependencies from autonomous changes due to respiratory events or sleep stages.

ST-time relative to the floating mean of the HR This feature is essentially analogue to the previous one, but considers timing effects due to the influence of $m_c(HR, \texttt{flmnLen})$.

At the end of `morphTiming()` the extracted features are written to the appropriate ARFF files.

6.4.7 Overall Shape: Deviations

The next four functions do not focus on special sections of the ECG wave, but aim at finding changes in the overall shape.

The first function of this group is `morphShape_Dev()`. The principle of this function is illustrated in Figure 6.49: First, it uses either all or all the healthy (from the annotation) ECG waves to compute a template. From this template measures are computed which characterize the ECG waves by means of histograms containing the frequency distributions of the ECG amplitudes. Second, in the feature computation step the deviation of each ECG wave from these measures is computed. The idea is that during SRBD events the ECG waves differ from these measures to a greater extend than during healthy phases.

Creation of the Templates

The complete recording is cut into separate ECG waves at the R-peaks. As the lengths of the ECG waves vary with the heart rate, all ECG waves are resampled to have the same length. This length is set to the *mean of all ECG waves*. This is done for two reasons:

134   Chapter 6. Detecting SRBD Events and Sleep Stages from an ECG Signal

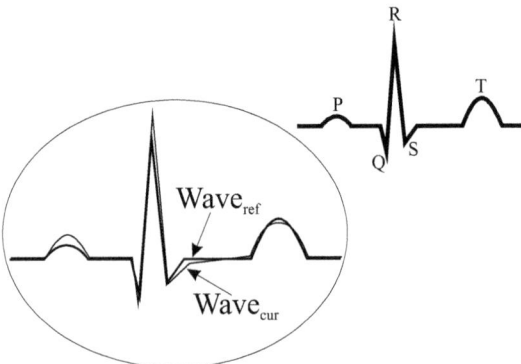

Figure 6.49: Principle of morphShape_Dev(): the deviation of each ECG wave is computed against a reference template.

1. Searching the longest or the shortest ECG wave is quite error prone as a) a single badly detected R-peak or b) an arrhythmia, AV-block, and so on, might completely spoil the result. Applying the mean is quite robust as single badly detected R-peaks are outbalanced by the large number of properly detected R-peaks.

2. Resampling the ECG wave means linearly stretching or squeezing it. But this is not physiologically correct as the ECG wave is not simply scaled with different heart rates, because some parts, e.g., the QRS-complex, do show only slight scaling effects, whereas other parts, e.g., the ST-segment and the QT-time (see Figure 3.12), are rescaled more extensively. Hence, setting the rescaling length to the mean reduces these errors.

Each of these resampled ECG waves is copied into a buffer which is used to compute the first template. A second buffer is created in exactly the same way, but only ECG waves from periods annotated as "normal respiration" are considered. This is to clean the template from the influences of respiratory events. Or from a different view point: putting together ECG from healthy and pathologic periods "blurs" the healthy template making it harder to see variations "sharply".

A "template buffer" is depicted in Figure 6.50. The blue "entanglement" is made up of the 90 ECG waves rescaled in length to $m(RR)$. The R-peaks are the boundaries on either side.

The next two templates are created from these buffers by computing the mean along values belonging to the same sample index in the buffer. The samples of the

6.4. Morphological Features

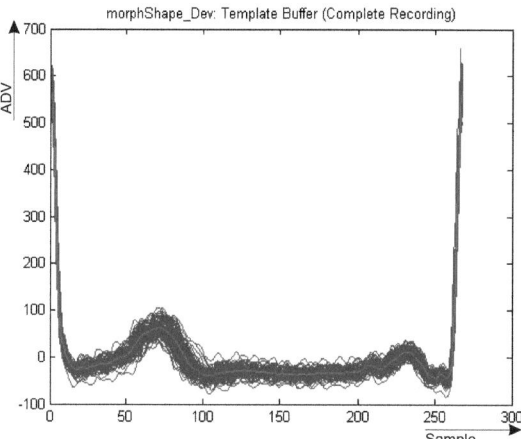

Figure 6.50: Template buffer for the complete recording created from 90 ECG waves which were split at the R-peak. The red curve in the "middle" is the mean of the values of the different ECG waves at a given index.

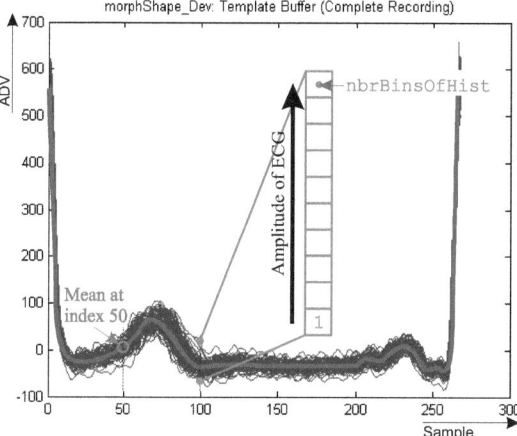

Figure 6.51: This is the same template as in Figure 6.50 with additional markers for illustration purposes: In green the derivation of the mean value of the ECG waves at a given index, e.g., 50. In orange the histogram of ECG wave values at index 100. For each index there is a dedicated histogram whose minimum and maximum bin value are defined by the corresponding extrema of the ECG waves. The number of bins of the histogram is given by `nbrBinsOfHist`.

136   Chapter 6. Detecting SRBD Events and Sleep Stages from an ECG Signal

ECG waves in the buffers are indexed from 1 to $m(RR)$ with RR being the distance from one R-peak to the next one. An illustration of the mean computation is given in Figure 6.51 in the green circle. Repeating this procedure for every index of the ECG wave results in the red curve.

Creation of Measures of Deviation

To compute the degree of deviation of a single ECG against the templates, EVA ml prepares two measures:

- the center values at a given sample index and

- the occurrence frequency of ECG amplitude values at a given (sample) index

These measures can be regarded as the *histogram* along a given index: all samples belonging to the same index are evaluated in a histogram which is spread equally spaced along the range of found values. Additionally, their frequency is counted. The number of histogram bins is set by the value nbrBinsOfHist in the processing configuration (see /10.2/) and defaults to 10. An illustration of the histogram is given in Figure 6.51 in the orange elements: the center values are the center of the histogram bins and the occurrence frequency for each amplitude range is the value stored in the histogram bin.

The computed "characterization of the reference ECG wave" used for computing the deviation of the each wave from the standard ECG wave are shown in Figures 6.52 and and 6.53. The weight is computed from two different components: the first component is the differences from the center values of a histogram to the amplitude of the current ECG wave at a given index. The second component is the frequency of all ECG amplitude values dropping into a given bin. The first component is shown in Figure 6.52 which shows the center values of the histograms along the rescaled ECG wave. In the Figure the histograms are created using ten bins.

The second component is shown in Figure 6.53 which shows the distribution of the frequencies with which amplitudes of all ECG waves drop into one of the ten bins along the amplitudes of the ECG waves.

Computing the Degree of Deviation

In this step the deviations of each ECG wave against the templates is computed. This is done in two different ways depending on the type of the template, i.e., whether the template is based on the histograms for center value and frequency or it is based on the means for a given index.

6.4. Morphological Features

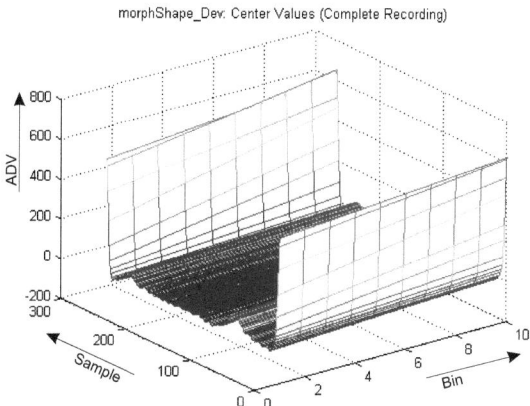

Figure 6.52: The center values of the histograms along the rescaled ECG wave created from the complete recording (see text for explanation). The coordinate axis starting in the middle of the Figure and running to the right indicates the bin number. The axis leaving the middle toward the left is the x-axis, i.e., time indicator, of the rescaled ECG wave. And finally, the upright axis is the ADV.

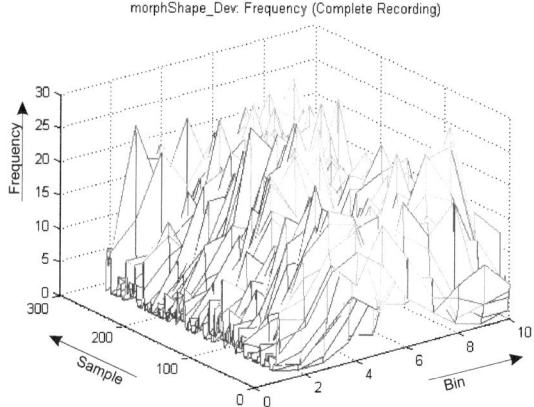

Figure 6.53: Frequencies of ECG wave amplitudes for the complete recording

138   Chapter 6. Detecting SRBD Events and Sleep Stages from an ECG Signal

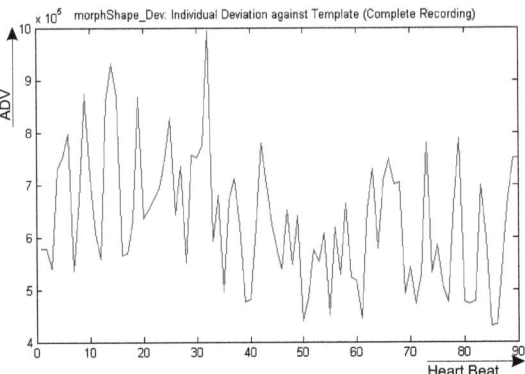

Figure 6.54: The deviation of each ECG wave is shown against the "weighted template" consisting of center values and corresponding frequencies. The template was created using all of the ECG waves, i.e., these annotated belonging to healthy phases and those annotated belonging to phases of pathological breathing.

In the first case the deviation for a given index is computed according to equation (6.11) The adding of 1 in the denominator of equation (6.11) is just to prevent the *Devision by Zero* error, if the frequency of a given bin is zero. The computed value dev is the deviation of a single ECG wave against the template. Accordingly, this value has to be computed for each ECG wave.

$$dev = \sum_{ind=1}^{m(RR)} \sum_{bin}^{\texttt{nbrBinsOfHist}} \frac{1}{freq(ind, n_{Bin}) + 1} \cdot (ECG(ind) - center(ind, n_{Bin}))^2 \tag{6.11}$$

In the case of the mean based templates the deviation dev_{mean} is computed according to equation (6.12).

$$dev_{mean} = \sum_{ind}^{m(RR)} (ECG(ind) - mean(ind))^2 \tag{6.12}$$

The next two Figures show the results of computing the deviation from the weighted template or from the mean of the ECG wave, respectively. The deviations in these Figures were computed against the template including healthy and disturbed breathing. Figure 6.54 depicts the deviation from the weighted template consisting of center values and corresponding frequencies and Figure 6.55 the deviations against the mean. A comparison of the shapes of the curves reveals that they resemble one another to some extent. This is not too surprising as computing the means of the

6.4. Morphological Features

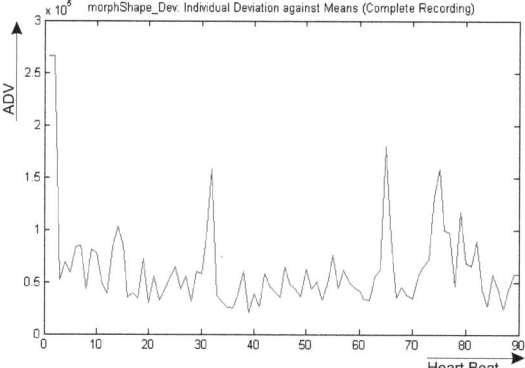

Figure 6.55: The deviation of each ECG wave is shown against the mean template. The template was created using all of the ECG waves, i.e., these annotated belonging to healthy phases and those annotated belonging to phases of pathological breathing.

ECG waves also creates a "weighted template" in a sense. The difference of the first approach is that it places a higher "penalty" on rare and far outliers.

During the next processing phase the deviations dev and dev_{mean} are computed based on the templates created from the ECG section belonging to phases of healthy breathing according to the annotations. Thus, the templates should be more "accurate" as they are not "blurred" by phases of pathologic breathing. Accordingly, these templates should be more sensitive to pathologic deviations of the ECG waves.

The computed deviations, i.e., histogram or mean based, are the features of this function. They are stored to the corresponding ARFF files.

6.4.8 Overall Shape: Independent Component Analysis

A basic introduction to the Independent Component Analysis (ICA) and a discussion about its application in the context of this work can be found in /10.5/.

The ICA Realization used: FastICA

There are several implementations of the ICA algorithm available. In the scope of this work the **FastICA** implementation was applied. It was designed by Aapo Hyvärinen [Hyvr07] at the Helsinki University of Technology. It is available for several computer languages, e.g., C++ and Phyton and Matlab, and can be downloaded freely. FastICA is a quite popular algorithm in the scientific world because of its convergence speed and its robustness.

140   Chapter 6. Detecting SRBD Events and Sleep Stages from an ECG Signal

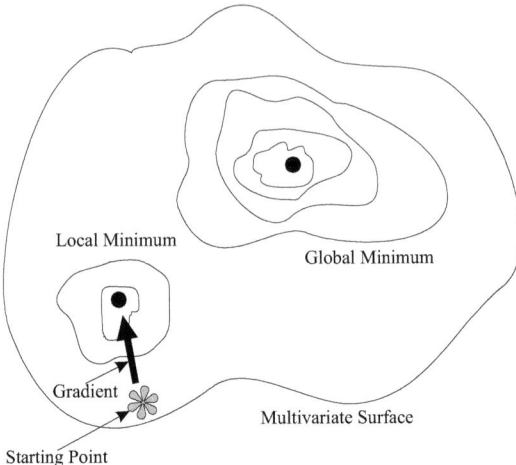

Figure 6.56: A reason why gradient descent algorithms tend to fail is shown here: if the (random) starting point of the iterative minimum approximation process happens to be chosen as in this Figure, the gradient which is computed to guide the next iteration does not point in the direction of the global but to the local minimum instead. Thus, the true minimum is not found.

It is based on the *maximization of nongaussianity principle* of the recovered signals (see /10.5.2/). The fixed-point algorithm uses the Newton procedure based on the kurtosis (see equation (10.8)) as convergence parameter.

The Newton procedure is an implementation of the gradient descent procedure (GDP), i.e., the direction of the next step coincides with the steepest gradient. During an iterative procedure the *global* minimum of a kurtosis based cost function is sought. In Figure 6.56 there is an graphical representation of a problem the GDP suffers: As the starting point is chosen arbitrarily, the algorithm tends to iterate into *local* minima [Bish 95]. In practice, calling the algorithm over and over again leads to different results – a behavior which is found in the EM based GMM (see /10.4/) as well.

The Idea and assumed Model

The idea behind using this concept in the context of this work is depicted in Figure 6.57. Considering how the ECG signal is generated (see /3.1/ and /3.1.1/), it is quite easy to imagine the ECG as a mixture of different events affecting different places or processes of the heart, e.g., the atria, the ventricles, and/or the repolarization, respectively. Exemplarily, during phases of respiratory events or arousals the normal

6.4. Morphological Features

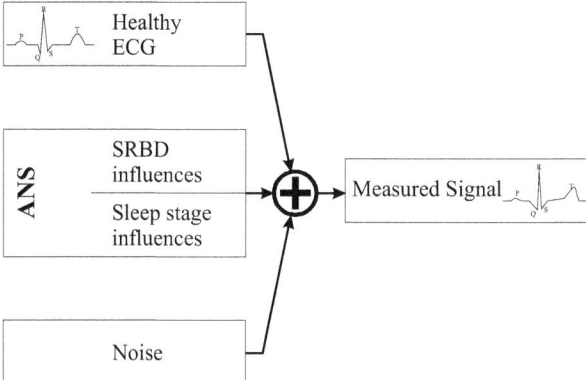

Figure 6.57: The ICA based Model: the measured ECG signal is a superposition from the "healthy ECG", influences from the ANS, and noise. The ICA reverses this mixing process and makes the various influences accessible individually. As these components embody the information about the dynamics of the ANS, e.g., driven by SRBD events and changes of sleep stages, their evaluation hints on the underlying processes.

ECG signal is superimposed by additional signal components. These additional components lead to variations in the ECG signal which can be separated by the ICA approach, i.e., the ICA reverses the mixing procedure based on the statistical properties of the individual/independent components (IC). The ICA approach is implemented in morphShape_CA().

A more effect orientated view on the ICA principle is illustrated in Figure 6.58. It shows modified ECG waves resulting from the various influences which are superposed to produce the recorded signal.

Configuration of the ICA Model

The ICA algorithm aims at finding as many independent components as observations are supplied to it, i.e., if three observations are supplied, three independent components are searched. But is the ICA capable of deciding how many ICs there are?

Figure 6.59 shows some typical "components" which are found when ICA is run on a large number (90) of ECG waves. "Large" is to be read as "many more than there are actually independent component". It can be noticed that none of the ICA components resembles the original ECG wave. This behavior of the ICA is called *Overlearning*. In this case the estimation of the components depends too much on

142   Chapter 6. Detecting SRBD Events and Sleep Stages from an ECG Signal

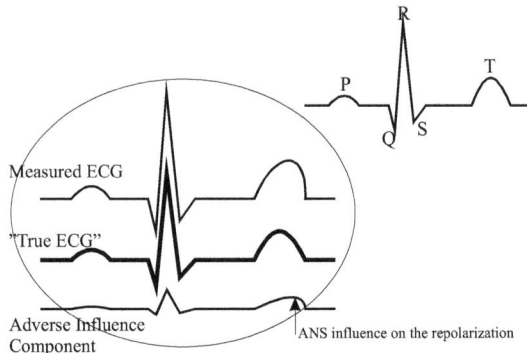

Figure 6.58: ICA – Principle of retrieving the SRBD information which is hidden in the recorded ECG signal: The measured ECG signal is a mixture of a healthy ECG and a component which is induced by SRBD events and arousals, respectively.

the single samples (of the ECG) and does no longer reveal the underlying processes [Kram 01]. This results in the finding that the ICA can not be used to determine the number of ICs, i.e., the number of contributing physiological processes.

To preestimate the number of independent physiological processes, the model presented in Figure 6.57 has to be reconsidered. It introduces the following contributors: the healthy ECG, influences from SRBD events and sleep stages, and noise. On the one hand the influences from the SRBD and the sleep stages directly affect the ANS which itself consists of the SNS and the PNS resulting in a total of two or four components. On the other hand the SRBD events directly affect the sleep stages and the ANS, thus, all these dynamics may be represented by a single component. Considering the noise component, it can be said that this component comprises the noises from the recording device and those from "anomalies" in the generation of the ECG. Accordingly, one or two independent components here. Summarizing, a total of three to seven independent components can be expected.

The upper assumed limit is supported by the (experimental) finding that the ICA starts to spoil the ECG wave from eight waves onwards (see Figure 6.59). To narrow down the range of expectable ICs, the ICA was run on a various number of ECG waves resulting in the following observations:

- Applying the preprocessing to the ECG signal reduces the number of found components by one. This means that the noise component *representing the adverse recording effects* can be canceled by preprocessing the ECG signal. The remaining contributor to the noise component has to be considered deriving from *the anomalies of the ECG generation*.

6.4. Morphological Features

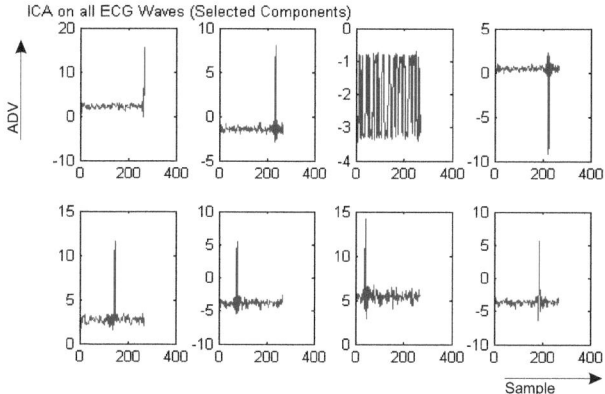

Figure 6.59: Results of running FastICA on "too many" components (some selected)

- FastICA retains the shape of a proper ECG wave in one of the components, if called with up to five ECG waves.

- The non-ECG components converge in shape, if called with more than three ECG waves, i.e., the underlying processes can no longer be distinguished.

Recalling the ICA model (see Figure 6.57) it is obvious that the information about SRBD events and sleep stages, respectively, has to be enclosed in the non-ECG components (see Figure 6.60b & c), as the ECG component (see Figure 6.60a) is considered "pure".

The SRBD events are said to be dominated by PNS influences (see p. 37) which is approved by the results of this work (see /7.4.1/). If so, the IC representing the SNS can be neglected and the ANS dynamics are represented by one single IC.

The noise component representing the anomalies of the ECG generation is likely to be governed by SRBD events and sleep stages alike. The latter is due to the influences of the sleep stages on the HR, the HRV, and the underlying physiological processes (see /2.4.2/). The noise component can be regarded as representing the longterm influences of sleep on the ECG generation. These influences are summarized by one single IC.

Given the model and the (experimental) findings, *the number of evaluated ICA components was set to three* by means of the configuration parameter nbrICAwaves. For further reference these three ICA components are named ECG, PNS, and noise.

144   Chapter 6. Detecting SRBD Events and Sleep Stages from an ECG Signal

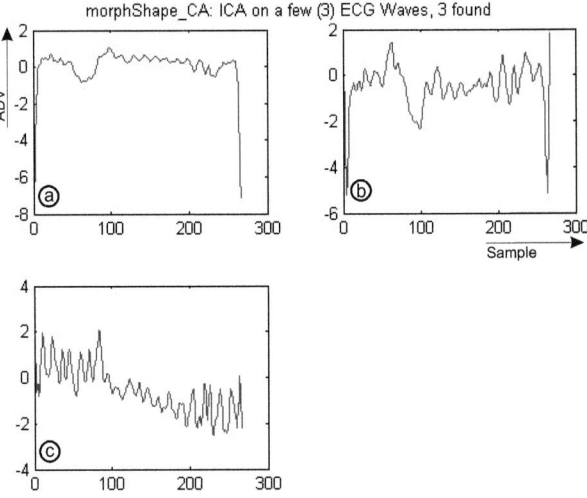

Figure 6.60: Results of the FastICA algorithm run on three ECG waves. Component (a) can clearly be distinguished as the ECG wave, even though it is turned upside down (ECG wave is split at the R-peak, see Figure 6.50). Component (b) resembles an (upside-down) ECG wave, but it features an additional peak, and component (c) is an "arbitrarily" shaped curve. According to the ICA model the components (b) and (c) encode the information about the occurrence of a SRBD event and the sleep stage.

6.4. Morphological Features

Applying FastICA

Applying the FastICA algorithm entails two ICA typical problems:

The Scaling Problem The components returned from ICA differ from the supplied input in their amplitude which includes the sign (see Figure 6.60a).

The Permutation Problem The components returned from ICA have no fixed assignment to any of the components in the input signal which means that the component containing the ECG wave may change with any call to the ICA algorithm.

This leads to the necessity that after each call to FastICA the returned components have to be rescaled to the amplitude of the input signal and reassigned to the categories "ECG", "PNS", and "noise". Thus, in the first processing step the ICA components are rescaled to have the same amplitude as the input signals by matching the minima and maxima.

In addition, FastICA sometimes fails to find the required number of ICs. The assumption that this behavior itself may well hint on the occurrence of a SRBD event or a change in the current sleep stage was not confirmed during the evaluation. To complete the feature vectors under these circumstances, the missing values are computed as the mean of their neighboring values, i.e., $m_c(.,3)$[12], during the postprocessing.

Implementation and Extracted Features

For the application of the native ICA algorithm the supplied ECG waves have to match two requirements:

- **The ECG waves must have the same length.** This requires the ECG waves to be rescaled along the time axis as the "lengths" of the ECG waves vary dependent on the HR. The rescaled ECG waves are stored in a buffer analog to the one in function morphShape_Dev() (see Figure 6.50).

- **The ECG waves must have zero mean.** This requirement is satisfied during the preprocessing by the DC-offset (highpass) filter. (Actually, the specific ICA implementation FastICA takes care of this requirement itself.)

After these preprocessing steps, the main processing loop along the ECG waves of the recording is entered. It starts with running FastICA on three ECG waves at

---
[12] The dot "." serves to denote the respective feature.

146   Chapter 6. Detecting SRBD Events and Sleep Stages from an ECG Signal

a time. For easier understanding of the following processing steps, the challenges of applying the ICA algorithm are summarized here:

1. FastICA may fail to produce the desired number of ICs.

2. It can not be predicted which output signal will represent the ECG wave, the PNS, or the noise component.

3. The scaling of the output components is completely random.

The subsequent processing determines the number of output components and orders the found components. If FastICA fails to produce the appropriate number of output components, the index of the current ECG wave is remembered for later postprocessing following the main processing loop (challenge 1). The ordering is done by computing the cross-correlation between the first of the three input ECG waves and all of the returned ICs. The cross-correlation is computed for the ICs themselves and for the ICs with inverted sign as the scaling factor can be negative as well. Subsequently, the results of the cross-correlation are sorted in descending order. The IC representing the ECG signal is expected to show the highest correlation and is placed first. The PNS component was chosen to be the second highest correlation result and the noise component the remaining IC (challenge 2). Finally, to counteract the random scaling, the amplitude of the IC representing the ECG wave is adjusted to match the one of the input ECG signal and the same scaling factor is applied to the other two ICs as well (challenge 3).

Figures 6.61 and 6.62 show the three resulting ICs. Their respective titles reveal their computed matching rank and whether the signal is inverted. In each of the Figures the blue curve is the original input signal and the red curve is the respective IC. It can be clearly seen that the signal with the highest matching rank, i.e., Figure 6.61, represents the ECG signal. Among the remaining components the one with the higher matching rank, i.e., Figure 6.62a, is assigned to the PNS component. Comparing Figure 6.61 and Figure 6.62a supports the ICA model as the differences (in comparison to the ECG wave) may well represent the influence of the PNS on the repolarization – especially in the area of the T-wave (see /3.5/). The last IC shown in Figure 6.62b is assigned to the noise component.

In the next step of morphShape_CA() the following features are derived from the ICs:

Energy of the PNS and noise components and their spectra According to the ICA model, these components concentrate the ECG disturbances introduced by either the PNS or the ECG generation noise.

6.4. Morphological Features

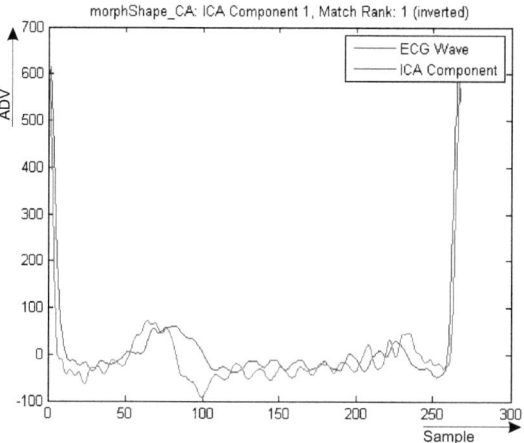

Figure 6.61: The IC with highest matching rank clearly represents the ECG wave.

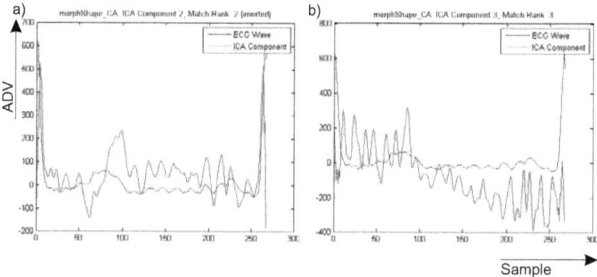

Figure 6.62: The ICA component 2 still resembles an ECG wave and is assigned to the PNS component. The last ICA component showing no resemblance to an ECG wave is assigned to the noise component of the ECG generation, i.e., spontaneous influences.

148   Chapter 6. Detecting SRBD Events and Sleep Stages from an ECG Signal

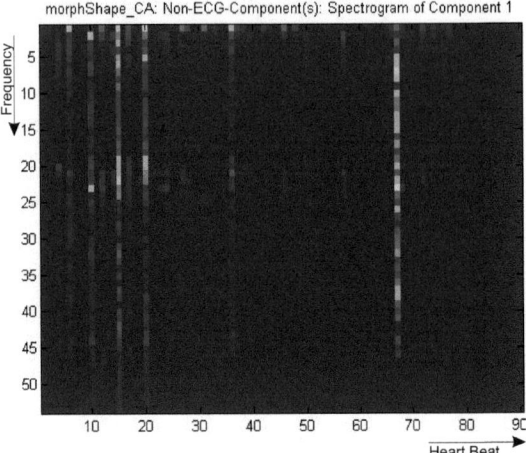

Figure 6.63: Spectrogram of the PNS component: on the x-axis there are the heart beats and on the y-axis there are the frequencies of the spectral components. The amplitudes of the spectral components are represented as "false-color".

As a measure of the degree of disturbance, MoD, the amplitudes of these signals are summed up according to equation (6.13) (nEc = "Non-ECG-Component", i.e., the PNS and the noise component). Hence, the result is not actually an "energy", but rather the "sum of voltages", physically speaking[13].

$$MoD = \sum_{n=1}^{m(RR)} nEc(n) \qquad (6.13)$$

Additionally, the spectrograms (see "false-color[14]" Figures 6.63 and 6.64) of these components are computed to evaluate the different physiological dynamics possibly introduced by ANS. The idea is that a dominating physiological effect may be visible at certain frequencies relating to the ANS time constants (see /3.3.1/). For each spectrogram `icaSpecNbrCoeffs` (which is set in the processing configuration) spectral coefficients are kept as features.

Comparing Figures 6.63 and 6.64 reveals that from a spectral point of view the two components are quite similar, even though they differ a lot in their shape. This may be due to the same (or closely linked) physiological processes.

---
[13]This is to keep the numerical values "low" and, thus, computation precision up.
[14]"False-color" means that the values of a displayed variable, i.e., the values of the DFT coefficients in this case, are represented by colors. Usually, low values are blue, mean values are green, and high values are yellow or white.

6.4. Morphological Features

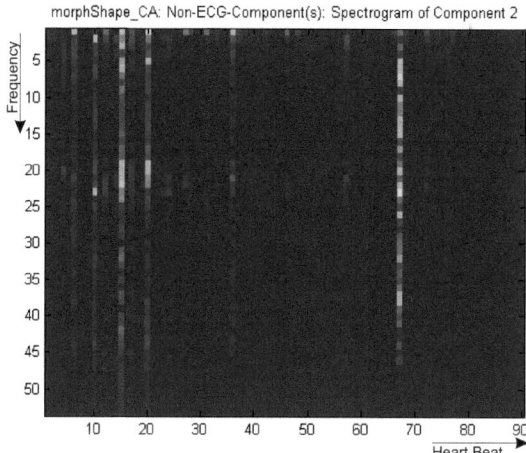

Figure 6.64: Spectrogram of the noise component

Cross-correlations between the original ECG wave or the overnight mean ECG wave, respectively, and the ICA derived ECG wave The idea behind these features is "the other way around" one of the previous concept: the "purer" the currently processed ECG wave, the more it resembles the ICA ECG wave which is assumed to be cleaned from adverse influences. And the higher their resemblance, the higher the correlation result which can be regarded – in the style of the previous feature – a "measure of pureness". The cross-correlation with the overnight mean ECG wave was included as a "degree of variance" measure to an individual set-point. Figure 6.65 shows the results of the cross-correlations of the ICA ECG component and the current ECG wave (blue) and the mean ECG from the wave buffer (red).

Running ICA on the difference between the current ECG wave and the overnight mean of all ECG waves This feature aims at differentiating the different adverse effects contributing to the dynamic changes of the ECG wave shape. The overnight mean is used as the subject's "normal" ECG wave as the mean evens the temporary deviations caused by, e.g., SRBD events. The currently processed ECG wave is reduced to these deviations by subtracting the mean from it. Hence, the subsequent call of FastICA tries to separate different types of adverse effects – and one of them may reflect the influence of respiratory events.

The feature computation is accomplished by creating a temporary buffer for two, i.e., (nbrICAwaves − 1), ECG waves which is filled with ECG waves from which

150   Chapter 6. Detecting SRBD Events and Sleep Stages from an ECG Signal

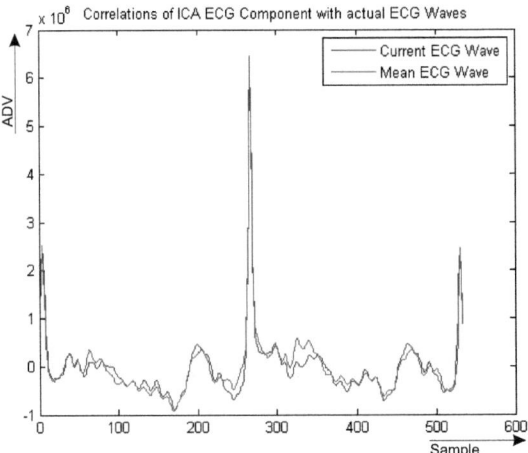

Figure 6.65: Correlations between the ICA derived ECG component and the currently processed ECG signal or the overnight mean ECG signal, respectively.

the overnight mean was subtracted. Subsequently, the ICA algorithm is applied to the temporary buffer. Afterwards, the amplitudes of the resulting components are summed up. In case that FastICA failed to determine all components, the missing values are replaced by their respective predecessors. The summed up amplitudes of the ICs are sorted in a descending manner and assigned to their respective feature vector. The requirements for the sorting step are already discussed above.

The curves in Figure 6.66 show the following: the blue one is the current ECG wave, the red one is the mean ECG wave, and the green one is their difference (only one component shown). The next two curves (black and yellow) depict the PNS and noise signals.

The two corresponding sums of the amplitudes of the ICs representing different types of adverse effects are shown in Figure 6.67.

Differences of the Energies of the components reflecting PNS and noise
This feature computes the difference of the energies of the two non-ECG-components, i.e., the PNS and noise components. It aims at finding the differential dynamics in these components. The "energies" are computed as in previous features as "sums of amplitudes". Figure 6.68 shows the results: in blue and green there are the energies of the non-ECG components and in red their difference.

The number of possible differences varies with the number of ICs determined by nbrICAwaves. In Figure 6.69 there is an illustration how to derive the number

6.4. Morphological Features

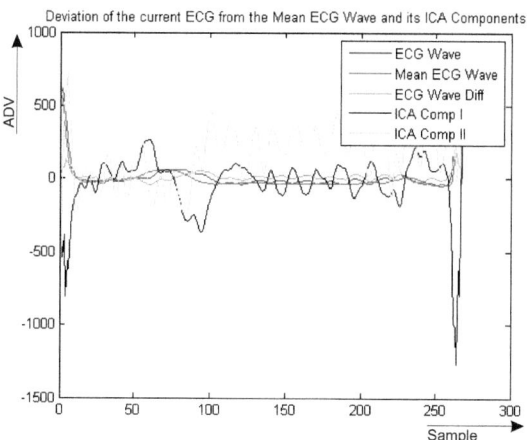

Figure 6.66: Deviation of the current ECG wave from the overnight ECG and the two different ICs representing PNS and noise

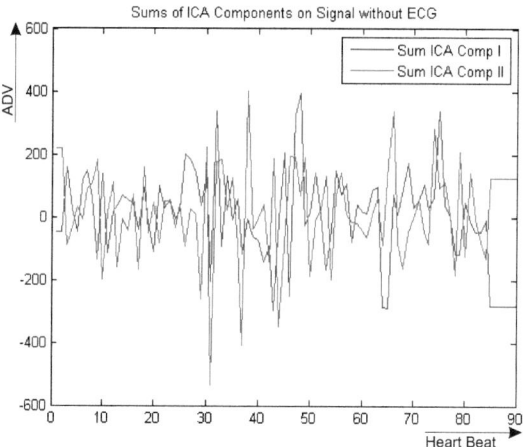

Figure 6.67: The sums of amplitudes for the two ICs representing either PNS or noise influences, respectively, for each heart beat; on the x-axis, there are the indices of the heart beats, and on the y-axis the values of the sums in ADV.

152   Chapter 6. Detecting SRBD Events and Sleep Stages from an ECG Signal

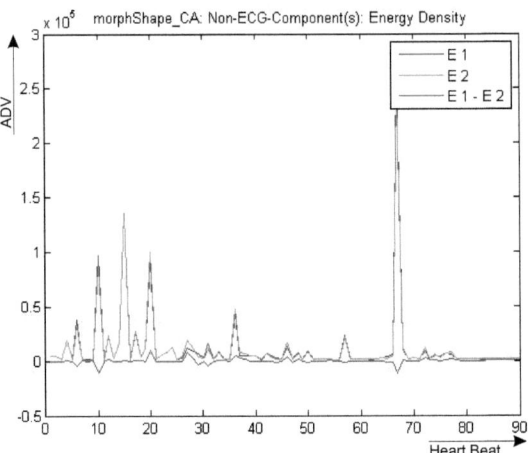

Figure 6.68: Dynamics of energies and their difference for the non-ECG components

of possible IC differences. As can be deducted that their number follows equation (6.14), where $n = \text{nbrICAwaves} - 1$. In the evaluated configuration of three ICs there is one difference computable.

$$nbr_{DiffComps} = \sum_{1}^{n-1} n = \frac{n(n-1)}{2} \qquad (6.14)$$

In the final step, all the features are written to the corresponding ARFF files. The number of the BtB features NoF_{BtB} obeys equation (6.15) and the corresponding equation for the number of RaK features NoF_{RaK} is shown as equation (6.16), where $nbr_{DiffComps}$ is defined in equation (6.14).

$$NoF_{BtB} = 2(nbrICAwaves - 1) + icaSpecNbrCoeffs \cdot$$
$$(nbrICAwaves - 1) + nbr_{DiffComps} + 2 \qquad (6.15)$$

$$NoF_{RaK} = 4(nbrICAwaves - 1) + 2 \cdot icaSpecNbrCoeffs \cdot$$
$$(nbrICAwaves - 1) + 2 \cdot nbr_{DiffComps} + 4 \qquad (6.16)$$

6.4. Morphological Features   153

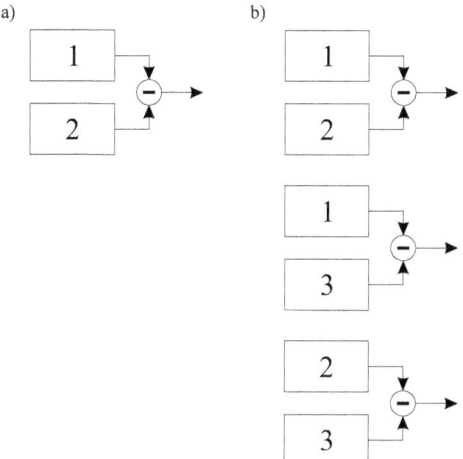

Figure 6.69: Illustration of deriving the possible number of IC differences: in case a) there are two non-ECG components resulting in one difference and in case b) there are three non-ECG components, e.g., PNS, noise, and an additional SNS component (see model), resulting in three computable differences.

6.4.9 Overall Shape: Spectral Transformations

The function morphShape_Spec() focuses on the evaluation of variations in the spectral features of the ECG waves. Different transformations, i.e., Discrete Fourier Transformation (DFT) and Discrete Cosine Transformation (DCT), are evaluated. While the DFT is a very common approach for general frequency analysis, the DCT is mainly used for redundancy based data compression, e.g., images (jpeg) and audio. It is evaluated in the context of this work with the notion of reducing the number of required coefficients for event classification.

As the R-peak dominates the ECG wave because of its amplitude, the transformations are applied on the ECG with (see Figure 6.70 black ECG curve) and without the R-peak (see Figure 6.70 red ECG curve) to explore its influence.

Creation of the ECG Buffer

The processing starts analog to the other functions dealing with the overall shape of the ECG wave with the creation of an ECG buffer. But in contrast to the other functions of this group morphShape_Spec() allows to select, whether the R-peaks are placed at the respective sides of the buffer, e.g., see Figure 6.50, or *centered in*

154   Chapter 6. Detecting SRBD Events and Sleep Stages from an ECG Signal

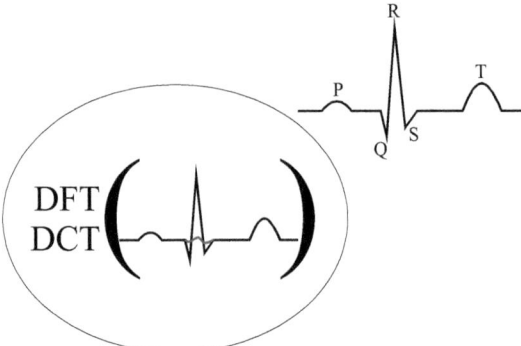

Figure 6.70: Creating the spectral transformations of the ECG wave

the middle of the buffer[15]. Placing the R-peaks in the middle of the buffer provides full control over the way the R-peak is extinguished and makes the extinction more demonstrative. Moreover, in this mode no rescaling is applied which preserves the initial morphology. Figure 6.71 shows the ECG data of the test set with centered R-peak.

Estimation of window length of data to cut out

Skipping the rescaling rises the question of the window length for the data to cut out as, nevertheless, for the subsequent feature evaluation using WEKA a constant number of features throughout a single input file is required. Hence, the ECG waves are cut from the continuous recording with the same length – ignoring the HR. Theoretically, to make sure that only a single ECG wave contributes to the features, the length of the data sample should equal the minimal distance of two R-peaks, i.e., the RR-interval at the highest heart rate.

This theoretical approach yields problems, if the patient shows arrhythmias or in the case of bad R-peak detections. In Figure 6.72 there are two more reasons: in Figure 6.72a there is an interval with an extraordinarily short R-peak distance which leads to an interval length that gathers too little data from the normal ECG waves. In Figure 6.72b an artifact influences the computation of the shortest R-peak distance leading to the same effect. In summary, this approach is error-prone and not robust enough.

---

[15]Selection is achieved by the value of the parameter `centerRPeakInBuffer` in the processing configuration file (see /10.2/)

6.4. Morphological Features

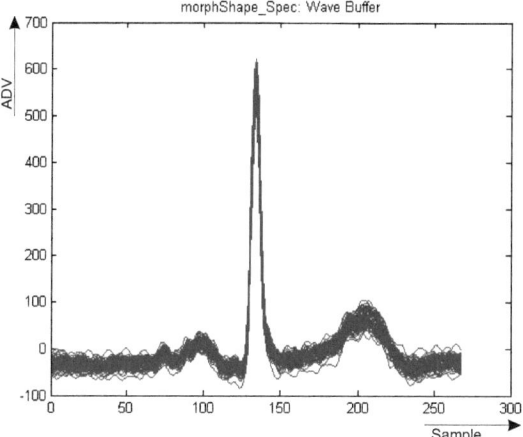

Figure 6.71: Centered buffer of ECG Waves

The finally chosen approach is to take the mean of all the R-peak distances. The mean of all of the R-peak distances is 224.17 samples and the mean of all of the R-peak distances without the period of artifacts (see Figure 6.72b) is 224.08 samples. The two values are literally equal which makes this approach very robust.

To evaluate the actual performance of this approach, Figure 6.73 shows an ECG wave with three different window lengths. In Figure 6.73a the length is equal to the mean of all of the R-peak distances of 224, in Figure 6.73b the minimal R-peak distance of 130 samples, and in Figure 6.73c a hypothetical value of 260 samples. The observation is: a) includes the complete ECCG wave, b) provides too little length and, accordingly, the ECG wave is not complete. The ECG wave in c) shows that in usual ECG waves there is a buffer of about 40 samples before the next R-peak enters the window.

These observations lead to the following conclusion: Computing the window length as the mean distance of two R-peaks is much more robust and practically perfect.

Extinguishing the R-Peak

Looking at an ECG wave it is obvious that the R-peak is the most dominant part of an ECG signal. Accordingly, it is likely to dominate the spectrum after each transformation which may suppress the information of the remaining ECG wave. To counteract this dominance, the transformations are applied to the ECG signal

156   Chapter 6. Detecting SRBD Events and Sleep Stages from an ECG Signal

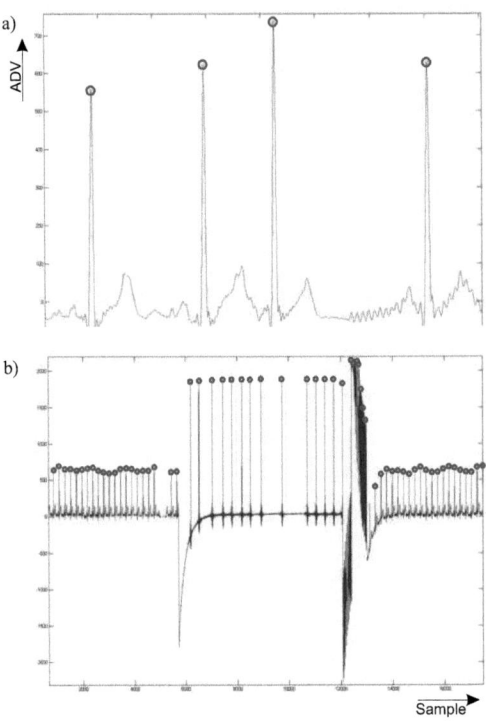

Figure 6.72: Estimating the minimal difference between two R-peaks

6.4. Morphological Features 157

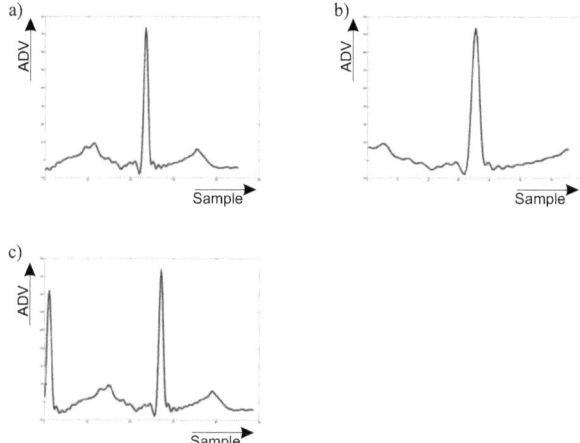

Figure 6.73: One ECG wave cut from the recording with different window lengths

without the dominating R-peak as well. This Section explains the extinction of the R-peak.

The method described here differs from the usual approach of applying the (decimal) logarithm or the square root. Why? First, looking at Figure 6.71 the following can be noted: the R-peak has an amplitude of 600 ADV, the T-wave of 100 ADV, and the P-wave of about 40 ADV. Applying the decimal logarithm yields the values 2.78, 2.00, and 1.60, and the square root 24.49, 10.00, and 6.32. Hence, the application of the logarithm reduces the ratio from T-wave to P-wave from 2.5 to 1.25, and the application of the square root to 1.58, which may reduce the classification powers of the derived features. Second, the features are morphology based and the application of any of the two functions affects the shape of the ECG waves.

When deleting the R-peak from an ECG wave, two questions arise. The first is: Which fraction of the ECG wave to delete from the ECG wave to delete the R-peak? And the second is: How to delete it?

Finding the limiters of the R-peak Figure 6.74 targets at answering the first question. In Figure 6.74a there is the original ECG wave (blue) and the signal with different fractions of the complete ECG wave length cut out to delete the R-peak: one fifth (red), one seventh (black), and one tenth (green): the red curve clearly deletes non R-peak parts. The black curve seems suitable concerning the Q-point, but a little too narrow at the S-point. The green curve is very close at the Q-point, but just keeps the Q- and S-point of the QRS-complex. In the end, one tenth of the RR interval was chosen as the fraction the R-peak covers.

Hence, the limiters, i.e., onset x_{onset} and offset x_{offset}, of the R-peak are computed according to equation (6.17) with the following parameters: The position of the current R-peak x_R, the mean length of the RR interval $m(RR)$ and the value of the parameter `percentageRpeak` from the processing configuration. As explained, the latter was heuristically found to be 10%.

$$x_{onset/offset} = x_R \pm m(RR) \cdot \text{percentageRpeak} \qquad (6.17)$$

In Figure 6.74b the resulting spectra due to the different fractions are compared (Colors are the same as in Figure 6.74a). As expected the blue spectrum is way over the others – indicator that most of the energy of the ECG signal is contained in the R-peak. The other spectra are fairly close to one another, but the green one seems to retain more information about the shape of the ECG wave.

Methods of extinguishing the R-peak To answer the second question of how to delete the R-peak, three different approaches of extinguishing the R-peak were implemented (see Figure 6.75):

- Setting ECG values to zero

- Linear interpolation

- Linear interpolation with moving-average-filtering (low pass)

Figure 6.75 shows (a part of) the complete ECG wave (blue) and different types of deleting the R-peak: Simply setting the ECG samples to zero (red), linear interpolation (black), and a moving average lowpass filter over the linearly interpolated signal (green).

The method of simply setting the ECG samples to zero has two disadvantages: the first one is that is leads to a kind of "phantom R-peak", if the ECG wave is not on the iso-electric potential, i.e., has a DC-offset. This problem can be fixed by using the DC offset compensation during pre-processing (see /6.1.2/). The second disadvantage is shared with the method of linear interpolation and it is that the – probably – sharp bends at either side are prone to violate the bandwidth limitation resulting in frequency aliasing, likely spoiling important information. As the method of linear interpolation in combination with the moving average lowpass filter does not show any of these disadvantages it is the one to be selected.

6.4. Morphological Features

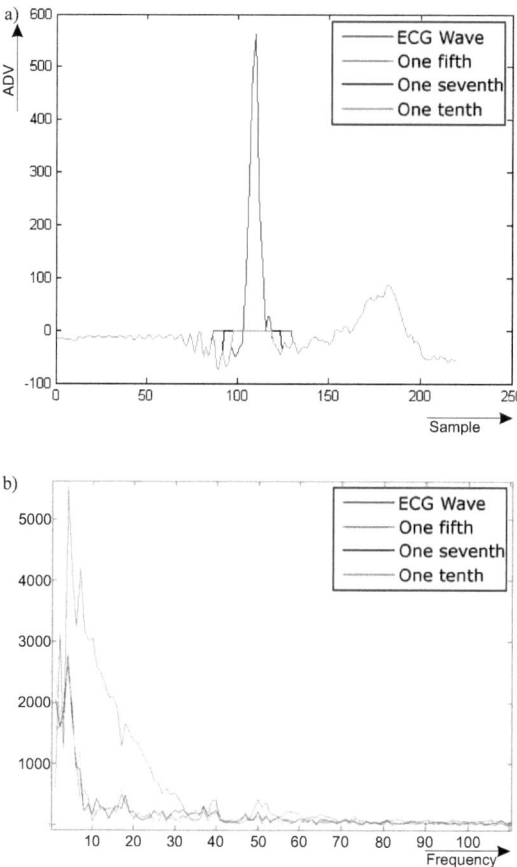

Figure 6.74: An ECG wave and different fractions of the complete ECG wave length applied to delete the R-peak: in a) the deleting of the R-peak in the time domain and in b) the corresponding spectra.

160   Chapter 6. Detecting SRBD Events and Sleep Stages from an ECG Signal

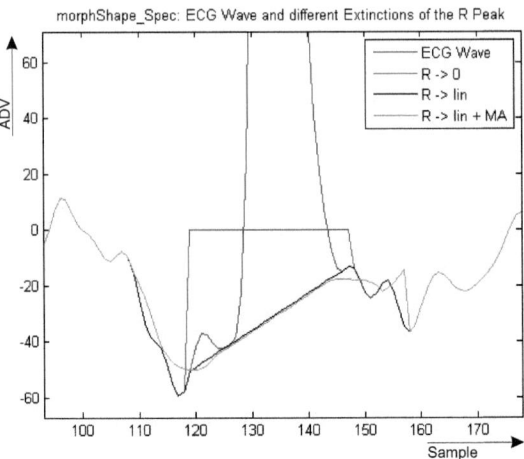

Figure 6.75: Different methods of extincting the R-peak

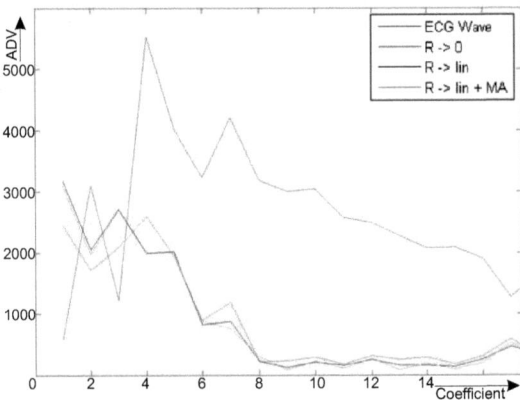

Figure 6.76: Original spectrum of the ECG wave and the spectra of the three different interpolation methods (On the abscissa, the coefficients are given, as the sample length does not equal the DFT length, i.e., sample length about 224 and sampling frequency 256 Hz, thus, one coefficient almost equals one Hertz.)

6.4. Morphological Features   161

Figure 6.76 evaluates the three methods in the frequency domain. It shows the spectra of the different interpolation methods in a zoomed view (The colors match the ones of Figure 6.75). As concluded in the discussion so far, the red spectrum shows some harmonics deriving from the rectangular approximation. But it comes as a surprise that the spectra belonging to the linear interpolation or to the moving average method, respectively, run in almost perfect parallel. Accordingly, it is potentially admissible to skip the moving average processing to save computation time in practical use. But, nevertheless, the smoothing with the moving average was activated for the processing the results discussed later on.

Windowing

The DFT assumes periodic signals, i.e., the DFT assumes that the small sample supplied to transform is repeated again and again. This assumption can not hold for biological signals as organic systems vary signals in frequency and shape. Accordingly, the DFT is not capable of computing the true spectrum, but one that is affected by leakage and high frequency components which are due to "jumps", i.e., non-continuity.

To overcome this draw-back, *windowing* functions are applied to the original signal. This means that the original signal is multiplied with a so called windowing function prior to being transformed. Window functions allow to control the extent of the "leakage" in the spectrum after the DFT. The leakage describes the phenomenon that the energy of a defined spectral component in the time domain signal becomes "smeared" over a range of frequencies in the spectrum, if the length of the extracted data block does not match a whole-number multiple of the assumed periodic time domain signal. The reduction of the "smear" effect is achieved at the expense of spectral resolution, i.e., the higher the reduction, the lesser spectral ranges can be distinguished. In other words: the application of a window function results in a "low pass filtering" of the spectrum (see Figure 6.77). This drawback of applying a windowing function derives from the following: The multiplication in the time domain becomes a convolution in the frequency domain. Convolution, however, can be considered as a kind of lowpass filtering with a moving window whose values are the impulse response of the windowing function.

The different windowing function differ in the degree of caused "blurring". As the frequency resolution is an important parameter in the scope of `morphShape_Spec()`, different windowing functions were considered and evaluated.

The easiest and "most natural" window function is the *rectangular window*. This window function is implicitly applied each time a block of data is cut out of a

162   Chapter 6. Detecting SRBD Events and Sleep Stages from an ECG Signal

sequence of samples "without applying any window at all" – it is characterized by keeping all values within the window untouched, i.e., multiplied by 1, and setting all other values to zero. It provides the highest frequency resolution at the expense of the biggest smearing.

All the windowing function – except Kaiser and Hamming Window – have in common that they are exactly zero at either end to prevent the influences of non-continuity in the signal.

Figure 6.77 shows a selection of the evaluated windowing functions. On the left side there is the signal in the time domain. In blue the original ECG signal, in red the window weighted signal and in black the windowing function itself (the later has been rescaled, because otherwise it would not have been clearly visible as windowing functions usually feature a value range from 0 - 1). On the right side there is the spectrum of the original signal in blue and the spectrum of the window weighted signal in red. The windowing functions which are shown are the Flat top window in row a), the Blackman window in row b), the Hamming window in row c), and the Kaiser window with $\beta = 2.5$ in row d).

As can be seen from the spectra the degree of "lowpass filtering" decreases from a) to d) which can be best seen by the increasing height of the peak representing the 50 Hz noise which is the European mains frequency (For the purpose of plotting Figure 6.77 the mains filter was disabled). The degree of lowpass filtering depends strongly on the width of the "bell function", i.e., the wider the bell function, the narrower the frequency domain representation of the bell function. And the narrower the frequency domain representation is, the lower the degree of "blurring" is which is caused by the moving averaging window.

In the case of the flat top window (in Figure 6.77a) the very narrow bell function leads to a complete suppression of the areas where the P- and T-wave are located. As the P-wave is expected to gain amplitude with the occurrence of an apnea due to an increase of intrathoracic pressure (see /3.4.1/) and as the T-wave is expected to be even more sensitive to abnormal behavior of the heart (see /3.5.4/ on p. 45), the extinction of these areas is not tolerable.

The reasoning for the flat top window applies almost completely to the Blackman window (see Figure 6.77b) and the Hamming window (see Figure 6.77c) as well: while both window functions seem to retain the P-wave, they suppress the T-wave like the flat top window does.

As the consequence of these evaluations the Kaiser window (see Figure 6.77d) was chosen for further processing as it obviously preserves most of the information. Even though it does not have zero values at either end, no increase in the high

6.4. Morphological Features

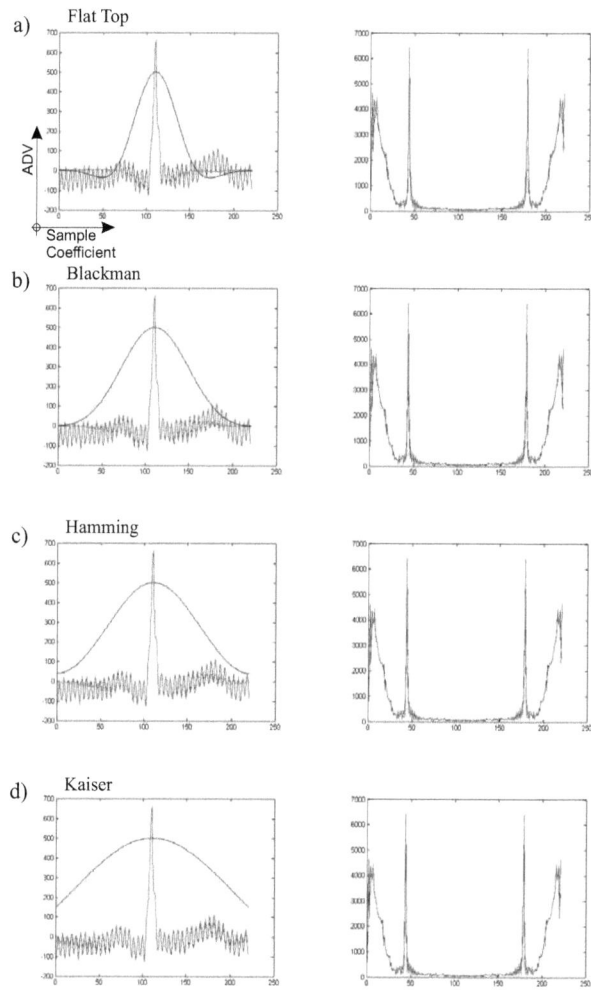

Figure 6.77: Different windowing functions and the their influence on the spectrum (the slight displacement of the 50 Hz mains noise peak results from running the DFT with a length of 221 on a signal which was sampled with 256 Hz)

164   Chapter 6. Detecting SRBD Events and Sleep Stages from an ECG Signal

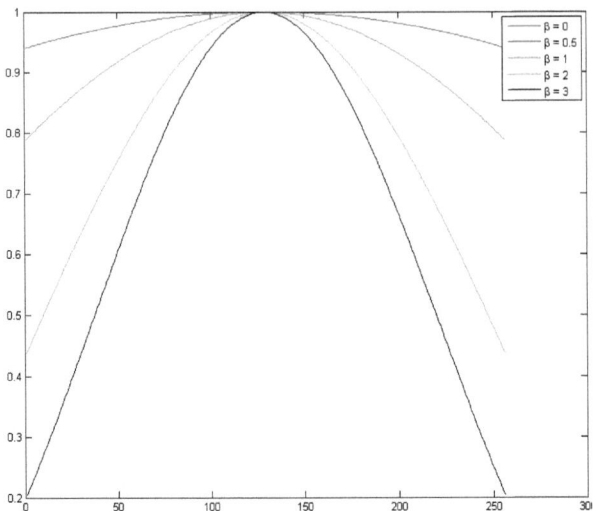

Figure 6.78: Kaiser window function for some values of the scaling factor β

frequency range due to the "jumps" can be observed. Moreover, the characteristic of the Kaiser window can be adjusted by means of the parameter β (see equations (6.18) and (6.19)).

The definition of the Kaiser window is given in equation (6.18), where I_0 is the zeroth order modified Bessel function.

$$w_n = \begin{cases} \dfrac{I_0\left(\beta\sqrt{1-(\frac{2n}{M}-1)^2}\right)}{I_0(\beta)} & 0 \leq n \leq M \\ 0 & \text{otherwise} \end{cases} \quad (6.18)$$

The parameter β affects the side lobe attenuation of the Kaiser window. Equation (6.19) defines which value to choose for β to achieve a required side lobe attenuation of $-\alpha$ dB in the design of a FIR filter. For the purpose of this work $\beta = 2$ was chosen which results in a side lobe attenuation of (almost) -30 dB.

$$\beta = \begin{cases} 0 & \alpha < 21 \\ 0.5842(\alpha-21)^{0.4} + 0.07886(\alpha-21) & 21 \leq \alpha \leq 50 \\ 0.1102(\alpha-8.7) & \alpha > 50 \end{cases} \quad (6.19)$$

Figure 6.78 shows five variations of the Kaiser window for different values of β. The window length M was set to 256 for plotting the Figure.

6.4. Morphological Features

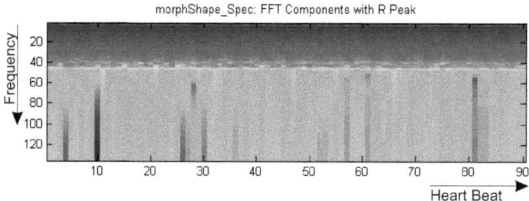

Figure 6.79: Spectrum resulting from running the DFT on the ECG wave with the R-peak

The chosen value for β creates a Kaiser window which is a compromise between the high spectral resolution of the rectangular window and the reduction of the leakage effect. As morphShape_Spec() aims at offering a high frequency resolution, the compromise tends to the rectangular window.

Applying the Transformations

To account for the comparatively slow speed of bodily functions, the resolution of the computed spectra can be increased by setting the value specResolution in the processing configuration accordingly. The increase of resolution is accomplished by means of zero-padding the data vector before applying the transformation. Zero-padding is chosen as it provides the advantage of increasing the spectral resolution of one *single* ECG wave without blurring, i.e., averaging, it over several ECG wave as would have been the case with increasing the length of the DFT window.

Subsequently, the transformations are executed. In the case of the DFT the window function is applied prior to the transformation which is not necessary for the DCT. The amplitude components for both transformations and for the DFT the phase components are kept as features.

The transformations are executed twice: Once on the ECG waves with the R-peaks and once on the ECG waves after the R-peaks have been extinguished (see next Section).

Figure 6.79 shows the spectrogram over the heart beats of the test data on the ECG signal with the R-peaks. As already mentioned EVA ml allows selecting the spectral resolution by setting the parameter specResolution to the desired value in the processing configuration. This feature addresses the fact that bodily functions are running at comparatively slow speeds. The effect is demonstrated in Figure 6.80 which shows the spectrogram for the ECG signal without the R-peaks. A comparison between Figure 6.80a and Figure 6.80b shows the effect of setting the

166   Chapter 6. Detecting SRBD Events and Sleep Stages from an ECG Signal

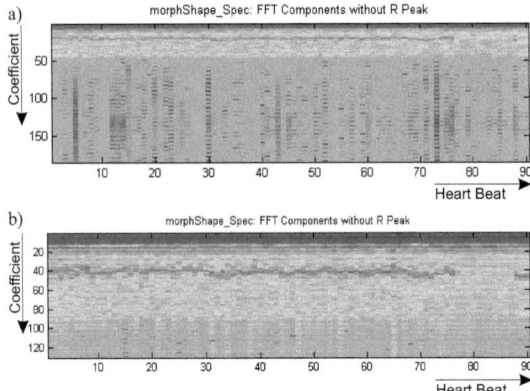

Figure 6.80: Spectrum resulting from running the DFT on the ECG wave without the R-peak: in a) the spectrogram in the standard resolution of one Hz; in b) the spectral resolution is increased by a factor of 2, i.e., $\frac{1}{2}$ Hz.

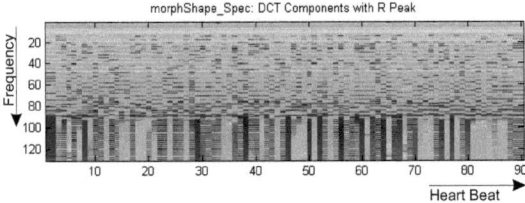

Figure 6.81: Spectrum resulting from running the DCT on the ECG wave with the R-peak

parameter `specResolution` to a value of 2: In b) the spectral resolution is twice as high which can be seen by the more pronounced second maximum at coefficient 40.

Postprocessing

In the postprocessing step the natural logarithm is applied to the amplitudes of all spectral components. This mimics a "dynamic gain adjustment" which means that the logarithm amplifies small amplitudes and attenuates higher amplitudes, i.e., it leads to a higher resolution of subtle changes of the amplitudes.

6.4. Morphological Features

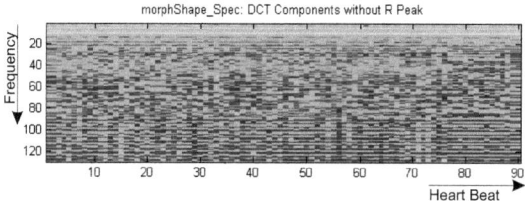

Figure 6.82: Spectrum resulting from running the DCT on the ECG wave without the R-peak

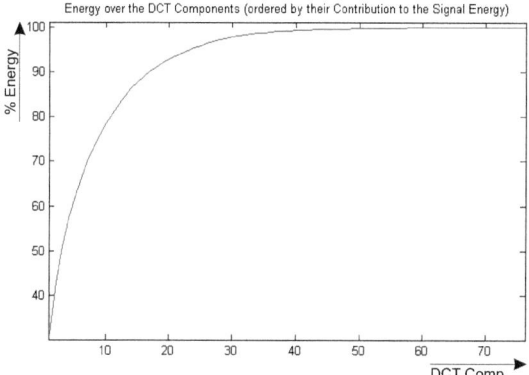

Figure 6.83: Number of DCT components and covered signal energy

Features of morphShape_Spec()

As explained the features are based on the spectral components of the transformations. Writing all components to the ARFF file might cause problems according to the "curse of dimensionality[16]" phenomenon.

Figure 6.83 shows the correlation between the number of DCT coefficients and the total of the signal energy they represent. It is clearly visible that about 30 coefficients contain "almost all energy". Accordingly, for the benefit of the later classification process the number of coefficients can be chosen between 20 and 30.

The number of coefficients of both transformations which are written to the ARFF files can be controlled by setting the parameters nbrFFTcomps and nbrDCTcomps, respectively, to the desired values. Both parameters were set to 20 in the applied processing configuration.

---

[16] The term was coined by Richard Bellman to describe "the exponential increase in volume associated with the adding of extra dimensions to a mathematical space" [Bell 09]

168   Chapter 6. Detecting SRBD Events and Sleep Stages from an ECG Signal

The BtB features consist of the amplitudes and phases for the DFT and the amplitudes for the DCT for each of the two cases of the ECG waves with and without the R-peaks. The total number of features can be calculated by equation (6.20).

$$nf_{BtB} = 4nbrFFTcomps + 2nbrDCTcomps \qquad (6.20)$$

The BtB features are mapped to the evaluation periods by the common approach of computing the mean and standard deviation within each evaluation period. Accordingly, there are twice as much features as can be seen by equation (6.21).

$$nf_{RaK} = 8nbrFFTcomps + 4nbrDCTcomps \qquad (6.21)$$

6.4.10 Overall Shape: Differences of Spectral Transformations

morphShape_SpecDiff is similar to morphShape_Spec in the aspect that it computes several spectra. But the spectra are computed from the signal which remains after a "purified" ECG signal has been subtracted from the ECG signal – hinted on in the name: *Spec*tral *Diff*erence. Thus, it is a combination of the part of morphShape_CA where FastICA is run on the signal without the ECG and morphShape_Spec. The main idea is that the remaining signal only contains influences deriving from disturbances of the normal ECG wave, i.e., impacts from SRBD events or changes in the sleep stage. The "purified", i.e., considered healthy, ECG wave which is subtracted from the currently processed ECG wave is computed as either the mean over the complete night $m(ECG)$ or as the mean of the last nbrLastECGwavesMean ECG waves $m_d(ECG, \text{nbrLastEVGwavesMean})$ – the later being more tolerant to long time changes. Figure 6.84 shows the principle.

Within morphShape_SpecDiff() the following steps are executed to extracted the features.

Creation of the ECG Buffer

The processing starts analog to the other functions dealing with the overall shape of the ECG by creating a buffer for all of the ECG waves whose length is set to the mean of the RR interval $m(RR)$. From this buffer the overnight mean of all ECG waves $m(ECG)$ is directly computed (see Figure 6.50).

6.4. Morphological Features

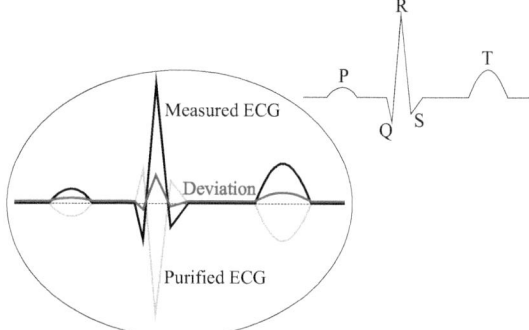

Figure 6.84: Principle of morphShape_SpecDiff(): From the measured ECG EVAml computes a "purified ECG" which is subtracted from the measured ECG. Subsequently, on the deviation the DFT is applied.

Subtracting the different means

The second mean $m_d(ECG, \text{nbrLastEVGwavesMean})$ is computed within the main processing loop from the last nbrLastEVGwavesMean ECG waves.

During the processing these two means are subtracted to purify the ECG wave from the "informationless standard ECG wave" which emphasizes the effects of the disturbances. Figure 6.85 shows the remaining signals after subtracting $m(RR)$ in the blue curve and $m_d(ECG, \text{nbrLastEVGwavesMean})$ in the red curve.

Applying the DFT

morphShape_SpecDiff() allows to select, whether a window function, i.e., the Kaiser window from morphShape_Spec(), is to be applied to the remaining signal prior to running the DFT. As default, this option is disabled to account for the reduction of spectral resolution that comes along the application of a window function[17].

As with morphShape_Spec() morphShape_SpecDiff() allows increasing the spectral resolution by setting the parameter specResolution[18] accordingly. Figure 6.86 shows the effect of increasing the spectral resolution: In Figure 6.86a the resolution is set to 1 Hz and in Figure 6.86b the resolution was set to half a Hz.

Finally, Figure 6.87 shows the phase of the spectrum (belonging to Figure 6.86a, i.e., at a spectral resolution of 1 Hz). The number of coefficients which are stored for

---
[17]The windowing can be selected by setting the parameter applyWindow in the processing configuration accordingly.
[18]The increase in spectral resolution is performed by zero-padding (see /6.4.9/)

170   Chapter 6. Detecting SRBD Events and Sleep Stages from an ECG Signal

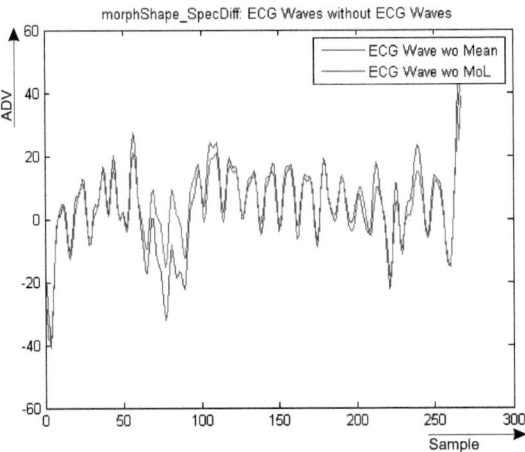

Figure 6.85: Remainders of an ECG wave after subtracting the overnight mean ECG wave (in the blue curve) and after subtracting the mean of the last (MoL) nbrLastECGwavesMean ECG waves (in the red curve).

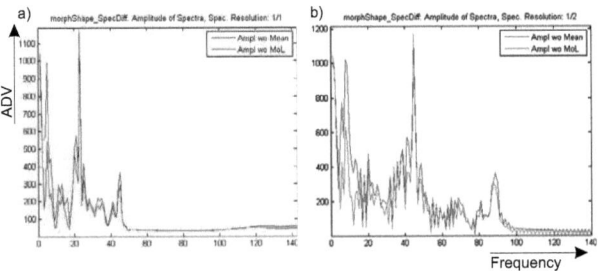

Figure 6.86: Magnitude of spectra for different spectral resolutions: in a) the resolution is 1 Hz and in b) it is half a Hz – accordingly the spectrum is stretched along the coefficients.

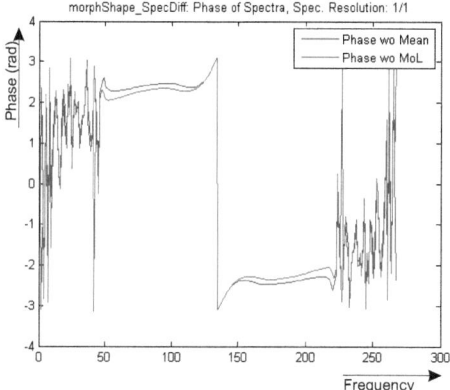

Figure 6.87: The phase of the signal

both amplitude and phase can be adjusted by setting the parameter nbrCoefsSpec in the processing configuration accordingly.

Features of morphShape_SpecDiff()

The BtB features consist of the amplitudes and phases for the DFT for the ECG waves with the different types of means subtracted. The total number of features can be calculated by equation (6.22).

$$nf_{BtB} = 4 \cdot nbrCoefsSpec \qquad (6.22)$$

The BtB features are mapped to the evaluation periods by the common approach of computing the mean and standard deviation within each evaluation period. Accordingly, there are twice as many features as can be seen by equation (6.23).

$$nf_{RaK} = 8 \cdot nbrCoefsSpec \qquad (6.23)$$

6.5 Summary and Preview

This Chapter provided the linkage between the medical basics of sleep and the ECG and the features which are extracted from the ECG recordings.

It introduced the AM which evaluates the HR fluctuations to assess the varying levels of ANS activity. The Section started with an in-depth explanation of the model itself and its (assumed) relation to the physiology of HR regulation.

For the morphological approach a total of nine feature sets was introduced. Each considers either an important distinctive point of the ECG, e.g., the R-peak, or the shape "as a whole", e.g., the deviation from a computed template.

For each of the feature sets, their main implementation steps were explained and the intermediate processing steps were visualized using Matlab plots.

The next Chapter will now present the results which were achieved during the classification process based on the computed features.

Chapter 7

Experimental Results

This Chapter presents the results of the successive processing steps during the evaluation of the ECG recordings. It starts with the detection of the distinctive ECG points (see /6.2/) and ends with a discussion of the classification results for each feature set, e.g., P-wave or R-peak.

The evaluation itself is split into three different steps: first, the most appropriate classifier for each combination of a feature set and a classification target, i.e., SRBD events or sleep stages, is selected by means of the *WEKA Experimenter*. It allows to evaluate different combinations of feature sets and classifiers (see /5.2.4/ and Figure 5.2e) in one run.

Subsequently, in the second step, for a detailed evaluation of the classification rates, *WEKA Explorer* is run for each feature set in four different setups which are combinations of the BtB and the RaK evaluation period and the two classification targets. This evaluation is performed applying the *patient-dependent* 10-folds method.

Finally, in the third step, the best feature-classifier-combinations are run on a *patient-independent* data set (see /7.5/) which allows to compare the classification rates between the training and test data set.

This Chapter ends with a discussion of the achieved results comparing them to the current state of the art (see /7.6/).

7.1 ECG Distinctive Points Detection

7.1.1 Types of Artifacts in the recorded ECGs

In everyday clinical PSG recording the quality of the recorded signals is limited — mainly by the subject him/herself, when he/she moves in bed. Within the evaluated

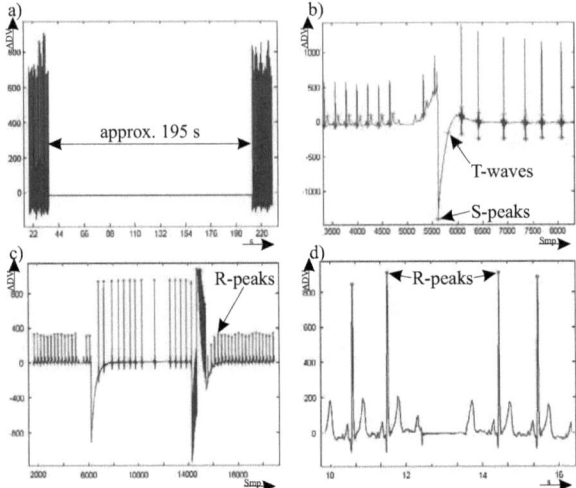

Figure 7.1: Different types of artifacts

files the percentage of annotated artifacts in the ECG signal is 0.2 ± 1.1 for one clinical partner and 1.3 ± 5.1 for the other. This Section gives an overview of the encountered artifacts and their consequences.

If there is a constant zero input signal for more than 30 seconds (which is the length of the search window), the R-peak detection takes very long, because the algorithm searches back and forth iteratively lowering the internal peak threshold. An example is shown in Figure 7.1a, where the amplitude of the signal remains zero for more than three minutes which is most likely due to an ECG electrode coming loose.

Figures 7.1b & c show examples for artifacts in the ECG recording which are most likely caused by the patient moving in bed. Even though the R-peak detection works properly in case b), the remaining distinctive ECG points could not be assigned correctly as they are not existent. This entails morphSTSegment() (see /6.4.4/) facing two problems: first, because there is no proper ST-segment, the features computed are of little use. Second, because there are too few samples in the extracted ST-segment, the polynomial approximation fails[1]. In case c), the R-peak detections works properly, but on improper data – accordingly, the found R-peaks will produce anomalies in the extracted features.

---
[1] To prevent this, morphSTSegment() detects this situation and inserts a horizontal segment of an appropriate length.

7.1. ECG Distinctive Points Detection 175

Figure 7.1d shows a recording with an AV-block which means that the sinoatrial node generates triggers to which the atria respond by producing a P-wave, but the excitation is blocked at the crossover to the ventricles which suppresses the remainder of the ECG wave (see /3.3.3/). AV-blocks are found at times in subjects suffering from sleep apnea. Even though AV-blocks are not considered features for the detection of SRBD events yet, their influence on the AM is canceled by the suppression of outliers.

7.1.2 R-Peak Detection

The evaluation of the performance of the R-peak detection was accomplished in two steps. First, the algorithm was tested on annotated data from Physionet. Second, the performance was visually tested on the actual data used for this work.

Assessment on Physionet Data

The Physionet data taken for evaluation purposes was originally provided for the "CinC Challenge 2000" for the challenge "Development and evaluation of ECG-based apnea detectors" which comprises the ECG recordings and corresponding R-peak annotations [Phys 04]. The R-peak annotations were generated automatically without manual editing. However, the threshold of the algorithm was adjusted while visually controlling the detected R-peaks to obtain best results.

The R-peak detection algorithm was tested on six recordings with a duration of 97 minutes each. The R-peak was considered correctly localized, if the detected position did not differ by more than one sample from the position given by the Physionet annotations.

Given these prerequisites, the achieved R-peak detection rate was $99.0 \pm 0.4\%$.

Visual Assessment on recorded Sleep Laboratory Data

The two Figures 7.2 and 7.3 may serve for the visual evaluation of the R-peak detection. Figure 7.2a shows a complete overnight recording with a very pronounced artifact (marked by the orange square). Even though this artifact appears "immense", Figure 7.2b reveals that only 20 heart beats are affected which is less than one per mill of a seven hour recording. Accordingly, it can be noted that isolated artifacts do not have great impact on the ECG point detection.

Figure 7.3 shows two cases with false R-peak detections. Figure 7.3a depicts a case where an artifact is misinterpreted as the R-peak as it represents the highest peak – accordingly the true R-peak is taken as the P-wave (being the highest point

176   Chapter 7. Experimental Results

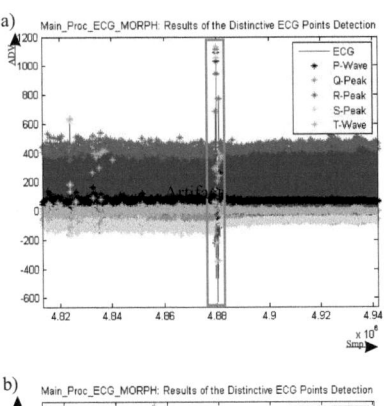

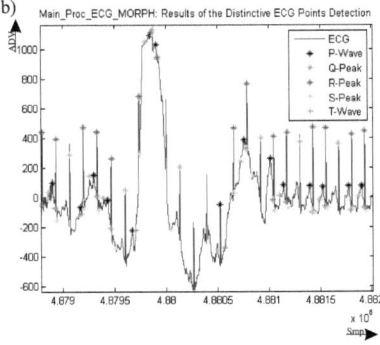

Figure 7.2: Peak-like Artifact (within the orange square) in the complete recording a) and the zoomed-in view in b)

7.1. ECG Distinctive Points Detection

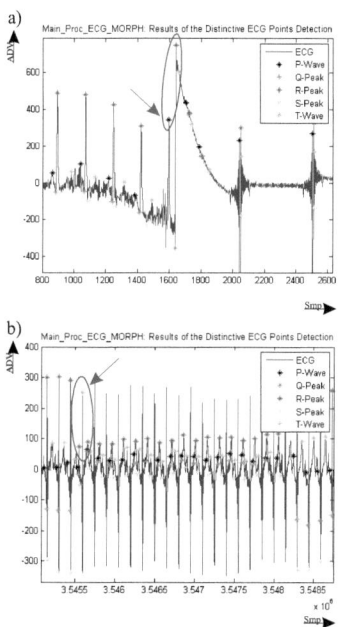

Figure 7.3: R-peak misclassifications

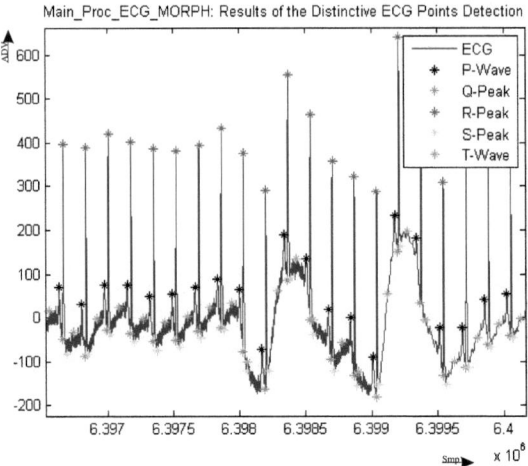

Figure 7.4: ECG distinctive points detection remains stable during most artifacts

"left to R-peak", see next Section). In Figure 7.3b the misdetection is caused by the continuously adapted threshold in conjunction with the application of physiological restraints: the very low S-peak (or just an artifact?) causes the threshold to be lowered. This adapted threshold results in an assignment of the short pulse just before the correct R-peak (both within the ellipse) to the false R-peak. The subsequent placement of a search window in a fixed distance from the detected "R-peak" leads a false detection of the following peaks. After a few false detections, though, the algorithm resynchronizes and correctly assigns the R-peaks.

Finally, Figure 7.4 shows that the distinctive point detection remains stable even during severe artifacts. Hence, it can be stated that the very good results of the R-peak detection found with the Physionet database can be visually approved.

7.1.3 Remaining Distinctive Points Detection

The detection of the remaining distinctive ECG points is very closely linked to the correct detection of the R-peak as can be expected from the description of the implementation principle (see /6.2/). As seen by the proper results in Figures 6.10 and 7.4 the implemented distinctive point detection algorithm works quite satisfying.

Figure 7.5 shows a case with a slightly descending ST-segment (see /3.5.1/) and (possibly) negative T-wave (see /3.5.4/). An expert asked whether the correct positions of the S-peak and the T-wave, respectively, could be at the positions

7.2. Running the Feature Extraction

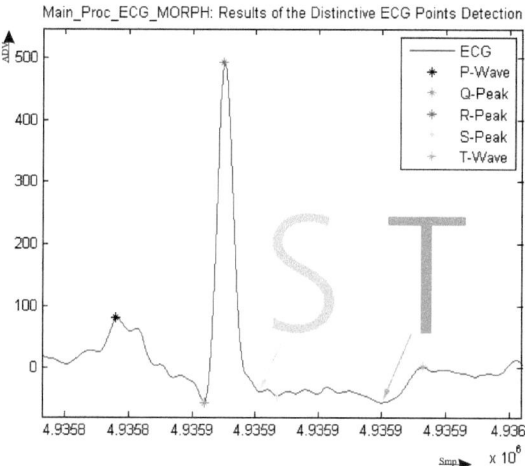

Figure 7.5: Case of a (possibly) unprecise S-peak and T-wave detection due to ischemic or chronic ST-depression in conjunction with a negative T-wave

indicated by the tips of the respective arrow with the consequence of indicating an ischemic reaction did not provide certainty. At the time index depicted the recording is annotated with "N", i.e., healthy, which contradicts an ischemic reaction due to a SRBD event. Further examination of the ECG showed that during periods with annotated SRBD events of type "H" or "O", respectively, the ECG looked according to standard, i.e., ST-segment ascending and T-wave positive. Furthermore, the subject's anamnesis did not reveal any present heart diseases. Summarizing these findings, the situation depicted in Figure 7.5 has to be considered incidental. Hence, the hypothesis that a SRBD event "unalterably" provokes ischemic reactions (see /3.5/) has to be rejected.

Concluding the evaluation of the distinctive ECG points detection, it can be stated that the visual checking proved proper point assignments, if the R-peak detection was successful for the respective ECG wave.

7.2 Running the Feature Extraction

From all the recordings acquired by the clinical partners (see /5.2.1/) five patients annotated in Nuremberg were chosen for evaluation purposes. This "cutback" was fed by the longish computation times required by EVA ml and especially WEKA, respectively: it took EVA ml two days per patient to compute the ARFF files and another six weeks were taken by WEKA to evaluate the six selected classifiers (see /10.7/), followed by two days for the detailed evaluation for each patient. In addition to the five evaluated patients another five patients were used to create the patient-independent data sets. The patients in this collective had an age of 47.6 ± 21.15 years, a BMI of 30 ± 10.4, and an AHI of 33.9 ± 95.7 ranging from 2.3 (practically healthy) to 98.8 (severely affected).

In contrast to most of the state-of-art works which rely on the Physionet database (see /4.2/), this work is based on a "proprietary" database. The reason therefor is mainly the higher degree of information the proprietary database provides: the Physionet database is based on intervals of one minute and labels each of them as "ill" or "healthy". The proprietary database provides annotations based on single events and includes their types, e.g., apnea or hypopnea. These are essential requirements as the approach pursued in this work aims at detecting exactly these characteristics.

The feature extraction was performed with EVA ml (see /10.2/). The software directly processes the 16-bit samples recorded at a sampling frequency of 256 Hz. The computed features – along with the experts' annotations (see /5.2.2/) – are written to ASCII files following the WEKA ARFF-file specifications.

Features were extracted on different time bases and with different classification targets. The two different time bases were chosen to gain insight into the physiological procedures and their respective response times. This knowledge is essential for the detection of single SRBD events. The two different classification targets reflect the two aspects of sleep quality, i.e., the AHI (see /2.5.6/) and the sleep architecture (see /2.4.2/). The different classification targets were selected by writing either the experts' SRBD event annotations or their sleep stage annotations to the respective ARFF files. The four evaluation sets are as follows:

1. Features are evaluated in intervals of 30 seconds[2] (RaK) with target class "SRBD event".

2. Features are evaluated on a beat-to-beat[3] (BtB) basis with target class "SRBD event".

3. Features are evaluated in the RaK interval with target class "Sleep Stage".

4. Features are evaluated in the BtB interval with target class "Sleep Stage".

EVA ml was run three times on the AM (see /6.3/) for all recordings. This was done because of the random behavior of the c-means initialization which may lead

---
[2] This is the standard evaluation period as proposed by Rechtschaffen and Kales (see /2.8.1/).
[3] The morphology based features are truly computed for each single beat, while for the Autonomous Model (see /6.3/) the shortest interval is about 75 seconds.

to different results every time the algorithm is invoked. This resulted in a total of twelve ARFF files for the AM.

EVA ml was run once on all functions extracting the morphology based features (see /6.4/). This is true as well for morphShape_ICA(), even though the applied approximation method showed the same "random behavior" which was already mentioned for the AM. This resulted in a total of four ARFF files for each morphologic feature set.

7.3 Selection of the Appropriate Classifiers

The evaluation of the classification rates started with the identification of the most appropriate classifiers for each combination of feature set and classification target. This task was accomplished applying the WEKA Experimenter. This data mining tools allows to define "experiments" which are subsequently performed automatically. An experiment is a set of ARFF files to analyze and a selection of classifiers which are to be applied. The result of an experiment is a selection of statistical parameters which allow to assess the performance of each classifier.

The following six classifiers, shortly introduced in /10.7/, were evaluated:

- Bayes Net

- RBF Network and Multilayer Perceptron, both function based classifiers

- IBk and KStar, both "lazy" classifiers

- Bagging, meta classifier wrapping a REP-Tree classifier

WEKA Experimenter uses configurations to control the evaluation process. A configuration basically consists of an "experiment" with associated evaluation settings. In the scope of this first evaluation a configuration consists of all ARFF files for a feature set (see /7.2/), the six classifiers mentioned, and the appropriate evaluation settings (see below). Due to excessive computational load WEKA Experimenter was run on a computer cluster of the RRZE (see /5.2.4/, p. 63) which allowed parallel processing.

The evaluation method for finding the most appropriate classifiers was set to the 10-folds method. 10-folds means that the data from each ARFF file is split into ten pieces with similar a-priori probabilities for each single class. Nine of these pieces are used to train the classifier and the tenth one is used as test data. This procedure is repeated ten times and the issued classification rate and error are the means of

	SRBD Events	Sleep Stage
Autonomous Model	IBk	KStar
Morphology	Bagging	Bagging

Table 7.1: Best classifiers with respect to feature set and classification target

all the folds. This method is considered "the evaluation method of choice in most practical limited-data situations" [Witt 05]. Consequently, the data for training and testing the classifier originated from the same patient, i.e., this approach is patient-dependent.

The results of the WEKA Experimenter were assessed for each of the five patients according to two statistical parameters : **percentage correct** and **kappa statistic** (see /10.1.2/). Percentage correct turned out to be useless for assessing the performance of the classifiers as it is dominated by the high a-priori probability of the SRBD event N, i.e., healthy breathing. In contrast, kappa statistic compensates for the very unevenly spread a-priori probabilities which is why it was chosen as indicator for the efficiency of the classifiers.

After combining the results for the five patients, the AM yielded kappa values of 0.35 ± 0.23 for SRBD events and 0.96 ± 0.02 for the sleep stages. Among the morphology based features the spectrum based features of morphShape_Spec() achieved kappa statistic values of 0.39 ± 0.17 for the respiratory events and 0.78 ± 0.04 for the sleep stages.

The best classifier was chosen by counting the number of wins given by the highest kappa value. The best classifiers with respect to feature set and classification target are shown in Table 7.1. It is remarkable that the Bagging classifier won 69% of the SRBD events and 84% of the sleep stages decisions resulting in a total of about 77% – which is essentially all the morphology based decisions. And even in the cases where Bagging did not actually win, it usually was a very good second best, i.e., the difference to the best one did not exceed three tenth percent in general.

During this first evaluation no dominant influence of artifacts on the classification rates could be noted as the patient with no artifacts annotated and the patient with the most artifacts (1.3%) both showed the worst classificatin results. This will be discussed in detail – along with the revelation of the true reason – in the next Section.

	Classified as			
a	b	c		
P_{aa}	P_{ab}	P_{ac}	a	
P_{ba}	P_{bb}	P_{bc}	b	Annotated as
P_{ca}	P_{cb}	P_{cc}	c	

Figure 7.6: Confusion Matrix

7.4 Evaluation of the different Feature Sets

The classification rates in the following Sections were determined applying the respective best classifier as listed in Table 7.1 with the WEKA Explorer. The evaluation method was set to 10-folds. The WEKA Explorer is capable of outputting confusion matrices (see Figure 7.6) and detailed statistical information, e.g., F-Measure, about the performance of a selected classifier.

The classification results are presented in Tables 7.2 and 7.3. These are condensed versions of the complete classification results which can be found in Tables 10.5 through 10.24 in the Appendix (see /10.8/). The condensed Tables are provided for easier comparison with the works presented in the state-of-art (see Chapter 4) as these do not differentiate between the different SRBD event types. They show the classification results for grouped events: obstructive, central and mixed apnea, and hypopnea are grouped as "apnea", and likewise S1 and S2 are grouped as "light sleep", S3 and S4 are grouped as "deep sleep". Wake and REM remain ungrouped. The F-Measure value is "grouped" according to the respective events by averaging the corresponding values. For the SRBD events, this includes the artifacts.

The Tables comprise the following values: the classification rates (CR) and the corresponding F-Measure (FM). The fact that these values sometimes seem to get "out of sync" derives from the way they are computed: CR is computed as the relative detection rate and FM is based on Type I and Type II errors. CR and FM are provided for the two different time bases "RaK", which represents the 30 seconds interval proposed by Rechtschaffen and Kales, and "BtB" which stands for beat-to-beat. All values are presented for an almost healthy patient (HP) (AHI: 5.4), for an "averaged over five" patient (AHI: 33.9), and for a diseased patient (DP) (AHI: 98.5).

Figure 7.6 shows a confusion matrix as output by WEKA. Based on the confusion matrix the classification rates for single events are computed according to equation (7.1a) and the classification rates for the grouped events – "b" and "c" in the example – follow equation (7.1b).

$$p_{single\,xx} = \frac{p_{xx}}{\sum_{n=1}^{3} p_{xn}} \tag{7.1a}$$

$$p_{group\,b\&c} = \frac{(p_{bb} + p_{bc}) + (p_{cb} + p_{cc})}{\sum_{n=1}^{3} p_{bn} + \sum_{n=1}^{3} p_{cn}} \tag{7.1b}$$

A best feature selection was performed for all feature sets to determine the respective features with the highest predictive capability. This was done to approve or reject the assumptions of the physiological ongoings introduced in Sections /6.3/ through /6.4.10/. Feature selection was performed on the *patient-independent* data set which was generated for the patient-independent evaluation (see /7.5/). The WEKA feature search was set to the feature evaluation approach *cfsSubsetEval* and the search method *BestFirst* using the *full training set*. *cfsSubsetEval* assesses the predictive ability for the target class of each attribute for itself and the degree of correlation between them. This evaluation method ends up with attribute sets which show a high correlation with the target class and almost none between one another, i.e., it suppresses cross-correlations. *BestFirst* operates on "greedy hill climbing with backtracking" [Witt 05]: it starts with no feature selected and adds them successively, keeping or discarding them according to their predictive power. The features were evaluated for the two evaluation intervals RaK and BtB to see, whether their predictive capabilities reflect fast and slow response times of the physiological mechanisms.

As the described settings suppress the correlations in the features, they likewise suppress any physiological correlations which may hint on secondary physiological cause-and-effect chains. Thus, only the primary or the most pronounced physiological effect is revealed.

7.4. Evaluation of the different Feature Sets

			AM	P	R	ST	T	Timing	Dev	ICA	Spec	SpecDiff
h	RaK	CR	**30.8**	0.0	0.0	0.0	0.0	0.0	0.0	0.0	0.0	0.0
		FM	**0.21**	0.17	0.17	0.17	0.17	0.17	0.17	0.17	0.17	0.17
	BtB	CR	**31.0**	0.0	3.2	2.5	0.6	0.0	0.0	0.0	5.9	2.2
		FM	0.26	0.28	0.29	0.17	0.28	0.28	0.25	0.19	**0.30**	0.25
∅	RaK	CR	**56.2 ± 20.7**	25.1 ± 32.9	33.4 ± 35.7	40.3 ± 38.9	27.9 ± 37.4	38.7 ± 39.2	31.7 ± 35.5	16.1 ± 28.0	42.8 ± 38.4	41.3 ± 37.7
		FM	0.4 ± 0.27	0.22 ± 0.07	0.22 ± 0.07	0.25 ± 0.11	0.23 ± 0.08	0.26 ± 0.13	0.22 ± 0.07	0.19 ± 0.02	0.27 ± 0.13	0.24 ± 0.10
	BtB	CR	**41.1 ± 13.2**	10.1 ± 14.3	25.4 ± 21.5	27.5 ± 25.5	19.0 ± 21.1	20.4 ± 24.0	10.1 ± 13.9	7.6 ± 12.7	40.9 ± 27.7	34.6 ± 25.4
		FM	**0.35 ± 0.12**	0.24 ± 0.06	0.29 ± 0.01	0.22 ± 0.06	0.27 ± 0.01	0.27 ± 0.01	0.22 ± 0.04	0.19 ± 0.01	0.33 ± 0.04	0.26 ± 0.01
d	RaK	CR	85.2	79.0	85.9	87.7	88.9	**91.5**	85.5	64.6	89.9	88.8
		FM	**0.59**	0.27	0.27	0.32	0.28	0.35	0.27	0.20	0.36	0.31
	BtB	CR	56.8	34.2	58.9	55.8	54.9	58.2	32.8	29.6	**70.3**	63.9
		FM	**0.43**	0.19	0.28	0.26	0.26	0.26	0.19	0.18	0.35	0.27

Table 7.2: Classification rates for the grouped SRBD events (h: (almost) healthy, ∅: averagely diseased, d: diseased, CR: classification rate (in [%]), FM: F-Measure

Table 7.3: Classification rates for the grouped sleep stages (h: (almost) healthy, ⌀: averagely diseased, d: diseased, CR: classification rate (in [%]), FM: F-Measure

7.4.1 Autonomous Model

The classification rates for the AM in Table 7.2 reveal two import findings which are almost universally valid for all the feature extraction functions:

- The evaluation in the RaK interval usually yields the better results which can be observed by comparing the classification results for the RaK and the BtB interval, respectively.

- The classification rates for the SRBD events dramatically increase with the subject's degree of disease. This is usually true for the DS and REM sleep stages as well, but contrary for the LS stages. These observations result from evaluating the classification rates for the HP (h), the averaged patient ($\varnothing$), and the DP (d).

Taking a look at Table 10.5 the reason for the second statement becomes evident: the HP has no M and C events (see Table 5.1) annotated and only a few O events, while for the DP there are quite a few, i.e., 0.7 - 8.4%, of these events. Recalling that these classification rates were found applying the 10-folds method, this observation can be concluded such that the classifier "saw" almost none of these events for the HP, hence, it could not "learn" them, whereas it had the chance to become "acquainted" with them for the DP. The strong correlation between the occurrence of an event type and the achieved classification rate has to be kept in mind when assessing the classifier's performance. However, the steep ascent of the classification rate along the event occurrence is quite striking.

For the SRBD detection all the features computed by the AM, i.e., the values describing the GMM like μ, σ (see p. 87), and the parameters for G_{Noise} (see /6.3.3/), are relevant. For the RaK interval the means[4] $m(.)$ are relevant, but not their standard deviations. Comparing these features with those relevant for the sleep stages (see below), it is remarkable that for the SRBD event detection only the rather statical parameters, i.e., the means, are relevant, whereas for the sleep stage detection the dynamic parameters, i.e., the standard deviations, are equally relevant. This is remarkable, because the more dynamic occurrence of SRBD events would be expected to be linked to the dynamic sensitive standard deviations and vice versa.

Reconsidering Figure 6.21a, the means $m(.)$ of the GMM are placed at the frequencies 0.2 Hz, 0.9 Hz, 1.3 Hz, and 1.5 Hz. The lowest frequency matches the period of the PNS which makes it most likely that the higher frequencies are the

---
[4] The BtB-values are mapped to the RaK-interval by applying the mean and standard deviation.

third, fifth, and sixth harmonics, respectively. If so, the SNS does not play a role. This finding is in perfect consent to the experts' assumption that short time variations of the HR are driven by the PNS [Koep 58]. Moreover, it matches the authors' finding in [Vano 95] that sleep is under PNS control. Considering the AM, this finding means that there is no SNS activity involved, and, accordingly, the generator G_{Symp} has no (or only very limited) influence.

When wondering why the means of the GMM, i.e., a value of "static character", are relevant to detect dynamic events or sleep stages, respectively, it has to be recalled that these means represent variations against the HR at rest, i.e., f_0, which is canceled by the FM-demodulation. This processing step makes the AM robust against longterm changes of the HR at rest as described in [Brin 02], where the author claims that the HR at rest is increased depending on the degree of the OSAS (see /2.5.4/).

In [Blas 03], it is explained that SNS activity remained at high levels up to 40 seconds after an acoustically provoked arousal. The authors' assumption was that SNS activity might accumulate, if apnea or hypopnea events are fired in close succession. Even though, the evaluation of the model frequencies suggests that only PNS influences are considered, this finding may affect the classification rate of the AM as the HR is always the result of both SNS and PNS. And as SNS influences tend to reduce the HRV, this directly affects the sensitivity of the GMM parameters.

The sigmas σ of the GMM generators are important values as could be expected from the AM. This holds true for all evaluation combinations except for the sleep stage detection in the BtB interval. As the σ values represent the "steadiness" of an generator, it is all too clear that these values are more important for the short term influences introduced by the SRBD events.

Another finding is that the GMM weights are more predictive than the corresponding amplitudes. The considered weights are those belonging to the higher frequencies. An increasing dominance of the higher frequencies entail higher frequency components in the ANS generator output which increases its dynamics. Thus, these weights can be understood as an indicator of a higher ANS activity which is connected to SRBD events or sleep stages W and REM (for N and DS the reasoning is inverse.)

The fact that the amplitudes are less relevant than the weights can be interpreted in the following way: the GMM separates the individual components, i.e., the contributing generators, from one another, whereas the absolute amplitude is the sum of these components which means that the information is "blurred": The closer the maxima of the spectra, i.e., the means μ of the GMM, are to one another, the more the sum, i.e., the absolute amplitude at a given point on the abscissa, differs from the individual components (see Figure 10.4).

The energy of the noise generator is considered for all evaluation combinations, but not as important as imagined. The noise generator captures "undefined", or non-specific influences on the HR and its variability which do not seem to be of great relevance. This finding confirms the importance of the distinctive generators which directly represent the ANS activity.

The evaluation of the AM shows that the most important features are those, which capture properties of the HR and the HRV. This finding confirms that the direct connection between them and the ANS makes them very strong indicator for the ANS activity.

Another finding of the AM evaluation is that a varying number of generators is used for the GMM, i.e., a varying number of maxima is found in the spectra. This seems to be an inter-subject variation. Thus, speculation may be: from a mathematical point of view the existence of higher harmonics entails a more "angled" waveform. In the AM scope this means that PNS activity is higher or more pronounced – on the expenses of the SNS. Recalling that high SNS activity levels entail low HRV, the interpretation of a higher number of generators is that this subject does not have long term stress and a lower mortality. However, according data was not available for verification.

It was mentioned that the feature extraction was run three times on the AM to find out, whether the random behavior of the c-means initialization method of the EM algorithm led to strong variations in the detection rate. Comparing the results, it can be stated that in one patient the difference was about 10%, but usually did not exceed 2 - 4%. Hence, it can be expected that on a large database this random behavior will not be relevant.

The AM approach is equally suited for both classification targets, but performs especially well for the sleep stage classification. It achieves better classification rates in the RaK interval. The AM outperforms the morphological approaches which emphasizes the important role of the HR and its variability as an indicator for the ANS.

7.4.2 P-Wave

In the literature, concerning the SRBD events, the predictive capability of the P-wave is usually considered negligible. This is commonly attributed to its small amplitude and the noise which is found in PSG ECG recordings. However, the classification values for the DP show that the P-wave is quite capable. It usually delivers better results in the RaK interval.

For the classification target SRBD and the RaK interval the means $m(P)$ and $m_d(P)$, the features describing the increase of load to the heart as maximum and minimum, the correlation between the P-wave amplitudes of subsequent evaluation periods, and the correlation between the P-wave and the R-peak amplitude are important.

For the classification target sleep stage in the RaK interval the relevant features are very much the same with two exceptions: first, only the maximum of the increased load to the heart feature is considered, and second, the correlation between the P-wave and the R-peak amplitude as mean, minimum and maximum is significant.

For the BtB evaluation only the mean $m_d(P)$ and the correlation between the P-wave and the R-peak amplitude is of interest for the classification and the crucial features for both classification targets are exactly the same.

The P-wave amplitude and its floating mean appear in both classification targets and evaluation intervals which means the dynamics of the amplitude are a significant indicator for load changes. As the RaK interval yields the better results and with the inclusion of the increasing load parameter in this evaluation interval, it can be concluded that the P-wave reflects the slowly increasing heart load during a SRBD event. Additionally, for the SRBD classification the minimum and the maximum of the increasing heart load feature were considered.

The same conclusion holds for the P-wave amplitude relative to the R-peak amplitude feature. Considering the predictive power of the R-peak amplitude alone and its predictive power when related to the P-wave amplitude (see next Section), it can be noted that the importance of this feature really derives from the correlation between both amplitudes. This, however, can only hold, if the dominating influence is coupled to the P-wave amplitude.

For the sleep stage classification only the maximum of the increasing load feature was considered in the way of an upper threshold. This explains why quite a proportion of the REM state was falsely assigned to LS or W: they show a similar variable load, whereas almost no false assignment to DS happened, because in this state physiological processes are quite stable.

The P-wave features clearly aim at detecting changes in the load condition of the heart. This predestines the P-wave features to detect SRBD events. Surprisingly, these features are quite powerful for the detection of LS in the DP as well.

7.4. Evaluation of the different Feature Sets

Even though, the results confirm the physiological assumptions about the P-wave, the P-wave derived features have to be considered weak in general which supports the claims found in the literature.

7.4.3 R-Peak

The R-peak based features usually perform better in the RaK interval which is true for SRBD event and sleep stage classification alike.

The total amplitude measured from the Q-peak to the R-peak is the only feature to appear for both targets and both intervals. This leads to infer that the amplitude of the R-peak itself is only of minor predictive power (see /7.4.2/ as well) and the sensitivity of this feature is mainly based on the dynamics introduced by the Q-peak amplitude. In cardiology, a pronounced negative Q-peak is considered to hint on an old cardiac infarct. Therefore, in the context of this work, the dynamics of the Q-peak amplitude may be due to varying oxygen supply, i.e., ischemia (see /3.5/).

The steepness of the QR-slope only appears for SRBD events in the RaK interval represented by its mean and standard deviation. Generally, the mean increases, while the standard deviation decreases during a SRBD event. With a simultaneously increasing QR-amplitude, this can only mean that the duration of the QR-delay remains constant or even decreases – driven by an increase of the HR. The decreasing standard deviation and the increasing HR seem to hint on the SNS activation during a SRBD event.

For classifying SRBD events and in the RaK interval, the features tracking the changes of the R-peak amplitude are most powerful. Among these features are the standard deviations of the R-peak amplitude and its floating mean $m_d(R,5)$. Further features in this group are:

- the increasing heart load feature (see /6.4.2/) in both versions, i.e., delayed and non-delayed

- the mean of the differences between the R-peak amplitudes of two subsequent evaluation periods $m(R_n - R_{n-1})$

- the difference between the R-peak amplitude and the delayed mean $m_d(R,5)$.

These findings suggest that SRBD events increase the R-peak amplitude dynamics. This assumption is further supported by the fact that the R-peak based features are especially strong for the detection of the REM sleep stage where high ANS dynamics are present.

The already known feature describing the relation of the P-wave to the R-peak amplitude is an important SRBD feature for both evaluation periods.

For the classification target sleep stage only a few of the R-peak features have to be evaluated: for the RaK interval the periods-of-increasing-load feature and the standard deviation of the relation between R-peak amplitudes of two subsequent evaluation periods. The periods-of-increasing-load feature performs significantly better in the delayed version. The standard deviation of this feature shows highest dynamics – lowest and *highest* values – during REM sleep which derives from the physiological strain of this sleep stage (see /2.4.2/).

For the BtB evaluation, $m_c(R,5)$ and the relation between P-wave and R-peak amplitude are required. Additionally, for both evaluation intervals the total QR-amplitude is of high predictive capability.

The overall performance of the R-peak feature set is in the center span of the morphology based feature sets. However, it may be increased by compensating the respiratory influences (see /10.3/) in future versions. Its main advantage is that it is reliably computable as the R-peak is the most dominant distinctive ECG point.

7.4.4 ST-Segment

For the detection of SRBD events in the RaK interval all the features describing the ascent or descent are important, i.e., the polynomial, the linear, and the gradient approach contribute to the classification. What is even more remarkable, is that these features have to be linearly independent as linearly dependent features are suppressed by the selected feature selection method.

Additionally, the feature counting the number of gradients under a threshold is considered. The values of the mean and standard deviation of this feature rise during SRBD events. Especially remarkable is the increase of this value during O events in the standard deviation. The transmural ischemia hypothesis is supported by the elevation feature contributing to the classification as well (see Figure 7.7): The mean of this value increases significantly during SRBD events, e.g., H and O, but remains in a limited range (about 15 - 21). The corresponding values for normal respiration (N) have a much higher dynamic ((about -13 - 22)). The standard deviation of this value likewise decreases. Both findings can be summarized in the following way: under the influence of a SRBD event the elevation rises to a constant value. According to the reasoning in /6.4.4/ this finding hints on fluctuations in the oxygen supply or varying repolarization curves (see Figure 3.10) due to varying ANS activity.

7.4. Evaluation of the different Feature Sets 193

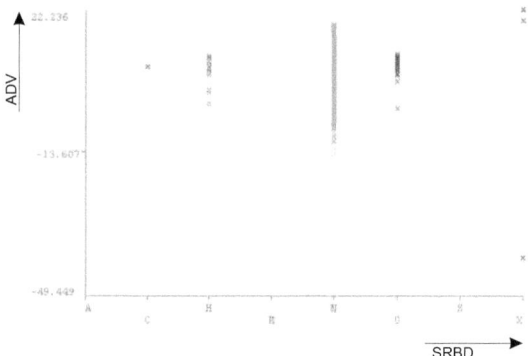

Figure 7.7: Distribution of the feature "ST-Elevation" over the SRBD events (plot created by means of the WEKA Explorer)

For SRBD evaluation based on a BtB interval the ascent and descent features are necessary as well. Additionally, the ST-amplitude relative to the floating means $m_d(S, 5)$ and $m_d(T, 5)$ as well as the depression feature are considered. ST-depressions are commonly found in SRBD patients. Varying repolarization due to ANS influences may trigger this behavior.

For the detection of the sleep stages in the RaK as well as the BtB interval all polynomial features, the linear ascent feature and the elevation or depression features are considered.

From the gradient based features only the first and the last segments are relevant. This may hint on changes in the repolarization process due to ANS driven funny current I_f (see /3.3.1/ and Figure 3.10) variations which would be a direct measure for the ANS activity.

The ST-segment derived features produce better results in the RaK interval which is true for both classification targets. The overall performance of the ST-segment features is located in the upper center span with an emphasis on the sleep stage detection.

7.4.5 T-Wave

The features derived from the T-wave reflect three different aspects: the direct amplitude variations, the trend, i.e., increase or decrease, of the T-wave amplitude, and the funny current I_f features which are directly linked to the ANS (see /3.3.1/). While the classification relevant features of the first two groups vary with the classification target and the evaluation period, the I_f features are always considered

194   Chapter 7. Experimental Results

– however, the amplitude and trend features are always higher in their predictive capability. Nevertheless, this may be taken as a prove of the sensibility of the repolarization process to changes in oxygen supply and ANS activity. This finding supports the model illustrated in Figure 6.43.

The directly amplitude related features show their highest relevance in the RaK interval for SRBD event detection. This is a consequence of the T-wave sensibility to fluctuations in the oxygen supply (see /3.5.4/). In this area, the T-wave amplitude relative to the reference is considered: the relation as standard deviation and the difference as mean and standard deviation. From the trend features, the negativeness and the accumulated negative trend of the T-wave amplitude are evaluated.

For the BtB evaluation the T-wave amplitude relative to the delayed floating mean $m_d(T, 5)$ and the negativeness of the T-wave are considered in addition to the I_f features. The assumption of ischemic influences (see /3.5.4/) due to SRBD events is supported by the fact that the negativeness of the T-wave appears in both evaluation periods and, additionally in RaK, the accumulated negative trend.

For the sleep stage classification almost the same features as for the SRBD events apply, except that for the RaK interval only the standard deviation of the T-wave amplitude relative to the reference and only the mean of the difference between both amplitude values are considered. This implies changes of the T-wave as an reaction to varying load conditions, as the T-wave features perform better for W and LS.

Considering the trend based features the negativeness of the T-wave amplitude is replaced by the number of subsequent decreasing T-wave amplitudes feature.

For the BtB evaluation, the only amplitude based feature is the T-wave relative to the reference feature, whereas all other relevant features are trend-based.

As already mentioned the I_f based features are important for both evaluation periods. This finding is especially remarkable as it supports the hypothesis that the T-wave model directly reflects the ANS activity state.

Generally, the T-wave features can not compete with the ST-segment based features, even though, these are very closely linked from a physiological view of point. Like other features, they perform better in the RaK interval.

7.4.6 Timing

Among the Timing based features the PQ-time and its relation to the floating mean of the HR are of general importance. The PQ-time represents the delay introduced by the AV-node. As even AV-blocks are quite common in SRBD patients, it does not surprise that this parameter is affected by SRBD events and the overall condition

7.4. Evaluation of the different Feature Sets 195

during the different sleep stages likewise. In an analog manner the results prove that the QT-time and ST-time are significant indicators for the ANS activity.

Somewhat more surprising is the fact that the QRS-time is found to be a relevant feature. The surprise results from the fact that the cardiac conduction system is designed to make the ventricle contract "all at once" to maximize blood output. The findings here prove that the cardiac conduction system is affected by the occurrence of SRBD events and sleep stages. These influences have already been assumed when discussing the steepness of the QR-ascent (see /7.4.3/).

For the detection of SRBD events in the RaK interval the means $m(PQ)$, $m(QRS)$, $m(\frac{QRS}{m_c(HR)})$, and $m(QT)$ are evaluated as well as the standard deviations of $\frac{QRS}{m_c(HR)}$, the QT-, and the ST-time. The relations between subsequent periods of QT- and ST-time, respectively, are evaluated only for this target-interval combination.

For the BtB interval, the features PQ-, $\frac{PQ}{m_c(HR)}$-, QRS-duration and the QT-time as well as its relation to $m_c(HR)$ are relevant. This proves the expected ANS influence on the AV-node conduction and the repolarization time.

For the sleep stage detection the same parameters are important for both evaluation periods – for the RaK interval mainly in the mean versions. The standard deviation is only considered for $\frac{QT}{HR}$, ST-, and $\frac{ST}{m_c(HR)}$-time. For the sleep stage detection $\frac{QT}{HR}$ is important as well. All of these features are related to the repolarization time. This links the duration of the repolarization to the general ANS activation due to the different sleep stages.

The fact that for both classification targets the timing parameters relative to the floating mean of the HR are of importance seems to hint either on processes gathering speed over periods of several heart beats (see Figure 3.8) or relative variations of these parameters in relation to the HR in the manner of Figure 3.12.

The feature $\frac{QT}{m_c(HR)}$, i.e., the QT-time relative to the current HR, is only required for the sleep stage detection. Figure 7.8 shows that this feature exhibits a much wider dynamic range for the REM stage which is characterized by a high ANS activity. Hence, the fact that the Timing based features achieve their maximum classification rates for S1 - S4, appears to indicate that these features capture the constancy of the HR.

A general observation is the following: for the SRBD detection the dynamic range of (almost) all features is much higher for N than during any of the apnea events, especially H and O. As an example, Figure 7.9 illustrates this behavior for the previous feature $\frac{QT}{m_c(HR)}$ which could be induced by rising activity of the SNS which is known to reduce the HRV.

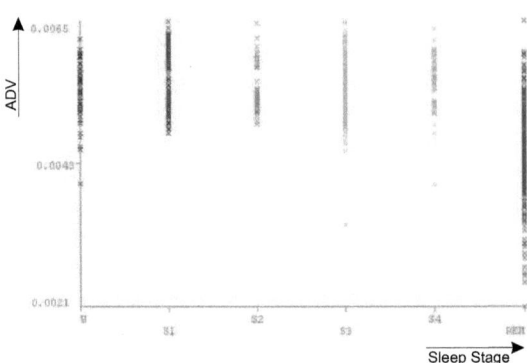

Figure 7.8: Feature values for $\frac{QT}{m_c(HR)}$ show a very high dynamic in REM.

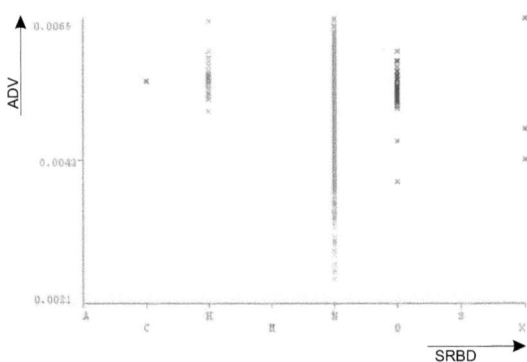

Figure 7.9: Values for $\frac{QT}{m_c(HR)}$ feature highest dynamic during N, while the dynamic decreases during the obstructive SRBD events O and H.

7.4. Evaluation of the different Feature Sets

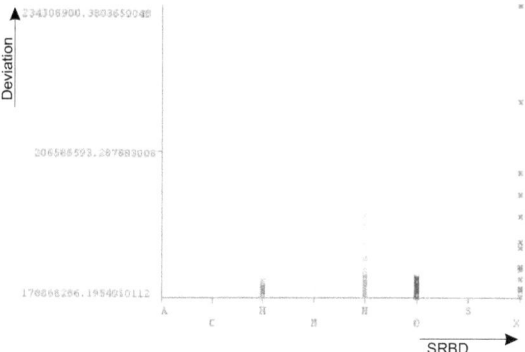

Figure 7.10: Distribution of the feature "Histogram based deviation against the overnight ECG buffer as mean" over the SRBD events

For the sleep stages, the distribution of the feature values is much more balanced, except for REM where many of the features show large value swings. These dynamics are even significantly higher than in W which is supposed to be akin.

The performance of the Timing based features for the SRBD event detection increases dramatically with the relative frequency of annotated SRBD events. Accordingly, they reach their maximum in the DP where they even outperform the AM.

7.4.7 Overall Shape: Deviations

One surprising fact about the morphShape_Dev() features is that the buffer built from all ECG waves as well as the buffer built from only the ECG waves during the healthy phases, i.e., those annotated N, are of importance. First, considering the feature selection method, this means that they are linearly independent. Second, the ECG waves must differ characteristically during SRBD events which supports the hypothesis of the morphological approach. Third, considering the a-priori probability of the healthy phases, it is even more remarkable that there is an obvious difference between both.

For the SRBD event detection in the RaK interval the histogram based deviations against the overnight ECG buffer as well as against the healthy phases based ECG buffer are evaluated as means. Additionally, the corresponding means to the previous ECG wave are analyzed.

Figure 7.10 illustrates the already formulated statement that in the RaK interval there is a generally higher dynamic for the feature values in N. This behavior can be attributed to two reasons: First, during any type of apnea event the ECG generation is "tenser" driven by SNS influences. Second, the values are simply wider distributed, because there are more instances annotated as N. The second assumption seems less probable for two reasons: first, the fact that both buffers of morphShape_Dev() are considered independently suggests significant differences in the ECG morphology during SRBD events. Second, the described behavior can be found even in subjects with increased frequencies of SRBD events. Hence, the reason for the generally higher dynamics in N derives from the different operating parameters of the ECG generation.

For the SRBD event detection in the BtB interval the same features as for the RaK interval are analyzed, but without the relation to the previous ECG wave as this feature is not available for this evaluation period.

For the sleep stage classification in the RaK interval the histogram based deviations against the overnight ECG Buffer as mean and against the healthy phases based ECG Buffer as mean and standard deviation. In this evaluation combination the deviation against the overnight mean ECG wave (see Figure 6.50, red curve) is considered as mean and standard deviation.

For the sleep stage classification in the BtB interval the only feature analyzed is the histogram based deviation against the healthy phases based ECG buffer. morphShape_Dev() achieves best results for the LS and REM sleep stages which are both assumed to exhibit high ANS activity. The healthy phases ECG buffer, however, is the ECG representation of the stable ECG phases which may, thus, be regarded the counterpart of high ANS activity. This contrast explains this feature.

Another observation is that the deviation based features show high dynamics for the artifacts (X). This is intuitively understandable as the ECG morphology during artifacts usually differ remarkably from a correctly recorded ECG wave.

The deviation based features perform better in the RaK interval. In comparison to the other feature sets the deviation features have to be deemed weak.

7.4.8 Overall Shape: Independent Component Analysis

The highest ranking feature for the SRBD event detection in the RaK interval is the difference between the "energies" of the ICA components reflecting PNS activity and noise as standard deviation. This is remarkable as only the difference is considered, but neither "energy" by itself. This can be interpreted as a change in the PNS activity accompanied by SNS activity which makes the ECG generation more "tense", thus, reducing noise. This assumption is supported by the results of morphShape_Dev() as well.

7.4. Evaluation of the different Feature Sets

The detection relies on some of the spectral coefficients (5, 7, 15, 9 Hz, ordered according to their predictive capability) of the first non-ECG component as well. According to the model (see Figure 6.57) this component reflects the PNS activity. As these spectral coefficients are only considered for the SRBD detection, this supports the hypothesis that the SRBD events trigger an additional component which provokes short term modulations of the ECG shape.

The idea that the ICA produces a kind of "purified" ECG wave in its ECG component is supported by the relevance of the "energy of correlation between ECG and the ICA purified ECG wave" feature as standard deviation. Indeed, the standard deviation emphasizes the dynamic character of this feature during SRBD events.

The feature which computes the energy of the ICA component resulting from running ICA on the difference between the current ECG wave and the overnight mean contributes to the classification as well. This fact also supports the assumption that SRBD events introduce systematic modifications to the ECG wave. This feature is considered as mean and standard deviation for the first component (PNS) and the second one (noise) as standard deviation alone. This finding can be interpreted as an increased activity in the PNS component.

For the SRBD event detection in the BtB interval the same features are considered with only one exception: the highest ranking feature of the RaK interval is replaced with the feature which computes the energies of the non-ECG components, i.e., those reflecting PNS activity and noise. This supports the ICA model directly.

The spectral coefficients of the PNS component considered in the BtB interval are those of higher frequencies (14, 20 Hz) whereas in the RaK interval lower frequencies are considered as well. This is due to a volatile behavior of the lower frequencies which requires the low pass filter effect introduced by the mapping to the RaK interval.

For the sleep stage detection in the RaK interval only two features are analyzed: the energy of the ICA components where ICA was run on the difference of the processed ECG and the overnight mean ECG wave. Both ICA model components, i.e., PNS activity and noise, are evaluated as standard deviations. As has already been mentioned, it is remarkable that the higher dynamic of the standard deviation is used to characterize the slower process of changing sleep stages. An explanation may be that the respective mean values do not show enough variation to be noted as significant.

For the detection of sleep stages on a BtB basis more features are relevant and they resemble those of the SRBD event detection. This hints on the detection of the arousal which is essential to sleep stage changes.

200   Chapter 7. Experimental Results

In detail the following features are revealed as relevant:

- The energy of the noise component which can reflect the long term regulation of the ECG generation according to the sleep stages (see /2.4.2/).

- The difference of the energies of the non-ECG ICA components, i.e., the difference between the PNS activity and noise.

- The energy of the correlation between the ECG and the ICA purified ECG wave.

- The energy of both components, i.e., PNS activity and noise, computed from the difference of the processed ECG and the overnight mean ECG wave.

The fact that ICA quite often fails to find all requested ICs supports the assumption that SRBD events themselves trigger a new process which means the ICs are only "visible" (or valid), *when* a SRBD event occurs. This process may be the reason for the 0.02 Hz indicating the "cyclic variation of the heart rate" (see /4.3/).

In general, the `morphShape_CA()` features produce better results in the RaK interval. Comparing the ICA approach to the others introduced in this work it is the least powerful one.

7.4.9 Overall Shape: Spectral Transformations

For the actual feature extraction the number of coefficients was reduced to 20 which was due to otherwise excessive computational load for the WEKA classifiers. This decision was supported by the fast decaying spectral coefficients as can be seen in Figure 6.74 for the DFT on the ECG signal without the R-peak. This suggests that the high coefficient values of the blue curve result from the R-peak. If so, its characteristics should be captured by the lower frequency coefficients as well.

In the following lists "DFT" means "amplitude of the DFT coefficient", "DCT" analog, and "Phase" stands for "phase of the DFT coefficient". An attached "-R" indicates the transforms with the R-peak extinguished (see p. 134). Most of the features mapped to the RaK interval are exploited as means. For the SRBD event detection (in both evaluation periods) the feature list ordered according to classification power is the following:

$$DFT \longrightarrow DCT \longrightarrow DFT-R \longrightarrow DCT-R \longrightarrow (Phase-R)$$

The phase information is only analyzed in the BtB interval.
For the sleep stage detection the ordered list looks like:

7.4. Evaluation of the different Feature Sets

$$DFT \longrightarrow Phase \longrightarrow DCT \longrightarrow DFT-R \longrightarrow Phase-R \longrightarrow DCT-R$$

These two lists can be summarized in the following way: The SRBD events are indicated by the amplitudes of the transform coefficients, mainly the DFT coefficients. The sleep stages are revealed by the properties of the DFT coefficients, i.e., amplitude and phase. In any case the better part consists of the transforms applied to the ECG waves including the R-peak. This finding confirms the considerable predicative capability of the R-peak itself (see /7.4.3/). It is surprising, though, that the low frequencies are more important than the higher frequency components representing the steep ascent of the R-peak.

As this spectral approach does not evaluate the HRV, but the shape of the ECG wave, it proves that the frequency components represented in the ECG signal vary which may be linked to the findings in morphShape_CA() where the results hint on an additional (ICA) component during SRBD events. This is most likely due to changes in the speed of the cardiac conduction system. Considering the dominance of the R-peak, this supports the finding that the QRS-duration (see /7.4.6/) from the Timing based features is an indicator for changes in the ANS balance.

The spectral transform features generally yield better results in the RaK interval, except only for LS in the HP and the DP. Comparing the classification results these features rank among the best ones of this work. The spectral features are responsible for most of the rare cases where the AM is outperformed.

7.4.10 Overall Shape: Differences of Spectral Transformations

Figure 6.86 shows that the spectrum "contains information" up to 45 Hz (F_{stop} of the preprocessing filter, see Table 6.4). However, to reduce the computational load[5], the number of coefficients was set to 20 (see previous Section). Likely, information was wasted here.

In the following lists "Mean" means "amplitude of DFT transform on overnight mean ECG subtracted from the ECG", "Phase" analog "phase of DFT transform on overnight mean ECG subtracted from the ECG". The features which result from the DFT on "mean of the last ECG waves subtracted from the ECG" are marked as "Last" and Last Phase", respectively. Almost all of the features are mapped to the RaK interval as means.

---

[5] The terminus "computational load" is meant to say that the classifiers got stuck which was counteracted by successively reducing the number of evaluated coefficients.

For the SRBD event detection in the RaK interval the upper 30.1% of the selected features are amplitudes, but the bigger part is made from the phase information. The feature list ordered according to classification power is the following:

$$Mean \longrightarrow Phase \longrightarrow Last \longrightarrow LastPhase$$

For the BtB interval the dominant upper 62.1% of the features are the amplitudes of the DFT coefficients. The ordered list is:

$$Mean \longrightarrow Phase \longrightarrow Last$$

For the sleep stage classification in the RaK interval the lower 66.6% of the features carry the coefficients' phase information.

$$Mean \longrightarrow Phase \longrightarrow Last \longrightarrow LastPhase$$

In the BtB interval the lower 58.8% of the features are made up from the phase information.

$$Mean \longrightarrow Phase \longrightarrow LastPhase$$

The evaluation of the features clearly shows that the overnight mean ECG is much better suited as a reference point than the mean of the last few ECG waves. This can be explained with the slowly increasing load to the heart during the SRBD event, i.e., the mean of the last ECG waves follows the significant variations of the ECG shape during a SRBD event too closely. Maybe an adaption of the considered number of ECG waves to the standard duration of a sleep stage would improve the results. However, in SRBD patients this is hardly possible as the standard sleep architecture (see /2.4.2/) is no longer valid.

For the detection of REM the higher frequency components (around 20) of the phase are sensitive whereas these features do not react to W. This behavior has already been observed by the shape deviation based features (see /7.4.7/) which can be interpreted in the way that REM introduces instabilities to the ANS which is in consent with the literature.

Comparing the spectral differences features to the spectral features it can be stated that the differential features do not perform as well. Recalling that the spectral features based on the ECG wave with extinguished R-peak did not play an important role, this can be intuitively understood. In fact, the classification results applying the differential features should be much worse as this time not only the R-peak is extinguished, but the "complete" ECG wave. This, however, is not true: the differential features are among the best performing feature sets and achieve classification rates which can compete with the spectral feature set.

7.4. Evaluation of the different Feature Sets 203

	AM	P	R	ST	T	Timing	Dev.	ICA	Spec.	Diff. Spec.
RaK	0.44	0.82	0.76	0.39	0.13	0.46	0.50	0.33	0.77	0.62
BtB	0.83	0.69	0.71	0.59	0.67	0.41	0.60	0.23	0.76	0.65

Table 7.4: Artifact detection rate for each feature set and evaluation period (given as F-Measures)

7.4.11 Detection of Artifacts

Along with the classification of SRBD events and sleep stages the detection of artifacts in the ECG signal was evaluated. The artifacts were grouped with the SRBD events as both event types show rather short durations compared to the sleep stages. Hence, the reasoning is that an artifact may prevent a proper SRBD event detection, but a quite reliable sleep stage detection is still feasible. Table 7.4 summarizes the achieved classification rates for each feature set.

Looking at the Table it becomes evident that both evaluation periods have equal wins. Comparing the given F-Measures, however, the more powerful evaluation period is (as a mean) the BtB interval. This can be assumed to be due to the mean duration of artifacts. It is highly remarkable that the AM which does not consider the shape of the ECG achieves such a high F-Measure. This is most likely due to the fact that during artifacts the R-peak detection fails entailing outliers in the σ values of the GMM approximation.

Even though none of the features was specifically designed to detect artifacts the classification results are promising. When assessing the classification rates, it has to be taken into consideration that only few artifacts were annotated. An increase of the classification rates as shown in Tables 7.2 and 7.3 can be expected. With a little effort a completely automatic processing of the ECG signal without any manual preprocessing (as it was done for the works mentioned in the State of the Art in Chapter 4) should be feasible.

7.4.12 Concluding the patient-dependent Classification Rates

Tables 7.5 and 7.6 show the best classification rates and the corresponding F-Measure along with most suitable feature set.

It is somewhat tricky to decide which the best feature set is as this depends on the chosen point of view. For the following assessment the "means of the grouped events" were chosen as markers as this reflects the averaged expectable performance. According to this benchmark the AM is the best feature set for both classification targets: for the SRBD event detection, the interval with the highest predictive

		Class. Rate [%]	F-Measure	Feature Set
RaK	O:	74.6	0.72	AM
	H:	86.4	0.74	Timing
	M:	60.2	0.54	AM
	C:	22.2	0.17	AM
	X:	83.3	0.83	AM
BtB	O:	47.8	0.46	AM
	H:	65.0	0.61	Spec
	M:	52.2	0.51	AM
	C:	11.1	0.20	R
	X:	61.0	0.69	P

Table 7.5: Condensed classification rates and F-Measures for the SRBD events and the most efficient feature set for the two evaluation periods (SRBD event N is not considered.)

		Class. Rate [%]	F-Measure	Feature Set
RaK	W:	90.3	0.91	AM
	S1:	65.7	0.64	AM
	S2:	94.5	0.93	AM
	S3:	84.5	0.83	AM
	S4:	98.0	0.96	AM
	REM:	89.2	0.91	AM
BtB	W:	96.2	0.96	AM
	S1:	74.7	0.69	AM
	S2:	97.3	0.97	AM
	S3:	92.5	0.93	AM
	S4:	99.0	0.99	AM
	REM:	96.9	0.97	AM

Table 7.6: Condensed classification rates and F-Measures for the sleep stages and the most efficient feature set for the two evaluation periods

7.4. Evaluation of the different Feature Sets   205

capability is RaK, and for the sleep stage detection, it is BtB. On the following ranks are:

- Spectral features

- Differential spectral features

- ST-segment

- Timing

This result matches the findings in the literature where the HR based features outrank the morphology based features. However, in contradiction to the literature, the morphological features are found to be good performers.

Evaluating the confusion matrices for *falsely classified* events, leads to the following conclusions: The by far biggest part of the falsely classified SRBD events is assigned to N. Considering the absolute percentage of the N event in the evaluated recordings and its accordingly high a-priori probability, this behavior is explained by the classifier going for the "safe", i.e., most likely, guess. In the case of the DP with his/her higher fraction of non-N annotations, the classifier tends to assign non-N events to other non-N events. For example, in the DP a lot of O events are classified as H which is due to the four fold higher a-priori probability of the H events. This assignment is fostered by the close physiological relation between O and H. This behavior would increase the "correctly detected" non-N events, if they were grouped prior to outputting the SRBD event type, i.e., if there were only two classes, namely N and non-N, as is the case in the literature (see Chapter 4).

Considering the sleep stage misclassifications the most frequent misclassification is the assignment of REM to S2. As this behavior is visible in the patient-independent data set (see /7.5/ below) as well, it is either physiologically driven or feature-immanent. This finding is somewhat surprising as W and REM are commonly considered "unequal brothers" (see /2.4.2/). The next Section will illuminate this matter in more detail. In the DP the dominant misclassification is the mapping of DS to LS, i.e., S3 is assigned to S2. Likely, this happens because of the higher a-priori probability of S2 (see Table 10.6, for example) and the generally fluent transitions from one sleep stage to another.

Concluding the classification result tables, there is one striking finding: the dramatic increase in correctly classified events with increasing occurrences of annotated events: on the HP the classification of the sleep stages is very good, whereas the classification of the SRBD events is quite poor – for the DP the findings are reciprocal. Recalling that these classification rates were derived applying the 10-folds method, i.e., a patient-dependent approach, the simple explanation is that the classifier could not train itself properly, if there are only few appropriate annotated instances.

To answer the question, how the classifiers perform, if there is more training data, the classification rates are reassessed in a patient-independent evaluation.

7.5 Patient-independent Evaluation

The general idea of the patient-independent evaluation is to train the classifier with the five patients evaluated in the previous Sections and to assess the trained classifier on a new patient. This approach is supported by the WEKA Explorer, but requires some prerequisites: the training data has to be merged into a single file and the number of features must match those of the test file. This is no constraint for the morphology based features as these produce a constant (processing configuration dependent) number of features. Consequently, for training the morphology based classifier, the five already evaluated patients were used as intended. However, the AM based processing of the ECG signal produces a varying number of features due to the number of maxima found in the spectrum (see /6.3.3/). Hence, for training the AM a set of four, including one new, patients was used.

To compensate for the high a-priori probability of the SRBD event N, the patient-independent data set for the SRBD event detection was created with the ratio between N and all other SRBD types set to 1 : 1. This was done by choosing all non-N instances and adding exactly as many N instances randomly chosen from the pool of N instances created from the five or four patients, respectively. As the sleep stages do not show this extremely unbalanced distribution, the complete annotations for the five or four patients were used for the patient-independent data set.

The test patient was found to exhibit an AHI of 63.3. To make sure that the test patient him/herself is not an outlier, his/her data was evaluated according to the already described patient-dependent 10-folds method. During this evaluation the relevant values were found to be within the same range as in a patient with a comparable AHI. The absolute occurrences of the respective events or sleep stages, respectively, are listed in Table 7.7.

The classification rates of the experiment are shown in Tables 7.8 and 7.9 for the grouped SRBD events or sleep stages, respectively.

The classification results show a striking decrease when compared to the patient-dependent evaluation. Reasons may be the small amount of training data in the patient-independent evaluation or the narrow adaption to the specific subject in the patient-dependent evaluation. To answer this question, more data needs to be

7.5. Patient-independent Evaluation

SRBD Event	abs %	Sleep Stage	abs %
N	51.6	W	10.5
O	18.4	S1	5.0
H	7.6	S2	53.4
M	19.3	S3	11.3
C	3.1	S4	8.7
X	0.0	REM	11.1

Table 7.7: Absolute occurrences of the SRBD events and the sleep stages in the test patient

evaluated (see Chapter 8). Further examination of these Tables leads to the following findings:

SRBD Event Detection The highest classification rate is achieved in the BtB interval by the deviation based features. However, on average, in the RaK interval 44.7% of the SRBD events are detected compared to 37.5% in the BtB interval. Hence, the RaK interval deems the more appropriate evaluation interval.

Sleep Stage Detection Three out of four sleep stages are best classified in the BtB interval. Only REM is best classified in RaK. Assessing the average classification rates, it is 26.4% in the RaK interval compared to 26.1% in the BtB interval. Hence, as the average classification rates are comparable and the BtB interval has more single wins, it is the more favorable.

These results confirm the seemingly paradox finding that the SRBD events which feature the higher dynamics compared to the sleep stages are better classified in the RaK interval, and vice versa. This is remarkable as about half of the SRBD events in the test patient are shorter or about the duration of the RaK interval. Accordingly, these events would be expected to be "blurred" by the mean functions which are used to map the BtB features to the RaK interval.

The one finding which is considerable is that in the patient-independent evaluation the morphology based feature sets outperform the AM. This may be due to the fact that there were lesser training data. However, considering the very good performance in the patient-dependent evaluation, this may as well be due to an adaption of the classifier to the special characteristics of a given patient.

		SRBD Events [%]	Sleep Stage [%]	
AM	RaK	41.9	W:	55.3
			LS:	41.6
			DS:	**11.1**
			REM:	5.5
	BtB	27.7	W:	49.5
			LS:	46.6
			DS:	3.9
			REM:	1.7
P	RaK	9.2	W:	83.5
			LS:	27.6
			DS:	0.0
			REM:	0.9
	BtB	3.1	W:	**94.4**
			LS:	17.0
			DS:	0.5
			REM:	0.1
R	RaK	64.4	W:	79.6
			LS:	27.8
			DS:	0.0
			REM:	32.7
	BtB	26.7	W:	61.2
			LS:	28.9
			DS:	17.2
			REM:	3.3
ST	RaK	62.9	W:	**94.2**
			LS:	6.2
			DS:	0.0
			REM:	0.0
	BtB	33.2	W:	48.2
			LS:	36.9
			DS:	1.9
			REM:	2.3
T	RaK	62.5	W:	74.8
			LS:	21.9
			DS:	3.5
			REM:	0.0
	BtB	54.4	W:	54.4
			LS:	41.5
			DS:	4.7
			REM:	2.5

Table 7.8: Classification rates of the patient-independent evaluation for the feature sets *AM* through *T-Wave*

		SRBD Events [%]	Sleep Stage [%]	
Timing	RaK	**79.2**	W:	55.3
			LS:	50.2
			DS:	1.0
			REM:	0.0
	BtB	41.4	W:	76.7
			LS:	25.0
			DS:	10.5
			REM:	3.6
Dev	RaK	76.7	W:	22.3
			LS:	15.9
			DS:	3.5
			REM:	**35.5**
	BtB	**100.0**	W:	21.3
			LS:	57.3
			DS:	**29.3**
			REM:	0.0
ICA	RaK	7.9	W:	51.5
			LS:	40.9
			DS:	2.0
			REM:	0.9
	BtB	24.6	W:	51.8
			LS:	43.3
			DS:	2.1
			REM:	0.6
Spec	RaK	27.9	W:	66.0
			LS:	29.5
			DS:	0.5
			REM:	2.7
	BtB	30.2	W:	80.5
			LS:	13.8
			DS:	0.8
			REM:	0.8
Spec Diff	RaK	14.0	W:	33.0
			LS:	**65.0**
			DS:	0.0
			REM:	13.6
	BtB	33.4	W:	29.1
			LS:	**69.4**
			DS:	1.5
			REM:	**8.2**

Table 7.9: Classification rates of the patient-independent evaluation for the feature sets *Timing* through *Differential Spectral Transformaion*

7.6 Discussion

In /3.3.1/ (see p. 38) a model to predict the HR considering PNS and SNS influences was introduced. Its authors implemented an autoregressive model approach. They summarized in their results that the PNS is responsible for the respiratory sinus arrhythmia and the HR fluctuations during SRBD events alike, while the influence of the SNS is negligible. These findings affirm the results which were achieved during the evaluation of the AM.

The different generators found during the evaluation of the AM were assigned to the PNS. The assessment of their center frequencies suggested that the spectrum consists of a base frequency and its harmonics. However, in the light of the just mentioned model, it may well be possible that there are supplemental PNS components in addition to the harmonics which are "blurred". To separate these blurred components, the spectral resolution has to be increased. As the spectral resolution increase entails a temporal resolution decrease, an overlapping mechanism analog to Figure 6.16 with a subsequent "likeliness estimator" must be implemented for a future version of the AM.

The classification results achieved during the evaluation are usually better in the RaK interval. The standard deviations of a given parameter turned out to be an important indicator for the occurrence of SRBD events and sleep stages alike. This finding is supported by the literature, e.g., [Vano 95], [Roch 99], and [Shio 97]. These findings raise hope that the performance of the BtB interval could be improved by considering the standard deviations of a given feature to its predecessor(s) and/or successor(s) as the standard deviations were only considered for the RaK interval in this work.

The QRS-complex as a morphological feature is rarely considered as a SRBD event marker. If so, usually the area is evaluated as a respiratory indicator (see /10.3/), e.g., [Mend 10]. In [Altu 09]), however, the QRS-complex duration was found to correlate with SRBD event induced bradycardia, but the authors did not use it for the classification of such events.

The evaluation of the data of this work revealed the QRS-time to be valuable indicator of SRBD events (see /7.4.6/) as well. As the fascicles of the cardiac conduction system are said to be "high-speed", the possible reason for the predictive capabilities has to be assumed in ischemic influences which impact the heart muscle.

Before a final assessment of this work's approach is presented, its motivation shall be recalled: the primary target of this work has been to develop a system which is capable of detecting *single* events and their *type*. As such, it quite differs

7.6. Discussion

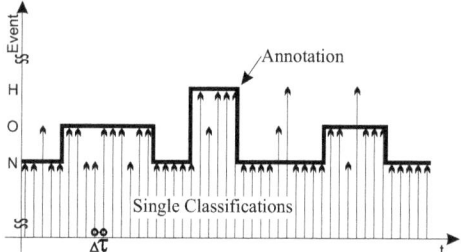

Figure 7.11: Comparision between annotations and evaluation period based single classifications

from the works presented in Chapter 4 which mostly aimed at assigning periods of one minute to either healthy or ill.

One basic requirement for the detection of *single events* is to have a higher temporal resolution than the duration of the events in focus. According to their definition SRBD events need to last at least ten seconds and may last up to a few minutes. In the case of the test patient for the patient-independent evaluation, for example, around 33% of the events lasted 10 - 19 seconds and around 12% lasted 40 - 49 seconds. To provide the required temporal resolution, the evaluation period τ was set to one heart beat (for the morphology based features). This period was the shortest evaluation interval possible as the described feature sets need one complete ECG cycle.

The consequences of this specification shall be explained with the help of Figure 7.11: The thick curve symbolizes the expert's annotations. Along the time axis the patient's annotated state changes from N to O, back to N again and so on. The small arrows in the distance τ from one another symbolize the evaluation period. For each evaluation period, there is a single classification. Consequently, a single event – as annotated by the experts – is represented by quite a few individual classifications – especially for the BtB evaluation interval. As illustrated, some of the arrows hit the thick curve whereas others do not, i.e., some of the single classifications match the experts' annotation and others fail. The classification rates provided in this Chapter are based on these single classifications.

A simple approach to improve the classification rates could be a majority decoder which outputs the class with the highest occurrence frequency during an evaluation interval. A more enhanced approach could be to apply physiological restraints to the single classifications considering the duration and occurrence pattern of SRBD events.

A more sophisticated approach could be based on the high temporal resolution which allows to separate each event into individual phases: SRBD events – and sleep stages alike – have a beginning, a center part, and an end which exhibit different properties represented by different values of the extracted features. To track these different parts of an event, further classes for these single phases should be introduced, e.g., bO, cO, and eO for the beginning, the center, and the end of an obstructive apnea event. Subsequently, some kind of "intelligence", e.g., a neural network or a Hidden Markov Model, would rebuild complete events from these single parts. This approach would improve the detection of transitions between the individual SRBD types. However, for this approach, the annotations would have to be revised – unless fixed fractions of the SRBD event duration are (automatically) assigned to these "sub-events".

The requirement of detecting the *types* of the SRBD events entails the following consequence: The classification results for the SRBD events in this Chapter are given as a classification rate for a "grouped event", i.e., the multi-classes problem is turned into a two-classes problem for easier comparison with the State of the Art. However, the individual SRBD events are grouped on basis of the confusion matrices according to equation 7.1b (see Tables 10.5 through 10.24) and subsequent averaging of the individual classification rates. The approaches in literature, however, separate healthy from diseased respiratory phases already during the training and testing, i.e., they are conceptually operating on the two-classes problem.

In the case of the SRBD event detection the multi-classes approach entails two main challenges:

- The individual SRBD classes show strong similarities in theory as well as in the recorded physiological signals to an extent which even confuses human experts. These similarities entailed the classification of O events as H in the DP as mentioned in /7.4.12/. In the scope of this work this is a misclassification whereas it would not matter for the two-class problem.

- It reduces the amount of training data for each single type. Recalling the strong dependency of the classification rates on the absolute percentage of annotated events, i.e., the a-priori probability, this demands for a much larger training data set.

A third requirement is implicitly made by the demand for a fully automated processing: an artifact detection. If the ECG recording in spoiled by an artifact, this period must be excluded from the processing and the operator has to be supplied with an according hint. In this approach the artifacts have been grouped with the

SRBD events as an individual type. None of the approaches in Chapter 4 addresses this problem.

Having pointed out the differences to the approaches in the literature, it should be obvious that this work's approach is quite different. This makes it hard to compare them. Just looking at the classification rates makes this work's approach drop behind. However, I hope to have proved that it has a lot of potential and reaches far beyond the so far described approaches.

This work has introduced two completely different approaches to process an ECG recording which are based on the shape (morphology) of the ECG and the dynamics of the HR. The introduction to the medical basics of SRBD and the ECG analysis helped to motivate the extracted features as indicators for the load changes to the heart. The achieved classification results prove that the desired target is indeed reachable.

7.7 Summary and Preview

This Chapter presented the achieved classification rates for each of the introduced feature sets (see Section 6.3 through 6.4.10). The feature sets were evaluated for both classification targets, i.e., SRBD events and sleep stages, and both evaluation periods, i.e., RaK and BtB.

At the beginning of the evaluation process various classifiers were assessed and the most appropriate ones were selected according to the classification target and the evaluation period. It was found that the classification of either the SRBD events or the sleep stages depends on the evaluation period which can be regarded as an adaption to the response times of the different physiological processes during a SRBD event or the sleep stages.

The results of the patient-dependent 10-folds evaluation were partly good to excellent – especially for the sleep stage classification. During this evaluation the HR based AM turned out to be the superior approach as could have been expected from the literature results. However, both spectral transformation feature sets were very successful as well, even though the selected number of coefficients did not cover the complete relevant spectrum.

As 10-folds method uses the same recording for the training and testing, the question arose, whether these results were simply due to a perfect adaption of the classifier to the characteristics of the analyzed patient. This question was answered during a patient-independent evaluation. As expected the classification rates dropped significantly. During this evaluation the morphology based feature sets – especially the spectral coefficients and the Timing based approaches – proved their strength and actually outperformed the AM.

Both evaluations – the 10-folds method and the experiment – showed a strong dependency of the classification rates from the absolute percentage of annotated events of a given type. The conclusion was that for further assessment of the classification power of the introduced feature sets larger data sets are required. Hence, a final rating is not possible yet.

The next Chapter will summarize the results of this work and relate them to the hypothesis, whether it is possible to derive sleep relevant parameters concerning SRBD events and sleep stages from a single lead ECG signal.

Chapter 8

Outlook

This work introduced a new approach aiming at the detection of *single* SRBD events and their *types*. At the same time the features were evaluated to detect the sleep stages as the sleep architecture is an indicator for the sleep quality. The results prove that this aim is principally feasible. Yet, for a practical application in, e.g., screening applications the introduced approaches have to be improved.

The decay of performance of the AM between the patient-dependent and the patient-independent evaluation is considerable. In [Jo04] the authors give evidence to the fact that the HRV is influenced by at least three different independent effects: vagal feedback from pulmonary stretch receptors, central medullary coupling between respiratory and cardio-vagal neurons, and arterial baroreflex sensors. These effects may feature a wide inter-subject variation. In this case, the AM can adapt perfectly to the subject's characteristics in the patient-dependent evaluation. However, in the patient-independent data set, these characteristics are not precise enough. If so, these effects need to be considered in the AM as well.

In this work, the ICA algorithm is applied for the separation of independent components in the morphology of the ECG signal. This approach did not fulfill the expectations. An analogue approach should be accomplished for the HR analysis. Combining the ICA approach and the AM could improve the AM as it may be possible to separate the above mentioned pulmonary and respiratory influences from those induced by SRBD events and sleep stages.

In the presented AM the spectra are approximated by a GMM. This GMM relies on the EM algorithm for the approximation. However, the EM algorithm quite often fails to create a proper GMM (see /10.4/) which leads to an interpolation (see Figure 6.22) of missing approximations. Thus, the extracted features do not necessarily reflect the subject's current state or dynamics. To improve the response of the model, other approximation algorithms can be explored, e.g., the radial symmetric base functions as they can be adapted to the properties of the mathematical function to be approximated. A much simpler approach for information retrieval would be to export the values of Figure 6.12 and therefrom derived features, e.g., a "sharpness" feature as a replacement for the GMM's σ values in the shape of $\frac{\Delta f}{ADV}$.

Another reason for the performance decay of the AM may be the lack of sufficient training data. For a fully automated generation of training data, however, one characteristic of the AM needs to be modified: the current AM adjusts the number of computed features to the given ECG recording. As only ARFF files with the same number of features can be merged, this characteristic of the AM requires a selection of appropriate ARFF files (see /7.5/). Hence, the processing of the AM needs some adaptation.

The evaluation of both spectral transformation based feature sets (see /7.4.9/ and /7.4.10/) was limited to the first 20 coefficients of the respective spectrum. Their quite promising performance suggests to run an additional evaluation on the full spectrum. An idea is not to evaluate consecutive coefficients, but only those seemingly containing relevant information. These coefficient ranges can be educed from Figures 6.74 and 6.86.

In the presented evaluations the features from the individual feature sets have only been evaluated separately. However, with the information about the most powerful features from each feature set at hand, new ARFF files can be created which comprise the best feature combinations. In the literature some authors mentioned that this approach yielded an improvement of the classification rates.

The information given in the medical introductory part allows to create further features, e.g., a double-peaked P-wave or AV-blocks. AV-blocks and arrhythmia are known to be linked to OSAS. Yet, they are not considered so far as they are not reliable markers, but merely an additional hint. However, if the job is (simply) to separate healthy from diseased subjects, these markers may well be considered. Regarding these markers long term ECG recordings are desirable as in OSAS subjects AV-blocks may occur during sleep, but vanish during wake state.

However, the current implementation of the distinctive ECG point detection is not suited for the detection of AV-blocks. The current implementation starts with the R-peaks and proceeds to the remaining points. Hence, successive P-waves which are characteristic for AV-blocks can not be found. The current implementation is well capable of distinguishing "missing R-peaks", but it can not tell failures of the sinu-atrial node from AV-blocks.

In the discussion of the last Chapter the difference between the "single events" EVA ml classifies and the "single events" a medical expert annotates was already explained (see /7.6/). Filtering EVA ml's decisions by a "physiology aware" filter and running this output through a neural network or a Hidden Markov Model should improve the overall classification results.

In [Roch 99] the authors claim that the differences between the corresponding nighttime and daytime parameters perform much better than the nighttime parameters themselves did. Accordingly, having daytime recordings as well is extremely valuable as it allows to compute subject specific set points. Considering these set points could increase the performance of the presented approaches, especially of the AM. However, the creation of a database combining daytime and nighttime recordings requires a more complex recording procedure which consists of a daytime holder ECG and a nighttime PSG recording.

For an efficient evaluation of all the different approaches the evaluation process has to be completely automated as the more or less manually conducted processing was way too time consuming and cumbersome. A fully automated evaluation process is essential for the heuristic search for the most suitable values in the processing configuration regarding the physiological timing.

Chapter 9

Summary

Among the fastest increasing sleep disorders are the so called "Sleep Related Breathing Disorders" (SRBD) whose central complaint are apneas. An apnea is the cessation of respiration during sleep. The lack of oxygen and the entailed short awakenings degrade sleep quality and cause cardiac sequel. As the usual diagnostic procedure is complex, this work is targeted at finding a way to retrieve the required information by evaluating an ECG signal.

As the SRBD event terminating arousals fragment the sleep, people suffering from SRBD commonly experience their sleep as non-restorative. 16% of male and 22% of the female study participants confessed daytime fatigue. Such study results make experts believe that more than the manifest 4% of the male and 2% of the female population actually suffer from sleep apnea.

Sleep is structured in six different sleep stages: wake stage, two light sleep and two deep sleep stages, and REM sleep. In general, the deep sleep stages are considered the period for the bodily recreation, and REM for the mental recreation. These stages alternate according to the sleep architecture. Its corruption by SRBD events is held responsible for the degeneration of sleep quality.

Apart from the daytime sleepiness which is held responsible for a large number of deadly car and machinery accidents the untreated continued suffering from SRBD entails severe damages to the cardio-vascular system.

As sleep disorders are complex, the diagnosis is complex as well: it starts with the exclusion of adverse habits, e.g., jetlag, organic disorders, and abuse of drugs and alcohol. If the SRBD persist, the patient is sent to a polysomnography (PSG).

A PSG is today's Gold Standard for diagnosing SRBD and assessing their severity. The procedure is expensive and requires experienced personnel. Moreover, patients supposed of suffering from sleep apnea often have to wait long times for their PSG. The approach of this work aims at simplifying the diagnostic procedure.

The standard therapy today are variations of the so called "continuous positive airway pressure" (CPAP) therapy where the patient is connected to an air pump via a mask.

The ECG signal is the electrical representation of the heart activity. It is generated as the superposition of the heart muscle fibers whose order of contraction is controlled by the cardiac conduction system. The signal is captured via electrodes which are attached around the patient's chest.

This work considers two main influences of SRBD events and sleep stages on the ECG: the heart rate variability (HRV) and morphological changes.

The heart rate is under the control of the autonomous nervous system (ANS) which consists of two antagonists: the sympathetic (SNS) and the parasympathetic nervous system (PNS). While the SNS increases the HR, the PNS decreases it. The arousals issue triggers to the SNS, thus, increasing the HR. An influence on the HR via the PNS is the sinus arrhythmia which is driven by the breathing.

The morphology of the ECG signal is altered by three means: the ANS, heart load changes, and ischemia driven effects. The ANS controls the repolarization process which is reflected in the T-wave and the ST-segment. SRBD events activate a vasoconstriction via the Euler-Liljestrand-Reflex which increases the "flow resistance" of the body. The heart counteracts this influence by increasing the output pressure. This additional load is reflected in the P-wave and the R-peak. The ischemic reactions are triggered by the oxygen lack which follows the SRBD event. The ST-segment and the T-wave are sensitive to ischemic influences.

Most of the approaches in the literature are based on a Physionet database for a Computers-in-Cardiology challenge. The subject's health state is supplied on a minute-by-minute basis and classified either as healthy or diseased. The approaches focus on the HR. Various mathematical methods like transformations, e.g., Fourier, Hilbert, and autoregressive models are applied to the HR series. Some of the approaches consider the shape of the ECG wave and extract features like the T-wave amplitude, the R-peak amplitude and the area under the R-peak to assess respiratory parameters. While the HR based approaches achieve classification rates from 80 - 96%, the results for the shape based approaches are usually poor. Accordingly, these results are summarized as "the main features are HR derived, but shape based feature may help improve classification rates".

As the approaches of this work aimed at detecting single SRBD events along with their types, the Physionet database was not applicable due to its limitations concerning temporal and event type resolution. Hence, for the purpose of this work a proprietary polysomnographic database including the full annotations about the on- and offset and the type of each event was recorded. Additionally, the artifacts in the ECG recording were annotated. The recordings were accomplished in the sleep laboratories of the clinical partners in Nuremberg and Marburg during the Bayrische Forschungsstiftung founded project "Sleep-Home-Monitoring".

The description of the ECG signal processing started with a short mention of adverse influences on the ECG signal during the recording. The effects discussed were the mains supply, DC-shifts, and general noise. The mains supply influence results in an additional frequency component of 50 Hz whose magnitude varies with the accurateness of the measurement setup. The DC-shifts are mainly caused by the patient moving in bed. Finally, the recording device itself introduces noise to the ECG recording. During the preprocessing of the ECG signal these adverse effects were eliminated by a combination of high- and lowpass filters. These filters featured very steep edges and linear phase to minimize the loss of morphologic information.

In the next processing step the distinctive ECG points were detected. The implemented algorithm started with the R-peaks and subsequently added the remaining distinctive points via a maximum/minimum-search.

Based on the medical introductions to SRBD and the ECG, new features were introduced which were to directly reflect activations or the status of the ANS, changing heart load conditions, and the influences of ischemia. These features were clustered in two groups – one based on the evaluation of the HR and the other considering the morphology of the ECG.

The HR is evaluated in the Autonomous Model (AM). The AM aims at reflecting the generation of the HR series. At the heart of the AM is a VCO which generates the frequency describing the HR (the shape of the output signal is not considered). This VCO is controlled by three arbitrary generators which symbolize the different influences on the HR.

These arbitrary generators are mapped to their physiological counterparts SNS, respiratory sinus arrhythmia, and noise. Hence, these generators are named G_{Symp} for the SNS and G_{Resp} for the sinus arrhythmia. The last generator G_{Noise} was intended to capture the remaining (or unspecific) influences which were not assigned a distinct meaning in the scope of the AM.

The AM algorithm mainly consists of two parts: first, there is the reverse-engineering of the HR generation to extract the output signals of the three generators. Second, the output signals are approximated by a GMM to characterize the properties of the generators.

The reverse-engineering of the AM consists of the following steps: computation of the HR series, FM-demodulation to compensate for the subject's personal HR at rest, computation of a template to track the dynamics of the generators along the evaluation periods, GMM approximation of the spectrum for each evaluation period to extract the changing characteristics of the generators, computing the signal energy of the generator G_{Noise}.

The GMM parameters are used to derive a measure for the HR and its stability as these parameters hint on HR fluctuations which are caused by SRBD events and the characteristics of each sleep stage. The HR is gathered from the mean values of the GMM and the stability from its standard deviations.

The morphological features evaluate the characteristics of single distinctive points, e.g., P and R, or the complete shape of an ECG wave. These points can be mapped to the dynamics of different body status indicators: the P-wave and the R-peak represent heart load changes, ischemic reactions are observable in the ST-segment and the T-wave, and the ANS influences are visible in, e.g., the Timing and the ICA based features. However, a feature set can usually be related to more than one indicator, e.g., the deviation based features can be mapped to any of the three indicators as the complete ECG wave is considered.

For each feature set various features are extracted. Among these features are usually the amplitude as absolute value or in relation to a reference. To capture the different response times of the physiological processes, some of the features consider past and future values of the currently processed feature. In addition to these common features each of the feature sets extracts specific attributes which relate to the characteristic way in which a distinctive point is sensitive to changes of one of the indicators, e.g., the ascent of the ST-segment or the negativeness of the T-wave.

In addition to the feature sets operating on one of the distinctive points or a segment of the ECG wave, there are four feature sets considering the overall shape. The deviation based features first create a reference and second compute the deviation of the current ECG wave from this template. The spectral transformation based feature sets either transform the complete ECG wave or the wave form which remains after an overnight mean was subtracted from the ECG wave. The ICA approach implements a model which is based on the assumption that a healthy ECG wave is superimposed by wave forms which represent SRBD event or sleep stage influences. Running the ICA algorithm on the recorded ECG wave shall separate these distinct wave forms from each other, so they can be evaluated individually.

The features were extracted in two different intervals: the first one was chosen with the target of the single event detection in mind resulting in a high temporal resolution of a beat-to-beat basis. The second evaluation interval was chosen according to the sleep laboratory standard interval of 30 seconds which was proposed by Rechtschaffen and Kales. Usually the beat-to-beat features were mapped to the 30 seconds interval by computing the mean and standard deviation of the respective value for this evaluation interval. However, additional features were created based on the consideration of previous evaluation intervals to capture long term dynamics in the physiological processes.

The feature extractor was implemented in a Matlab program named "EVA" (**E**CG **V**aluation **A**pplication). The ECG signal was read as 16-bit samples which were extracted from the proprietary data files of the polysomnography recorder. The feature extractor wrote the computed features along with the experts' annotations directly in the ARFF file format. This format is appropriate to be further evaluated in the WEKA data mining suite.

The R-peak detection performance was tested on Physionet test files with a total of 582 minutes. Given that the detected and the annotated R-peak position must not differ by more than one sample, the detection rate was $99.0 \pm 0.4\%$. The assessment of the remaining distinctive ECG point detection was performed visually on the database used for this work. Numerous random samples proved it comparably successful.

The further evaluations were performed using the WEKA data mining suite on five patients featuring an AHI from 5.4 - 98.5. At first, the best classifier for each combination of classification target and evaluation interval was sought using the 10-folds method. The evaluated classifiers were Bayes Net, RBF Network, Multilayer Perceptron, IBk, KStar, and Bagging (REP-Tree classifier). The classification results were assessed based on the kappa statistic. For the AM the best classifiers were IBk for the SRBD events and KStar for the sleep stages. For all morphology based feature sets the selected classifier was Bagging.

In a patient-dependent evaluation the SRBD event classification rate for AM was 85.2% in the RaK interval and 56.8% in the BtB interval. Concerning the sleep stages the AM achieved classification rates from 89.2 - 99.0% (depending on the sleep stage) in the RaK interval and 95.5 - 99.0% in the BtB interval. The evaluation of the produced feature values proved that the model had to be updated: the frequencies of the found generators rather fit the PNS than the SNS. The AM turned out to be most powerful feature set.

The morphology based feature sets achieved a classification rate of 91.5% in the RaK interval and of 70.3% in the BtB interval for the SRBD events. Concerning sleep stage classification this group of features achieved 81.1 - 92.7% in the RaK interval and 71.2 - 92.7% in the BtB interval. It is quite remarkable that this feature group obtained a classification rate of up to 86.4% for obstructive hypopneas.

Subsequently, a patient-independent evaluation was performed. For this purpose a database was created from the five patients evaluated so far with exactly as many N instances as the sum of all other SRBD events. The evaluation resulted in a classification rate of 79.2% for the timing based features in the RaK interval and 100% for the deviation based features in the BtB interval. For the sleep stage classification, the following results were achieved: wake state with 94.4% in the BtB interval using P-wave features, light sleep with 69.4% in the BtB interval using differential spectrum based features, deep sleep with 29.3% in the BtB interval, and REM with 35.5% in RaK interval, both using the deviation based features. Thus, these results were dominated by the morphological feature sets, while the AM dropped behind.

The discussion showed that the approach presented in this work was hardly comparable to existing approaches. While some findings matched the ones found in the literature, the classification rates achieved could not compete with the results of the state-of-the-art. Further steps to improve the classification rates were discussed.

The Outlook proposed further approaches to compensate for the decay of the classification rates from the patient-dependent to patient-independent evaluation: the consideration of further influences on the ANS balance and a replacement for the GMM.

A very important step is to have the evaluation process fully automated, so it can easily be run on more data for a more profound statistical evaluation.

Chapter 10

Appendix

This Chapter provides some background information on tools and mathematical principles which are used in this work.

10.1 Criteria for Rating the Concordance

This Section will give a short introduction to the "Kappa Coefficient" κ and its derivatives. The κ coefficient is a method of rating the concordance between two "opinions". It is based on the comparison between two different options, e.g., annotations and classifications, which are based on the same information.

This Section is based on [Grou 07] and [Weib 04].

10.1.1 Kappa Coefficient

The "Kappa Coefficient" κ was originally suggested by Jacob Cohen in 1960. His idea was to rate the concordance between two raters based on their "real competence" without considering "accidental agreements". Therefore, his coefficient aims at computing a "chance corrected concordance".

Consider two possible classes:

- **A** representing any abnormality during sleep, i.e., any event like apnea, hypopnea, and so on (which is quite tolerable as all events more or less entail the same sequels)

- **N** representing normal respiration

Given two raters (R_1 and R_2) and the these two classes Table 10.1 shows the possible combinations and their probabilities.

	$R1_A$	$R1_N$	
$R2_A$	p_{AA}	p_{AN}	$p_{A.}$
$R2_N$	p_{NA}	p_{NN}	$p_{N.}$
	$p_{.A}$	$p_{.N}$	$p_{..}=1$

Table 10.1: Permutation matrix of a two-class-problem

The probabilities p_{ij} in Table 10.1 have the following meaning: $i = j$ means that both raters have assigned an event to the same class, either **A** or **N**, whereas $i \neq j$ means that an event has been assigned to different classes by the raters.

The Kappa coefficient κ is defined as given in equations (10.1). In these equations p_o means the "observed concordance" and p_e means the "expected concordance". The expected concordance p_e represents the chance driven agreements in the annotations.

$$\kappa = \frac{p_o - p_e}{1 - p_e} \tag{10.1a}$$

with

$$p_o = p_{AA} + p_{NN} \tag{10.1b}$$

$$p_e = (p_{AA} + p_{AN}) \cdot (p_{AA} + p_{NA}) + (p_{NA} + p_{NN}) \cdot (p_{AN} + p_{NN}) \tag{10.1c}$$

The values for κ range from -1 to +1. $\kappa = +1$ means that there is perfect concordance between the two raters, likewise $\kappa = -1$ means that there is none at all. The special case of $\kappa = 0$ indicates that the concordance could have been achieved by random classification, i.e., both raters chose their class assignments without any skill.

This coefficient shows the so called *"Kappa Paradox"*: the value of κ strongly depends on the values of p_{NA} and p_{AN} and may vary significantly – about twofold – even if the true concordances, i.e., p_{AA} and p_{NN}, are constant. Moreover, the value of κ depends on the probability distribution of the classes. Hence, κ is considered a reliable measure of concordance only if the values of $p_{..}$ are "balanced", i.e., symmetric and of comparable dimension.

10.1.2 Modified Kappa Coefficient

To overcome the restrictions of κ, the so called "modified Kappa Coefficient κ_{mod}" was introduced. The equations of κ_{mod} are given in (10.2) with p_o being the same as in equation (10.1b).

10.2. Introduction to EVA ml

κ	Degree of Concordance
< 0.20	weak
0.21 - 0.40	light
0.41 - 0.60	moderate
0.61 - 0.80	good
0.81 - 1.00	very good

Table 10.2: Judging the degree of raters' concordance from the value of the kappa coefficient κ

$$\kappa_{mod} = \frac{p_o - p_c}{1 - p_c} \qquad (10.2a)$$

with

$$p_c = p_{AA}^2 + p_{NN}^2 \qquad (10.2b)$$

The benefit of κ_{mod} is that p_c includes only those parts of the marginal distribution which actually contribute to p_o, i.e., the observed concordance [Kuts 05].

Judging the Concordance by the Value of Kappa κ

The value range of κ (and κ_{mod}) varies from -1 to 1. But as $\kappa = 0$ means that any concordance in the annotations is purely accidental, negative values of κ are seldom which effectively limits the value range of κ to 0 - 1. To help interpret the remaining value range, Table 10.2 gives a rough rating which value of κ hints on which degree of raters' concordance.

The values given in Table 10.2 vary somewhat in literature.

10.2 Introduction to EVA ml

EVA ml is the feature extractor which was implemented in the scope of this work. An explanation of the extracted features is presented in Chapter 6. "EVA ml" is an acronym for "**E**CG e**V**aluation **A**pplication implemented in **M**atlab". The applied Matlab version is 7.4.0 (R2007a).

This Section provides a description of EVA ml. It begins with the selection of the processing options which EVA ml allows to select in two ways: the most common ones are selectable from the GUI. Additional options which control the behavior of the algorithms are available via the processing configuration (see /10.2.2/). Subse-

228   Chapter 10. Appendix

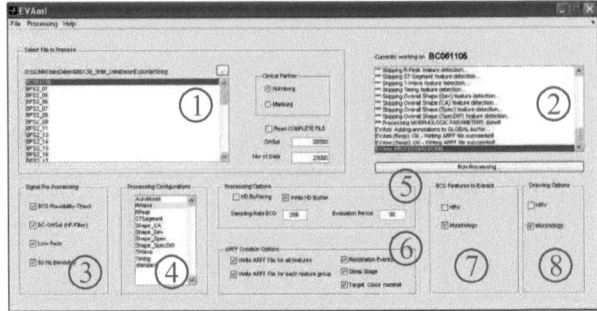

Figure 10.1: GUI of EVA ml having processed the morphological features of the P-wave

quently, there is an explanation of the successive processing step along a flow chart. Finally, an illustration of the various output options is presented.

10.2.1 The GUI of EVA ml

EVA ml provides a GUI which makes most of the features and some of the primary processing options conveniently available. An example of the GUI of EVA ml is displayed in Figure 10.1.

EVA ml's GUI is separated into eight areas. The first one (see Figure 10.1-1) is the file selection area. EVA ml automatically scans the selected input folder for processable ECG files and displays them within the list box. A file is selected by clicking on it. Either of the two clinical partners' annotations can be selected by setting the radio button to either "Nuremberg" or "Marburg". The last option in this area allows selecting, whether only a part of the file, specified by offset and number of data samples, or the complete file is to be read.

Area 2 (see Figure 10.1-2) is dominated by the progress and status indicator. The "Run Processing" button starts the processing of the ECG data.

The available preprocessing filters can be chosen in area 3 (see Figure 10.1-3): a high pass for DC-offsetting, a low pass for noise reduction, and a notch filter to cancel mains supply influences (see /3.1.2/ and /6.1/). The option "ECG Plausibility Check" scans the ECG data for artifacts, and emits the positions and the duration of the events.

In addition to the general processing options which are accessible via the GUI, further processing options for a specific feature set are set in a *.epc file (see /10.2.2/). This is an ASCII file (American Standard Code for Information In-

10.2. Introduction to EVA ml

terchange) which contains the processing parameter values. EVA ml automatically scans a preselected configuration folder and displays the available configuration files in area 4 (see Figure 10.1-4). A configuration file is selected by clicking on its name.

The upper two options in area 5 (see Figure 10.1-5) concern the HD Buffering. It allows to "snapshot" the processing state after the preprocessing and the distinctive point detection (see /6.2/). In subsequent processing calls this snapshot can be read back to spare processing time (about an hour for an eight hour recording).

If "Write HD Buffer" is selected, the snapshot of the preprocessed data is written to the HD under the name evaBF_*FileName*.ebf (EVA ml Buffer File), where *FileName* is the name of the currently selected file.

If "HD Buffering" is selected, EVA ml reads a previously stored snapshot skipping the preprocessing. If no snapshot is available for the selected file, processing is aborted issuing an according message.

The lower two options in area 5 specify the properties of the ECG recording, i.e., the sampling rate, and the evaluation period for the RaK ARFF files (see Section 10.2.3). These two options default to the sampling rate of the recordings made during the BFS project and an evaluation period of 30 seconds which was defined by Rechtschaffen and Kales.

Area 6 (see Figure 10.1-6) allows to select the output ARFF files (see p. 201). EVA ml can write ARFF files for two different classification targets, namely SRBD events and sleep stages. Additionally, the target class can be nominal, e.g., "Monday", "Tuesday" and so on, and numeric, e.g., "78". This option is intended to match the target class type expected by a given WEKA classifier.

Area 7 (see Figure 10.1-7) allows selecting the group(s) of features which should be extracted from the ECG – choosing "HRV" invokes the AM and choosing "Morphology" invokes the generation of morphology based features.

During the processing of the ECG signal EVA ml can plot diagrams which illustrate intermediate processing results (see /6/). The plotting of the diagrams can be selected for each group of features separately in area 8 (see Figure 10.1-8).

10.2.2 Processing Configurations

In addition to the general processing options available through EVA ml's GUI a compilation of more feature set specific processing options can be adjusted in the *configuration files*. One of these files can be selected via the GUI (see Figure 10.1-4). The feature set specific processing options consist of, e.g., thresholds for the detection of maxima, the number of spectral coefficients to write to the ARFF file, and the number of values to incorporate into the floating means.

Function	Number of Processing Parameters
hrvAutonomousModel()	20
morphPWave()	1
morphRPeak()	1
morphSTSegment()	5
morphTWave()	5
morphTiming()	1
morphShape_Dev()	1
morphShape_CA()	3
morphShape_Spec()	6
morphShape_SpecDiff()	5

Table 10.3: The processing functions and their numbers of processing parameters

The configuration files are ASCII files with the file extension *.epc ("EVA Processing Configuration"). Each line of the file contains either a comment or a value for one of the processing parameters. Comment lines start with '%' which is likewise the Matlab indicator for a comment. The lines containing processing parameter values have the following structure: $F\_P\ V$ where F is the name of the function the value belongs to, e.g., morphPWave(), P is the name of the parameter, e.g., flmnLen, and V is its value, e.g., 5.

In total, there are 48 parameters for all feature sets. Table 10.3 gives an overview of the number of configuration parameters for each feature set.

10.2.3 EVA ml processing Vital Data

As EVA ml provides a large scale of processing options, the following explanation only applies, if all the features are enabled. A flowchart is shown in Figure 10.2.

The first processing step is the **reading the processing configuration** from the currently selected configuration file (see /10.2.2/).

In the next step EVA ml **reads the data to process**. By default, the ECG and the selected exert's annotations are loaded. If the ARFF option "Sleep Stages" is selected, the corresponding hypnogram (see /2.4.2/) is loaded as well.

During the **preprocessing** step (see /6.1/) the selected filters (see Figure 10.1-3) are applied. Any displacement between the ECG and the annotations (and the hypogram) due to the filtering is compensated.

The **labeling of the distinctive ECG points** creates the basis for the following processing steps. As can be noticed in Figure 10.2 there is a slight difference for the two processing branches: for the AM this parameter is r-peaks resulting in the extraction of only the R-peaks, whereas for the morphological features the argument

10.2. Introduction to EVA ml

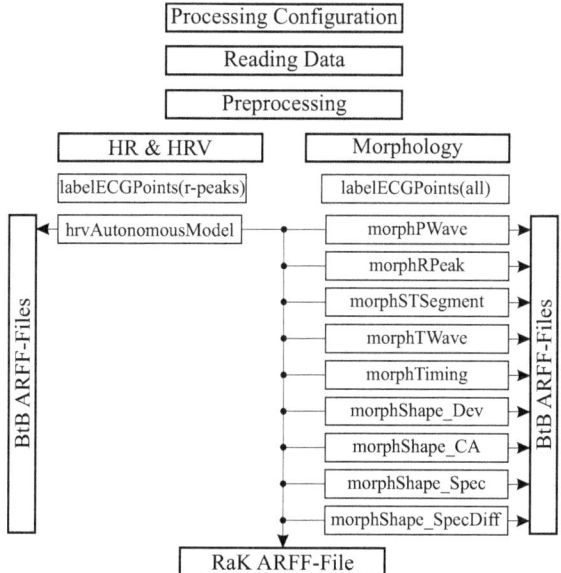

Figure 10.2: Flowchart of EVA ml

is all meaning all of the distinctive ECG points are to be extracted. As the detection of the ECG points may last up to two hours in an overnight recording with half of the time for the R-peak detection and the other half for the remaining points this feature helps to speed up processing, if only the AM is chosen.

The procedure is controlled by labelECGPoints(). labelECGPoints() returns a data vector the same length as the vector of ECG samples. At the beginning the output vector is initialized with the character "I" standing for "intermediate" which labels any point between the distinctive points. Subsequently, the individual detection functions for each distinctive point are called which replace an "I" by their respective label, i.e., for example "R", "P", and so on (see /6.2.1/, Figure 6.9).

Following the initial processing steps the **feature extraction** is handled by the approach specific functions. For each feature set there is one corresponding function. These functions take the preprocessed ECG signal, the labeled distinctive points, and the annotations. Additional parameters are sampling frequency and the duration of the evaluation period (see Figure 10.1-5).

The features for "each feature group", i.e., BtB based, are directly written to an function specific ARFF file. The features for "all features", i.e., RaK based, are stored in an internal buffer which will be written to an ARFF file after the processing of all selected feature sets.

The extracted features are written to various **output ARFF files**. According to the options selected in the GUI (see Figure 10.1-6) the ARFF files are written for any of the two classification targets and any of the two evaluation intervals.

Respiratory Events and Sleep Stages   To evaluate the classification rate of either the SRBD events or the sleep stages, their respective annotation can be selected to be grouped with the extracted features in the WEKA instances[1].

"All features" and "each feature group" ARFF Files   EVA ml allows to write the extracted features to ARFF files for two evaluation intervals: "each feature group" means that the features are extracted based on a beat-to-beat (BtB) interval, i.e., the features are extracted for each heart beat. These ARFF files are directly written by the respective feature extracting function, e.g., `morphPWave()` or `morphRPeak()`. Hence, there is an ARFF file for each selected feature extracting function.

By contrast, the "all features" option gathers the features from all selected feature extracting functions in a buffer and writes them to a single ARFF file at the end of the processing. These features are based on the RaK interval entered in EVA ml's GUI (see Figure 10.1-5).

Nominal and Numerical Target Classes   WEKA provides classifiers for nominal and numerical classes. Nominal means that a class consists of a few discrete values and the "values" are names. The days of the week are an example for a nominal class which consists of seven discrete values ("Monday" - "Sunday"). Numerical means that the target class is a numerical value or a range of values, e.g., the temperature.

EVA ml provides this option to fully benefit from the large package of WEKA classifiers. If "numerical" is selected the upper case letters, e.g., "N" and "A", denoting the different SRBD events are replaced by the respective numerical value according to the ASCII code, i.e., "N" is 78 and "A" is 65.

---

[1] A WEKA instance is a row vector containing the values of the feature and the class.

10.3 ECG derived Respiration

As the respiration influences the HR via the PNS (see /3.3.1/), the first idea to compensate for these influences in the scope of the AM (see /6.3/)was the following: derive the respiration directly from the ECG, compute its frequency and control ratio (see equation (6.1)), use these properties to mask them.

The medical basis for this approach is the amplitude modulation of the amplitudes of the R-peaks caused by the respiration. This phenomenon is entailed by the tilting of the heart in the chest by the periodically expanding lungs. More details can be found in /3.4.2/.

This approach starts with the amplitude demodulation of the ECG signal. This is performed by `BreathEnvelopeADM()`. In the first step this function detects the maxima of the input signal, i.e., the R-peaks, and starts a decaying exponential function at each of them. While the input signal is lower than the present value of the exponential function – which is usually true for all amplitudes between the R-peaks – this signal keeps decaying. This decay is to catch subsiding amplitudes of the R-peaks, e.g., caused by respiration. The timing parameters are computed in such a manner that from one R-peak to the next one the exponential function drops to approximately 80% of the starting value which presents a good compromise between the tracking of the changing R-peak amplitudes and the ripple produced. The moment the next R-peaks occurs the input signal is higher than the present value of the exponential function and the procedure starts over again. This behavior simulates the electronic amplitude demodulation approach, e.g., in radio tuners. For the demodulation of the lowest amplitude of an ECG signal, (usually) the Q-peak, the same procedure is performed with inverted signs.

In the next step the output signal of the amplitude demodulation process is filtered to cancel the ripple. Initially, a low pass filter kernel is computed which consists of a Blackman windowed sinc function. It features a cut-off frequency of 0.56 Hz and a transition band width of 0.6 Hz. More information on the design of this filter can be found in [Smit 99].

The final step of the amplitude demodulation process is the resynchronization of the filtered signal, as it is delayed by the application of the filter. The result is shown in Figure 10.3a: The blue curve is the input ECG signal. The red curve runs along the highest amplitudes, i.e., the R-peaks, and the pink curve runs along the lowest amplitudes, i.e., the Q-peaks. The "offset" to the highest or lowest amplitudes, respectively, is due to the low pass filtering: it performs a kind of meaning between the maxima, i.e., the R-peaks, and the lowest amplitudes of the decaying exponential functions.

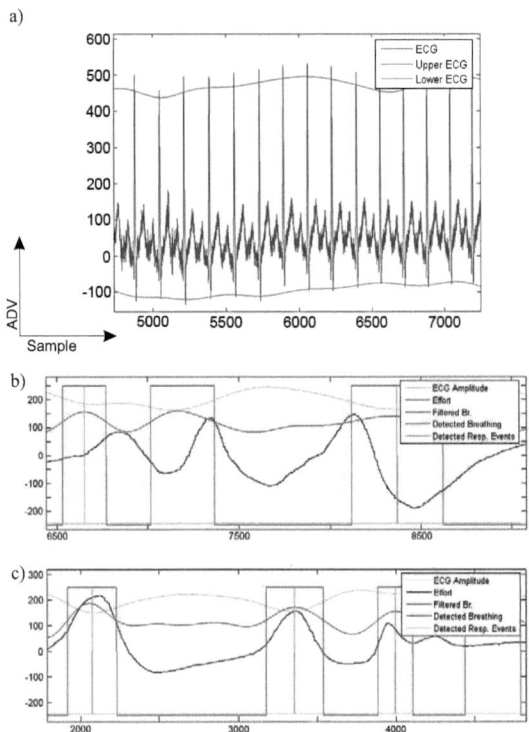

Figure 10.3: Principle and (visual) results of deriving the respiration from the ECG: a) The blue curve represents the ECG signal and in different tones of red the upper and lower amplitudes of the R-peaks after the AM demodulation are plotted. (The demodulated amplitudes are not running along the peaks and the base due to an implicit lowpass filtering.) b) & c) Visualizations of the results of the ECG derived respiration in comparison to the measured respiration as the sum of thoracic and abdominal respiratory effort (see PSG, /2.8.1/): The green spikes indicate where inspirations were detected by the algorithm and the black curve is the measured inspiration. Accordingly, b) illustrates a period of the ECG signal where the respiration was not detected very well, whereas c) illustrates an almost perfect reconstruction. (More details in the text)

Subsequently, `BreathDetectRespiration()` computes the respiration from the demodulated signal. According to parameters supplied during the function call this function applies the first or second derivation to extract the respiration. Finally, physiological restraints (concerning frequency and duration between events) are applied.

These different processing steps are illustrated in Figures 10.3b & c: The cyan curve is the total ECG amplitude, i.e., form the Q-peak to the R-peak, as computed by `BreathEnvelopeADM()`. The black curve is the measured respiration as the sum of thoracic and abdominal respiratory effort – both of them are provided by the Weinmann PSG system (see /2.8.1/). The blue curve is the computed intermediate respiration signal which is evaluated to produce "estimated respiration events". The estimated respiration events are plotted as the red square curve. The duty cycle of the red curve was intended to reflect inspiration and expiration durations. Finally, the green spikes indicate the estimated respiration events which passed the physiological filtering, i.e., these are the detected respiration events.

Accordingly, Figure 10.3b illustrates an episode of the ECG signal where the respiration was not detected very well, whereas Figure 10.3c illustrates an almost perfect reconstruction on an earlier (by the sample indices) episode of the same ECG signal.

Altogether, the results of extracting the respiration from the ECG amplitude alone were not satisfying. Most likely, they could have been improved by taking into consideration the sinus arrhythmia (see /3.3.1/) as well. However, the reason why this approach was finally rejected was the following: the general approach of compensating the parasympathetic influences by the generator G_{Resp} in Figure 6.11 was tested by matching the measured respiratory effort (from the PSG system) to the swings of the sinus arrhythmia induced HRV. This test did not succeed, i.e., the respiration introduced HRV was not in phase with the measured respiratory effort.

10.4 Principle of the Gaussian Mixture Model Approximation

The purpose of the Gaussian Mixture Model (GMM) is to reduce the amount of information necessary to describe a curve by approximating it with a set of Gaussian distributions (see [Niem 03] and [Schu 95]).

The black curve in Figure 10.4 consists of 201 single values. If these values are fed directly into a classifier, two problems occur:

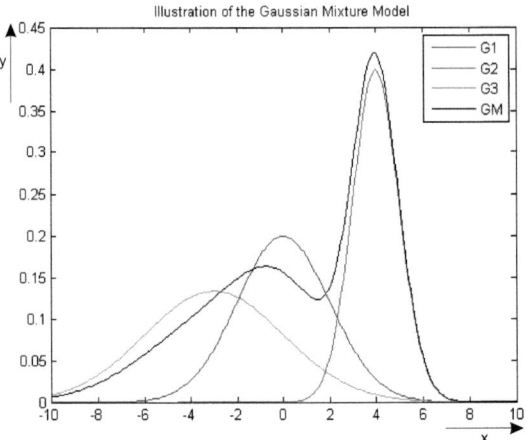

Figure 10.4: Principle of a GMM: Superposition of different Gaussian distributions to approximate a given curve, i.e., a computed spectrogram for the different evaluation periods in the context of this work

1. The high number of features makes it likely that the classifier becomes "cursed by dimensionality", i.e., it gets stuck.

2. The classifier does not "see" the construction principle of the curve which makes it somewhat hard to distinguish, how a second curve differs from this one.

In a GMM approximation, the same curve consists of mere nine parameters. How that? First, the general description of a Gaussian distribution is given in equation (10.3). This means that the complete curve can be completely specified with just two parameters – μ and σ.

$$f(x; \mu, \sigma) = \frac{1}{\sqrt{2\pi}\sigma} e^{-\frac{(x-\mu)^2}{2\sigma^2}} \tag{10.3}$$

Second, if a set of Gaussian distributions is summed to produce the black curve, e.g., the function $g()$, this can be written as shown in equation (10.4). In this equation, w_n is the weight of the nth Gaussian distribution, i.e., the degree to which this function contributes to $g()$, μ_n is the mean of the nth Gaussian distribution, i.e., the position of its axis of reflection, and σ_n is the variance of the nth Gaussian distribution, i.e., its width.

$$g(x; \mu_1, \ldots, \mu_n, \sigma_1, \ldots, \sigma_n) = \sum_{1}^{n} w_n \frac{1}{\sqrt{2\pi}\sigma_n} e^{-\frac{(x-\mu_n)^2}{2\sigma_n^2}} \tag{10.4}$$

10.5. Independent Component Analysis – ICA

Curve	μ	σ	w
blue	0	2	0.5
red	4	1	1.0
green	-3	3	0.7

Table 10.4: Properties of the different (exemplary) Gaussian distributions

The curves in Figure 10.4 have the properties given in Table 10.4. If they are summed up according to equation (10.4), the black curve results. But this time only nine (!) values suffice to describe the complete curve. Moreover, this mathematical description boosts a "kind of understanding" for the structure of the curve.

In practice, the EM algorithm is applied to decompose the given function $g(\ldots)$ into a combination of Gaussian distributions $f(x; \mu, \sigma)$. Usually, the decomposition can not approximate the target function perfectly and an approximation error remains. For more details see [Witt 05]. Figure 6.56 hints on one of the concerns in the application of the approximation algorithms.

10.5 Independent Component Analysis – ICA

This Section gives an overview of the Independent Component Analysis (ICA). It introduces the basic problem the ICA aims at solving and hints on the basic principles. A very profound introduction to the ICA and the related mathematics can be found in [Hyvr 01].

10.5.1 Introduction

The standard introductive example of the ICA is the *cocktail party problem*: at this party the guests are talking to one another simultaneously. If this situation was recorded with several microphones, each of them would percept all of the speakers with different levels of loudness as a mixture depending on the spacial properties of the party room. In this situation the ICA strives at demixing the speakers in such a manner that each speaker's voice can be separated from the others'.

From a more technical view: Several independent sources emit their output signals which need to be measured. Unfortunately, it is not possible to access the output of the sources separately – it is even impossible to access the mixture matrix, but only the mixture of the signals is accessible. This is why this situation is called the "Blind Source Separation" problem. The ICA aims at reversing the mixture process and delivering the independent source signals, i.e., providing an answer to the following question:

"... What could be a function from an m-dimensional space to an n-dimensional space such that the transformed variables give information on the data that is otherwise hidden in the large data set. That is, the transformed variables should be the underlying factors or components that describe the essential structure of the data. It is hoped that these components correspond to some physical causes that were involved in the process that generated the data in the first place ..." ([Hyvr01], p. 2)

10.5.2 Basic mathematical Principle

The assumption of the ICA is that the presumably *statistically independent* signals can be separated, if they differ in their statistical properties. The only requirement is that their probability density function (pdfs) is *non-Gaussian*.

The mixed signal can be derived from the individual signals in the following manner (see equation (10.5)):

$$m = \mathbf{M} \cdot s \qquad (10.5)$$

where m is the vector of the measurable mixed signals, M is the mixture matrix, and s is the vector of the individual signals. Accordingly, to perform the separation of the signals the reverse operation described by equation (10.6) has to be computed.

$$s = \mathbf{M}^{-1} \cdot m \qquad (10.6)$$

Hence, the job of the ICA can be defined as finding the inverse mixture matrix M^{-1}. For finding M^{-1} the ICA relies on a measure of statistical independence: the "kurtosis" κ. It is defined according to equation (10.7a).

$$\kappa = E\{(m - \mu_m)^4\} - 3 \cdot E\{(m - \mu_m)^2\}^2 \qquad (10.7a)$$

where

$$\sigma = E\{(m - \mu_m)^2\} \qquad (10.7b)$$

$$\mu_m = \frac{1}{N}\sum_{i=1}^{N} m_i \qquad (10.7c)$$

10.5. Independent Component Analysis – ICA

Equation (10.7b) defines the standard deviation (variance) and equation (10.7c) the mean with N being the number of elements. For a zero mean, i.e., $\mu_m = 0$, and a normalized pdf, i.e., $\sigma = 1$ the equation simplifies to:

$$\kappa = E\{m^4\} - 3 \tag{10.8}$$

The kurtosis provides a measure of the degree to which the pdf is Gaussian:

- $\kappa = 0$ means the pdf is Gaussian (for examples, see the green, red, and blue curves in Figure 10.4)

- $\kappa < 0$ means the pdf is sub-Gaussian, i.e., flat (example: uniform distribution)

- $\kappa > 0$ means the pdf is super-Gaussian, i.e., peaked (example: Laplace distribution)

One of the principles of performing the ICA is the *maximization of Gaussianity*. This can be considered as inversion of the *Central Limit Theorem*. The Central Limit Theorem states that the pdf of any mixture of random variables is more Gaussian than any of its components. At the limit, if an infinite number of components is mixed, their joint pdf is Gaussian. Having the kurtosis as a measurement of Gaussianity the algorithm unmixes the components in such a manner that their joint pdf is least Gaussian.

There are several implementations of the ICA algorithm. The most popular are:

- FastICA

- JADE (Joint Approximate Diagonalization of Eigenmatrices)

- infomax (Information Maximization)

More details on the ICA and its limitations – especially the *scaling problem*, *permutation problem*, and the requirements concerning the input signals can be found in ([Clif06], p. 157 - 167).

Is the ICA applicable?

Usually, ICA is run on signals which were recorded from *different microphones simultaneously*. However, this differs from the way the ICA is applied in this work: morphShape_CA() applies the ICA on ECG signals which were recorded from *one "microphone"*, i.e., *one set of ECG electrodes, successively*. This puts into question, whether the ICA can be applied at all. The answer is provided in the following:

Separation of ECG and different noises [Voss 08] shows the practical application of the ICA on ECG signals to remove noises, e.g., electrical potential of the respiratory muscles, motion artifacts. The different noise types were "artificial signals" which were generated according to mathematical definitions. Thus, the ICA derived components, i.e., ECG and noise, could be compared to the original signals. The results of this work proved that the different types of influences on the ECG recording can be separated as long as they differ sufficiently in their pdfs.

ECG as ergodic process The generation of the ECG signal is controlled by the cardiac conduction system (see /3.1/ and Figure 3.2). This process surely shows some inter-subject variations and the frequency varies with physical activity. However, the analyzed ECG recording arises in a *single* subject and the creation of the ECG buffer (see Figure 6.50) cancels frequency influences. Hence, the ECG generation process can be considered a stable process.

Stable process are called *ergodic processes* in statistical terminology. In ergodic processes the observation of different realizations of a process can be replaced by the continuous observation of a *single realization* of the process. The consequence of this property is that the statistical parameters of the process do not have to be calculated by considering numerous realizations of the process, but can be calculated from a series of samples of the observed process.

Spectral separability There is evidence in [Davi 07] that even a *underdetermined ICA*, i.e., (theoretically[2]) too little independent data to retrieve all components, may decompose all components, if they are spectrally separable. Given that the heart beats (approximately) once a second and the ANS features time constants of about 3 - 40 seconds, these components should be distinguishable by the ICA .

Temporal structure of the ECG According to [Hyvr 01] the requirement of the spectral separability for the independent signals can be "softened", if the signals feature a "temporal structure". In this case, the covariance matrix provides additional information for the ICA. The ECG signal represents such "time structured data", i.e., the samples can not be reordered without loss of information.

In any case, even if the ICA should fail to separate all independent components of the ECG signal, the ICA may still reveal "interesting features" ([Davi 07], p. 1821) – and this may quite well be all that is of interest in the context of this work.

---

[2]Concerning a complete theoretical solution to this problem research is still going on; yet, most researches seem to believe that there should be a solution. However, the proof so far is only available for spectrally disjunct signals and may require an infinite number of samples.

In the end, the results (see Chapters 6 and 7) prove that the ECG component is reconstructed correctly. Hence, the assumptions leading to the application of the ICA hold true.

10.6 Definitions of applied Means

Throughout this work three different "types" of means are applied in various contexts. They are defined here in an overview:

$$m(f) = \frac{1}{|f|} \cdot \sum_{n=1}^{|f|} f(n) \qquad (10.9a)$$

$$m_c(f(x), l) = \frac{1}{l} \cdot \sum_{n=x-\frac{l-1}{2}}^{x+\frac{l-1}{2}} f(n) \qquad (10.9b)$$

$$m_d(f(x), l) = \frac{1}{l} \cdot \sum_{n=x-l+1}^{x} f(n) \qquad (10.9c)$$

$m(f)$ defined in equation (10.9a) is the "standard mean", i.e., it is the mean value of all samples of the vector f. $m_c(f(x), l)$ (see equation (10.9b)) and $m_d(f(x), l)$ (see equation (10.9c)) are both "floating means" which means they represent the mean value of a section of data. Hence, the value of the "floating means" depends on the position of the sections which is why the function parameter is $f(x)$ with f being the data vector and x the position within this vector. The difference between $m_c(f(x), l)$ and $m_d(f(x), l)$ is the relative position of the data sample $f(x)$: for $m_c(f(x), l)$ this value is centered in the data section, whereas for $m_d(f(x), l)$ this value is the last within the data section, i.e., $m_d(f(x), l)$ is **d**elayed. In both equations "l" defines the length of the data section. As the indices into the data vector have to be integer values, "l" is an odd number.

Usually, if the exact position of the means $m_c(f(x), l)$ and $m_d(f(x), l)$ is of no importance (in the context of the description), the exact position x is left out. In these cases, $m_c(f, l)$ and $m_d(f, l)$ refer to $m_c(f(x), l)$ and $m_c(f(x), l)$, respectively.

10.7 Applied Classifiers

WEKA classifiers from different families were applied to figure out, whether there are (types of) classifiers which are "more suitable" for the problem. This Section will give a short introduction to the applied classifiers and their properties. This Section is mainly based on [Witt 05], [Schu 95], and [Niem 03].

10.7.1 Bayes Networks

Naive Bayes classifiers are based on Bayes's rule of *conditional probability*. In theory, their application is only "allowed", if the events, i.e., the attributes in the ARFF file, are statistically independent. Even though, this assumption does not hold true for many "real life" classification tasks they are applied to, they are known to show good results.

More information on the WEKA BayesNet classifier and its settings can be found in [Bouc 08a]. General information on Bayes Nets is provided in [Moor 01] and [Char 91].

10.7.2 RBFNetwork and MultilayerPerceptron

These classifiers belong to the family of function classifiers. Classifiers of this family are characterized by the fact that they "can be written down as mathematical equations in a reasonably natural way" [Witt 05], i.e., they are (mathematical) functions.

"RBFNetwork implements a Gaussian radial basis function network" [Witt 05]. The radial basis functions are used to map the distance between two points, i.e., one point in the input space and one in the output space, into a measure of similarity. The center values and the width – in the case of the Gaussian function the mean and the variance values – are learned during the training phase. RBFNetwork provides a hidden layer between the input and the output space whose output is put to a logistic regression in the case of nominal classes which is true for the chosen settings of EVA ml. A drawback of the RBFNetwork classifier is that it considers every attribute equally important, i.e., each attribute is given the same weight. Accordingly, it can not deal efficiently with irrelevant attributes – something the Multilayer Perceptron can.

"Multilayer Perceptron is a neural network that trains using back-propagation" [Witt 05]. The principle mechanism of back-propagation is the following:

- Apply input values.

- The output of the neural network is related to the *expected, i.e., known,* output. The deviation is considered the error.

- This error is back-propagated to the input optimizing the weights of the neural nodes with a gradient descent mechanism.

10.8. Detailed Classification Results

This back-propagation process is responsible for the improved capabilities of the Multilayer Perceptron in dealing with irrelevant attributes.

10.7.3 IBk and KStar

These two classifiers belong to the family of "lazy classifiers". They owe their name to the fact that they do nothing but store the training instances during the training phase. Their work cycle starts with the initiation of the classification.

"IBk is a k-nearest-neighbor classifier" [Witt 05] which uses the Euclidean distance measure. A k-nearest-neighbor classifier is essentially a nearest-neighbor classifier which assigns a test instance to the same class as the *nearest neighbor* in the training set. For an improved noise resistance this classifier does not considering just *one* nearest neighbor but k of them.

"KStar is a nearest-neighbor classifier with a generalized distance function which is based on transformations." [Witt 05] These transformations are made of a "sequence of predefined elementary operations".

10.7.4 Bagging

Bagging belongs to the family of the meta learning algorithms. Their characteristic is that they take an existent classifier, e.g., a decision tree, and improve its learning capability by internally training several decision tree classifiers from several pieces of the training data. If it comes to classifying a test instance, this instance is supplied to all the internal, i.e., "bagged", decision trees and the final classification is produced by a majority decision, i.e., the class receiving the most votes from the internal decision trees is the one selected.

The idea behind this concept is that the structure of these internal decision trees – most likely – varies due to noise or slight changes in the statistical properties of each of the training data pieces. During the classification process these slight variations in the internal decision trees annihilate one another and make the decision process more robust.

In the context of this work the "bagged" classifier is a REP-tree. This is a fast tree-learner deleting branches according to "reduced error pruning" [Witt 05].

10.8 Detailed Classification Results

This Section presents the Tables containing the detailed classification results for each feature set. For each of the feature sets there are two Tables, i.e., one for each of the classification targets. An explanation and discussion of these values is given in /7.4/.

The Tables 10.5 through 10.24 show the following parameters: the absolute percentage of each event type as annotated by the medical experts, i.e., the number of annotated events of a given type divided by the complete number of all events, the classification rate of a given event type as given by equation (7.1a), and the corresponding F-Measure for the healthy (AHI: 5.4) and the diseased (AHI: 33.9) subject, respectively. These values are provided for the two different evaluation intervals, i.e., BtB and RaK.

10.8. Detailed Classification Results

10.8.1 Autonomous Model

		abs %	Class. Rate [%]	F-Measure
healthy	RaK	N: 97.4	97.4	0.98
		O: 0.2	0.0	0.00
		H: 2.3	33.3	0.29
		M: 0.0	(undefined)	0.00
		C: 0.0	(undefined)	0.00
		X: 0.2	0.0	0.00
	BtB	N: 97.0	97.6	0.98
		O: 0.2	0.0	0.00
		H: 2.5	35.3	0.35
		M: 0.0	(undefined)	0.00
		C: 0.1	0.0	0.00
		X: 0.2	50.0	0.25
∅	RaK	N: 76.3 ± 24.0	87.4 ± 10.3	
		O: 7.2 ± 8.3	41.1 ± 26.8	
		H: 14.0 ± 16.1	44.5 ± 15.3	
		M: 1.9 ± 4.1	18.4 ± 27.8	
		C: 0.2 ± 0.3	4.9 ± 8.1	
		X: 0.4 ± 0.4	40.2 ± 24.2	
	BtB	N: 78.0 ± 19.4	83.1 ± 14.8	
		O: 6.8 ± 7.6	32.2 ± 23.5	
		H: 13.0 ± 12.4	38.2 ± 12.2	
		M: 1.5 ± 3.0	28.1 ± 26.7	
		C: 0.4 ± 0.4	4.7 ± 5.3	
		X: 0.4 ± 0.5	60.5 ± 21.7	
diseased	RaK	N: 41.6	76.3	0.76
		O: 8.1	37.0	0.37
		H: 40.9	71.7	0.70
		M: 9.3	60.2	0.54
		C: 0.2	0.0	0.0
		X: 0.0	(undefined)	0.0
	BtB	N: 51.3	59.7	0.59
		O: 8.4	47.8	0.46
		H: 32.7	50.6	0.50
		M: 7.0	52.2	0.51
		C: 0.7	7.1	0.09
		X: 0.0	(undefined)	0.0

Table 10.5: Detailed SRBD event classification results for the Autonomous Model features. Further explanation is given in /7.4.1/.

		abs %	Class. Rate [%]	F-Measure
healthy	RaK	W: 27.3	90.3	0.91
		S1: 4.3	37.0	0.37
		S2: 29.9	89.9	0.88
		S3: 4.2	84.5	0.83
		S4: 14.3	98.0	0.96
		REM: 20.0	89.2	0.91
	BtB	W: 31.2	96.2	0.96
		S1: 4.3	74.7	0.69
		S2: 28.9	95.1	0.95
		S3: 4.6	92.5	0.93
		S4: 15.3	99.0	0.99
		REM: 15.8	96.9	0.97
∅	RaK	W: 28.2 ± 8.8	88.2 ± 3.9	
		S1: 5.1 ± 2.2	49.7 ± 11.5	
		S2: 40.3 ± 12.0	90.3 ± 2.8	
		S3: 8.1 ± 2.7	82.0 ± 6.9	
		S4: 7.8 ± 6.3	86.1 ± 14.2	
		REM: 10.6 ± 5.5	85.1 ± 3.6	
	BtB	W: 30.3 ± 8.5	96.1 ± 1.7	
		S1: 5.1 ± 2.0	76.5 ± 5.5	
		S2: 39.5 ± 12.3	96.0 ± 1.3	
		S3: 8.0 ± 2.6	93.1 ± 2.0	
		S4: 7.9 ± 6.4	97.3 ± 2.5	
		REM: 9.2 ± 3.9	94.9 ± 1.5	
diseased	RaK	W: 16.3	86.6	0.88
		S1: 4.7	61.7	0.64
		S2: 59.7	94.5	0.93
		S3: 8.8	72.7	0.74
		S4: 1.0	70.0	0.55
		REM: 9.6	88.5	0.87
	BtB	W: 18.6	95.5	0.95
		S1: 4.9	80.9	0.82
		S2: 59.0	97.3	0.97
		S3: 9.0	92.5	0.92
		S4: 1.0	95.0	0.93
		REM: 7.5	95.1	0.93

Table 10.6: Detailed sleep stage classification results for the Autonomous Model features. Further explanation is given in /7.4.1/.

10.8.2 P-Wave

		abs %	Class. Rate [%]	F-Measure
healthy	RaK	N: 97.4	100.0	0.99
		O: 0.2	0.0	0.0
		H: 2.3	0.0	0.0
		M: 0.0	(undefined)	0.0
		C: 0.0	(undefined)	0.0
		X: 0.2	0.0	0.0
	BtB	N: 97.2	100.0	0.99
		O: 0.2	0.0	0.0
		H: 2.3	0.0	0.0
		M: 0.0	(undefined)	0.0
		C: 0.1	0.0	0.0
		X: 0.1	61.0	0.69
∅	RaK	N: 76.3 ± 24.0	90.9 ± 13.2	
		O: 7.2 ± 8.3	5.7 ± 10.4	
		H: 14.0 ± 16.1	21.3 ± 32.9	
		M: 1.9 ± 4.1	6.1 ± 10.6	
		C: 0.2 ± 0.3	0 ± 0	
		X: 0.4 ± 0.4	30.2 ± 35.6	
	BtB	N: 79.3 ± 18.1	94.9 ± 7.6	
		O: 6.5 ± 7.4	3.5 ± 5.0	
		H: 12.2 ± 11.4	8.4 ± 15.5	
		M: 1.3 ± 2.7	0.5 ± 0.9	
		C: 0.5 ± 0.5	0 ± 0	
		X: 0.2 ± 0.3	59.9 ± 11.7	
diseased	RaK	N: 41.6	70.8	0.71
		O: 8.1	1.2	0.02
		H: 40.9	74.9	0.65
		M: 9.3	18.3	0.25
		C: 0.2	0.0	0.0
		X: 0.0	(undefined)	0.0
	BtB	N: 55.7	82.5	0.70
		O: 7.5	0.4	0.01
		H: 29.8	35.9	0.40
		M: 6.1	1.5	0.03
		C: 0.9	0.0	0.0
		X: 0.0	(undefined)	0.0

Table 10.7: Detailed SRBD event classification results for the P-wave features. Further explanation is given in /7.4.2/.

			abs %	Class. Rate [%]	F-Measure
healthy		RaK	W: 27.3	80.3	0.76
			S1: 4.3	0.0	0.00
			S2: 29.9	66.6	0.59
			S3: 4.2	4.4	0.08
			S4: 14.3	80.9	0.72
			REM: 20.0	34.4	0.40
		BtB	W: 29.6	64.2	0.55
			S1: 4.3	0.5	0.01
			S2: 28.5	46.4	0.42
			S3: 4.2	1.7	0.03
			S4: 14.3	34.9	0.37
			REM: 19.1	20.3	0.24
∅		RaK	W: 28.2 ± 8.8	65.3 ± 18.1	
			S1: 5.1 ± 2.2	2.2 ± 3.8	
			S2: 40.3 ± 12.0	75.7 ± 10.0	
			S3: 8.1 ± 2.7	12.4 ± 6.8	
			S4: 7.8 ± 6.3	49.6 ± 30.9	
			REM: 10.6 ± 5.5	21.2 ± 16.3	
		BtB	W: 29.7 ± 8.6	55.6 ± 15.7	
			S1: 5.0 ± 2.2	1.3 ± 1.3	
			S2: 39.1 ± 11.7	68.7 ± 16.8	
			S3: 8.0 ± 2.7	4.1 ± 1.8	
			S4: 7.7 ± 6.1	21.1 ± 16.5	
			REM: 10.5 ± 5.2	11.6 ± 6.0	
diseased		RaK	W: 16.3	42.7	0.47
			S1: 4.7	2.1	0.04
			S2: 59.7	91.7	0.77
			S3: 8.8	6.8	0.12
			S4: 1.0	0.0	0.00
			REM: 9.6	10.4	0.16
		BtB	W: 18.5	42.3	0.51
			S1: 4.9	3.0	0.05
			S2: 57.6	93.2	0.76
			S3: 8.5	4.5	0.08
			S4: 1.0	0.0	0.00
			REM: 9.5	8.9	0.14

Table 10.8: Detailed sleep stage classification results for the P-wave features. Further explanation is given in /7.4.2/.

10.8.3 R-Peak

		abs %	Class. Rate [%]	F-Measure
healthy	RaK	N: 97.4	100.0	0.99
		O: 0.2	0.0	0.00
		H: 2.3	0.0	0.00
		M: 0.0	(undefined)	0.00
		C: 0.0	(undefined)	0.00
		X: 0.2	0.0	0.00
	BtB	N: 97.2	99.8	0.99
		O: 0.2	0.0	0.00
		H: 2.3	3.7	0.07
		M: 0.0	(undefined)	0.00
		C: 0.1	0.0	0.00
		X: 0.1	56.1	0.66
∅	RaK	N: 76.3 ± 24.0	92.0 ± 10.8	
		O: 7.2 ± 8.3	19.0 ± 24.4	
		H: 14.0 ± 16.1	22.0 ± 34.6	
		M: 1.9 ± 4.1	2.9 ± 5.0	
		C: 0.2 ± 0.3	0 ± 0	
		X: 0.4 ± 0.4	15.4 ± 30.8	
	BtB	N: 79.3 ± 18.1	93.6 ± 8.2	
		O: 6.5 ± 7.4	13.3 ± 16.2	
		H: 12.2 ± 11.4	18.0 ± 22.4	
		M: 1.3 ± 2.7	6.2 ± 5.4	
		C: 0.5 ± 0.5	8.4 ± 8.7	
		X: 0.2 ± 0.3	58.0 ± 11.3	
diseased	RaK	N: 41.6	74.9	0.77
		O: 8.1	3.7	0.07
		H: 40.9	79.8	0.67
		M: 9.3	8.6	0.13
		C: 0.2	0.0	0.00
		X: 0.0	(undefined)	0.00
	BtB	N: 55.7	80.8	0.76
		O: 7.5	4.2	0.07
		H: 29.8	57.5	0.54
		M: 6.1	10.1	0.16
		C: 0.9	11.1	0.20
		X: 0.0	(undefined)	0.00

Table 10.9: Detailed SRBD event classification results for the R-peak features. Further explanation is given in /7.4.3/.

		abs %	Class. Rate [%]	F-Measure
healthy	RaK	W: 27.3	88.2	0.83
		S1: 4.3	4.3	0.07
		S2: 29.9	77.6	0.76
		S3: 4.2	17.8	0.28
		S4: 14.3	86.2	0.83
		REM: 20.0	78.8	0.76
	BtB	W: 29.6	72.8	0.70
		S1: 4.3	10.2	0.16
		S2: 28.5	66.4	0.67
		S3: 4.2	3.8	0.07
		S4: 14.3	58.8	0.57
		REM: 19.1	56.7	0.53
∅	RaK	W: 28.2 ± 8.8	79.4 ± 7.1	
		S1: 5.1 ± 2.2	8.3 ± 6.2	
		S2: 40.3 ± 12.0	82.3 ± 6.6	
		S3: 8.1 ± 2.7	18.9 ± 7.7	
		S4: 7.8 ± 6.3	55.6 ± 36.7	
		REM: 10.6 ± 5.5	38.7 ± 24.9	
	BtB	W: 29.7 ± 8.6	68.2 ± 9.7	
		S1: 5.0 ± 2.2	8.6 ± 4.9	
		S2: 39.1 ± 11.7	73.9 ± 10.4	
		S3: 8.0 ± 2.7	9.5 ± 4.3	
		S4: 7.7 ± 6.1	37.2 ± 26.9	
		REM: 10.5 ± 5.2	27.5 ± 17.1	
diseased	RaK	W: 16.3	74.4	0.73
		S1: 4.7	4.3	0.07
		S2: 59.7	93.2	0.82
		S3: 8.8	15.9	0.24
		S4: 1.0	0.0	0.00
		REM: 9.6	18.8	0.30
	BtB	W: 18.5	70.7	0.72
		S1: 4.9	13.7	0.20
		S2: 57.6	91.6	0.80
		S3: 8.5	8.9	0.14
		S4: 1.0	0.0	0.00
		REM: 9.5	18.1	0.27

Table 10.10: Detailed sleep stage classification results for the R-peak features. Further explanation is given in /7.4.3/.

10.8.4 ST-Segment

			abs %	Class. Rate [%]	F-Measure
healthy		RaK	N: 97.4	100.0	0.99
			O: 0.2	0.0	0.00
			H: 2.3	0.0	0.00
			M: 0.0	(undefined)	0.00
			C: 0.0	(undefined)	0.00
			X: 0.2	0.0	0.00
		BtB	N: 97.2	99.9	0.99
			O: 0.2	0.0	0.00
			H: 2.3	2.7	0.05
			M: 0.0	(undefined)	0.00
			C: 0.1	0.0	0.00
			X: 0.1	56.1	0.00
∅		RaK	N: 76.3 ± 24.0	92.1 ± 10.6	
			O: 7.2 ± 8.3	24.4 ± 33.7	
			H: 14.0 ± 16.1	28.4 ± 35.1	
			M: 1.9 ± 4.1	11.5 ± 19.9	
			C: 0.2 ± 0.3	0 ± 0	
			X: 0.4 ± 0.4	9.6 ± 19.3	
		BtB	N: 79.3 ± 18.1	94.5 ± 7.8	
			O: 6.5 ± 7.4	17.0 ± 24.8	
			H: 12.2 ± 11.4	19.1 ± 20.2	
			M: 1.3 ± 2.7	7.4 ± 12.8	
			C: 0.5 ± 0.5	0.3 ± 0.5	
			X: 0.2 ± 0.3	48.3 ± 6.9	
diseased		RaK	N: 41.6	75.8	0.79
			O: 8.1	0.0	0.00
			H: 40.9	83.7	0.72
			M: 9.3	34.4	0.41
			C: 0.2	0.0	0.00
			X: 0.0	(undefined)	0.00
		BtB	N: 55.7	81.8	0.75
			O: 7.5	2.4	0.04
			H: 29.8	49.2	0.48
			M: 6.1	22.2	0.30
			C: 0.9	0.0	0.00
			X: 0.0	(undefined)	0.00

Table 10.11: Detailed SRBD event classification results for the ST-segment features. Further explanation is given in /7.4.4/.

		abs %	Class. Rate [%]	F-Measure
healthy	RaK	W: 27.3	91.7	0.91
		S1: 4.3	6.5	0.11
		S2: 29.9	83.6	0.77
		S3: 4.2	33.3	0.42
		S4: 14.3	88.2	0.86
		REM: 20.0	70.3	0.73
	BtB	W: 29.6	86.9	0.87
		S1: 4.3	7.7	0.13
		S2: 28.5	72.7	0.66
		S3: 4.2	6.5	0.11
		S4: 14.3	77.5	0.69
		REM: 19.1	49.6	0.53
∅	RaK	W: 28.2 ± 8.8	82.9 ± 8.0	
		S1: 5.1 ± 2.2	5.5 ± 3.2	
		S2: 40.3 ± 12.0	85.0 ± 4.3	
		S3: 8.1 ± 2.7	25.6 ± 8.8	
		S4: 7.8 ± 6.3	64.9 ± 37.7	
		REM: 10.6 ± 5.5	44.0 ± 18.4	
	BtB	W: 29.7 ± 8.6	74.1 ± 13.0	
		S1: 5.0 ± 2.2	5.9 ± 4.1	
		S2: 39.1 ± 11.7	78.0 ± 8.0	
		S3: 8.0 ± 2.7	11.1 ± 7.1	
		S4: 7.7 ± 6.1	38.9 ± 34.5	
		REM: 10.5 ± 5.2	25.4 ± 14.0	
diseased	RaK	W: 16.3	82.3	0.78
		S1: 4.7	8.5	0.16
		S2: 59.7	91.7	0.83
		S3: 8.8	26.1	0.33
		S4: 1.0	0.0	0.00
		REM: 9.6	19.8	0.29
	BtB	W: 18.5	69.2	0.68
		S1: 4.9	4.9	0.08
		S2: 57.6	91.5	0.80
		S3: 8.5	11.5	0.18
		S4: 1.0	0.3	0.01
		REM: 9.5	14.3	0.22

Table 10.12: Detailed sleep stage classification results for the ST-segment features. Further explanation is given in /7.4.4/.

10.8.5 T-Wave

		abs %	Class. Rate [%]	F-Measure
healthy	RaK	N: 97.4	100.0	0.99
		O: 0.2	0.0	0.00
		H: 2.3	0.0	0.00
		M: 0.0	(undefined)	0.00
		C: 0.0	(undefined)	0.00
		X: 0.2	0.0	0.00
	BtB	N: 97.2	100.0	0.99
		O: 0.2	0.0	0.00
		H: 2.3	0.7	0.01
		M: 0.0	(undefined)	0.00
		C: 0.1	0.0	0.00
		X: 0.1	51.2	0.68
∅	RaK	N: 76.3 ± 24.0	91.6 ± 12.9	
		O: 7.2 ± 8.3	10.0 ± 14.1	
		H: 14.0 ± 16.1	23.2 ± 35.6	
		M: 1.9 ± 4.1	5.7 ± 9.9	
		C: 0.2 ± 0.3	0 ± 0	
		X: 0.4 ± 0.4	1.9 ± 3.9	
	BtB	N: 79.3 ± 18.1	95.1 ± 7.0	
		O: 6.5 ± 7.4	7.0 ± 7.0	
		H: 12.2 ± 11.4	14.9 ± 19.7	
		M: 1.3 ± 2.7	3.8 ± 5.8	
		C: 0.5 ± 0.5	2.7 ± 2.4	
		X: 0.2 ± 0.3	40.8 ± 19.5	
diseased	RaK	N: 41.6	70.3	0.76
		O: 8.1	1.2	0.02
		H: 40.9	83.0	0.67
		M: 9.3	17.2	0.24
		C: 0.2	0.0	0.00
		X: 0.0	(undefined)	0.00
	BtB	N: 55.7	83.8	0.76
		O: 7.5	3.5	0.06
		H: 29.8	49.7	0.49
		M: 6.1	10.5	0.16
		C: 0.9	5.7	0.11
		X: 0.0	(undefined)	0.00

Table 10.13: Detailed SRBD event classification results for the T-wave features. Further explanation is given in /7.4.5/.

		abs %	Class. Rate [%]	F-Measure
healthy	RaK	W: 27.3	89.6	0.89
		S1: 4.3	13.0	0.22
		S2: 29.9	82.0	0.73
		S3: 4.2	2.2	0.04
		S4: 14.3	85.5	0.79
		REM: 20.0	50.5	0.55
	BtB	W: 29.6	83.5	0.80
		S1: 4.3	6.9	0.12
		S2: 28.5	69.9	0.62
		S3: 4.2	3.7	0.06
		S4: 14.3	66.7	0.62
		REM: 19.1	37.2	0.42
∅	RaK	W: 28.2 ± 8.8	75.3 ± 12.9	
		S1: 5.1 ± 2.2	9.5 ± 5.0	
		S2: 40.3 ± 12.0	82.9 ± 6.0	
		S3: 8.1 ± 2.7	15.4 ± 11.1	
		S4: 7.8 ± 6.3	63.3 ± 36.1	
		REM: 10.6 ± 5.5	21.7 ± 17.3	
	BtB	W: 29.7 ± 8.6	67.4 ± 13.8	
		S1: 5.0 ± 2.2	6.4 ± 4.0	
		S2: 39.1 ± 11.7	74.9 ± 10.0	
		S3: 8.0 ± 2.7	6.8 ± 4.8	
		S4: 7.7 ± 6.1	36.0 ± 31.5	
		REM: 10.5 ± 5.2	17.9 ± 11.8	
diseased	RaK	W: 16.3	76.8	0.72
		S1: 4.7	14.9	0.21
		S2: 59.7	92.3	0.82
		S3: 8.8	15.9	0.25
		S4: 1.0	0.0	0.00
		REM: 9.6	12.5	0.20
	BtB	W: 18.5	61.8	0.61
		S1: 4.9	5.2	0.09
		S2: 57.6	91.2	0.78
		S3: 8.5	3.6	0.07
		S4: 1.0	0.0	0.00
		REM: 9.5	11.5	0.18

Table 10.14: Detailed sleep stage classification results for the T-wave features. Further explanation is given in /7.4.5/.

10.8.6 Timing

			abs %	Class. Rate [%]	F-Measure
healthy		RaK	N: 97.4	100.0	0.99
			O: 0.2	0.0	0.00
			H: 2.3	0.0	0.00
			M: 0.0	(undefined)	0.00
			C: 0.0	(undefined)	0.00
			X: 0.2	0.0	0.00
		BtB	N: 97.2	100.0	0.99
			O: 0.2	0.0	0.00
			H: 2.3	0.0	0.00
			M: 0.0	(undefined)	0.00
			C: 0.1	0.0	0.00
			X: 0.1	56.1	0.68
∅		RaK	N: 76.3 ± 24.0	92.5 ± 10.5	
			O: 7.2 ± 8.3	21.5 ± 29.8	
			H: 14.0 ± 16.1	25.1 ± 36.7	
			M: 1.9 ± 4.1	16.1 ± 27.9	
			C: 0.2 ± 0.3	0.0 ± 0.0	
			X: 0.4 ± 0.4	11.6 ± 23.1	
		BtB	N: 79.3 ± 18.1	94.0 ± 8.3	
			O: 6.5 ± 7.4	7.4 ± 10.1	
			H: 12.2 ± 11.4	15.6 ± 20.8	
			M: 1.3 ± 2.7	7.7 ± 13.3	
			C: 0.5 ± 0.5	0.0 ± 0.0	
			X: 0.2 ± 0.3	46.6 ± 8.9	
diseased		RaK	N: 41.6	76.3	0.81
			O: 8.1	0.0	0.00
			H: 40.9	86.4	0.74
			M: 9.3	48.4	0.53
			C: 0.2	0.0	0.00
			X: 0.0	(undefined)	0.00
		BtB	N: 55.7	80.8	0.76
			O: 7.5	1.9	0.04
			H: 29.8	50.5	0.49
			M: 6.1	23.1	0.29
			C: 0.9	0.0	0.00
			X: 0.0	(undefined)	0.00

Table 10.15: Detailed SRBD event classification results for the Timing features. Further explanation is given in /7.4.6/.

		abs %	Class. Rate [%]	F-Measure
healthy	RaK	W: 27.3	92.0	0.89
		S1: 4.3	8.7	0.14
		S2: 29.9	76.3	0.72
		S3: 4.2	13.3	0.19
		S4: 14.3	76.3	0.74
		REM: 20.0	68.4	0.70
	BtB	W: 29.6	87.4	0.85
		S1: 4.3	7.5	0.11
		S2: 28.5	59.0	0.55
		S3: 4.2	5.1	0.08
		S4: 14.3	56.5	0.52
		REM: 19.1	40.7	0.43
∅	RaK	W: 28.2 ± 8.8	82.8 ± 7.9	
		S1: 5.1 ± 2.2	7.3 ± 6.1	
		S2: 40.3 ± 12.0	81.7 ± 7.7	
		S3: 8.1 ± 2.7	15.5 ± 4.5	
		S4: 7.8 ± 6.3	53.1 ± 33.4	
		REM: 10.6 ± 5.5	38.0 ± 23.2	
	BtB	W: 29.7 ± 8.6	73.4 ± 16.1	
		S1: 5.0 ± 2.2	4.5 ± 2.4	
		S2: 39.1 ± 11.7	73.4 ± 12.5	
		S3: 8.0 ± 2.7	5.9 ± 3.6	
		S4: 7.7 ± 6.1	28.4 ± 21.0	
		REM: 10.5 ± 5.2	24.3 ± 14.2	
diseased	RaK	W: 16.3	86.6	0.79
		S1: 4.7	17.0	0.24
		S2: 59.7	92.2	0.83
		S3: 8.8	15.9	0.23
		S4: 1.0	0.0	0.00
		REM: 9.6	13.5	0.28
	BtB	W: 18.5	76.1	0.71
		S1: 4.9	5.2	0.09
		S2: 57.6	92.0	0.80
		S3: 8.5	1.2	0.02
		S4: 1.0	0.3	0.01
		REM: 9.5	6.5	0.11

Table 10.16: Detailed sleep stage classification results for the Timing features. Further explanation is given in /7.4.6/.

10.8.7 Overall Shape: Deviations

		abs %	Class. Rate [%]	F-Measure
healthy	RaK	N: 97.4	100.0	0.99
		O: 0.2	0.0	0.00
		H: 2.3	0.0	0.00
		M: 0.0	(undefined)	0.00
		C: 0.0	(undefined)	0.00
		X: 0.2	0.0	0.00
	BtB	N: 97.2	100.0	0.99
		O: 0.2	0.0	0.00
		H: 2.3	0.0	0.00
		M: 0.0	(undefined)	0.00
		C: 0.1	0.0	0.00
		X: 0.1	34.1	0.48
∅	RaK	N: 76.3 ± 24.0	90.0 ± 12.7	
		O: 7.2 ± 8.3	13.6 ± 18.8	
		H: 14.0 ± 16.1	24.1 ± 34.8	
		M: 1.9 ± 4.1	5.4 ± 3.9	
		C: 0.2 ± 0.3	0.0 ± 0.0	
		X: 0.4 ± 0.4	9.6 ± 19.3	
	BtB	N: 79.3 ± 18.1	95.2 ± 7.2	
		O: 6.5 ± 7.4	3.1 ± 4.5	
		H: 12.2 ± 11.4	7.8 ± 12.6	
		M: 1.3 ± 2.7	0.7 ± 1.2	
		C: 0.5 ± 0.5	0.0 ± 00.0	
		X: 0.2 ± 0.3	41.1 ± 5.3	
diseased	RaK	N: 41.6	70.6	0.74
		O: 8.1	0.0	0.00
		H: 40.9	79.8	0.66
		M: 9.3	16.1	0.23
		C: 0.2	0.0	0.00
		X: 0.0	(undefined)	0.00
	BtB	N: 55.7	83.5	0.71
		O: 7.5	1.4	0.03
		H: 29.8	29.6	0.34
		M: 6.1	2.1	0.04
		C: 0.9	0.0	0.00
		X: 0.0	(undefined)	0.00

Table 10.17: Detailed SRBD event classification results for the deviation features. Further explanation is given in /7.4.7/.

		abs %	Class. Rate [%]	F-Measure
healthy	RaK	W: 27.3	77.2	0.71
		S1: 4.3	2.2	0.04
		S2: 29.9	62.5	0.58
		S3: 4.2	2.2	0.04
		S4: 14.3	75.7	0.74
		REM: 20.0	38.7	0.41
	BtB	W: 29.6	56.6	0.49
		S1: 4.3	0.5	0.01
		S2: 28.5	43.9	0.39
		S3: 4.2	0.5	0.01
		S4: 14.3	36.2	0.38
		REM: 19.1	14.6	0.18
∅	RaK	W: 28.2 ± 8.8	70.7 ± 14.9	
		S1: 5.1 ± 2.2	8.9 ± 7.4	
		S2: 40.3 ± 12.0	77.6 ± 9.8	
		S3: 8.1 ± 2.7	17.5 ± 13.8	
		S4: 7.8 ± 6.3	55.4 ± 34.4	
		REM: 10.6 ± 5.5	21.0 ± 11.6	
	BtB	W: 29.7 ± 8.6	50.1 ± 22.4	
		S1: 5.0 ± 2.2	1.6 ± 1.5	
		S2: 39.1 ± 11.7	68.4 ± 17.6	
		S3: 8.0 ± 2.7	3.2 ± 2.4	
		S4: 7.7 ± 6.1	20.2 ± 18.4	
		REM: 10.5 ± 5.2	7.7 ± 5.0	
diseased	RaK	W: 16.3	54.3	0.57
		S1: 4.7	21.3	0.29
		S2: 59.7	89.0	0.78
		S3: 8.8	11.4	0.18
		S4: 1.0	0.0	0.00
		REM: 9.6	20.8	0.30
	BtB	W: 18.5	23.0	0.29
		S1: 4.9	1.2	0.02
		S2: 57.6	90.9	0.72
		S3: 8.5	1.1	0.02
		S4: 1.0	0.0	0.00
		REM: 9.5	2.1	0.04

Table 10.18: Detailed sleep stage classification results for the deviation features. Further explanation is given in /7.4.7/.

10.8.8 Overall Shape: Independent Component Analysis

		abs %	Class. Rate [%]	F-Measure
healthy	RaK	N: 97.4	100.0	0.99
		O: 0.2	0.0	0.00
		H: 2.3	0.0	0.00
		M: 0.0	(undefined)	0.00
		C: 0.0	(undefined)	0.00
		X: 0.2	0.0	0.00
	BtB	N: 97.2	100.0	0.99
		O: 0.2	0.0	0.00
		H: 2.3	0.0	0.00
		M: 0.0	(undefined)	0.00
		C: 0.1	0.0	0.00
		X: 0.1	9.8	0.17
∅	RaK	N: 76.3 ± 24.0	90.7 ± 15.4	
		O: 7.2 ± 8.3	2.2 ± 4.8	
		H: 14.0 ± 16.1	15.0 ± 28.1	
		M: 1.9 ± 4.1	0.0 ± 0.0	
		C: 0.2 ± 0.3	0.0 ± 0.0	
		X: 0.4 ± 0.4	5.8 ± 11.6	
	BtB	N: 79.3 ± 18.1	96.4 ± 6.0	
		O: 6.5 ± 7.4	1.4 ± 2.9	
		H: 12.2 ± 11.4	6.7 ± 13.1	
		M: 1.3 ± 2.7	0.1 ± 0.2	
		C: 0.5 ± 0.5	0.0 ± 00.0	
		X: 0.2 ± 0.3	9.5 ± 2.8	
diseased	RaK	N: 41.6	64.4	0.60
		O: 8.1	0.0	0.00
		H: 40.9	64.5	0.57
		M: 9.3	0.0	0.00
		C: 0.2	0.0	0.00
		X: 0.0	(undefined)	0.00
	BtB	N: 55.7	86.2	0.71
		O: 7.5	0.2	0.00
		H: 29.8	30.0	0.36
		M: 6.1	0.4	0.01
		C: 0.9	0.0	0.00
		X: 0.0	(undefined)	0.00

Table 10.19: Detailed SRBD events classification results for the ICA features. Further explanation is given in /7.4.8/.

		abs %	Class. Rate [%]	F-Measure
healthy	RaK	W: 27.3	77.2	0.72
		S1: 4.3	2.2	0.04
		S2: 29.9	56.2	0.53
		S3: 4.2	4.4	0.08
		S4: 14.3	57.9	0.54
		REM: 20.0	36.8	0.38
	BtB	W: 29.6	75.1	0.65
		S1: 4.3	0.6	0.01
		S2: 28.5	51.6	0.48
		S3: 4.2	0.5	0.01
		S4: 14.3	40.4	0.39
		REM: 19.1	20.2	0.25
∅	RaK	W: 28.2 ± 8.8	51.7 ± 25.3	
		S1: 5.1 ± 2.2	3.5 ± 6.8	
		S2: 40.3 ± 12.0	68.2 ± 19.9	
		S3: 8.1 ± 2.7	3.7 ± 3.3	
		S4: 7.8 ± 6.3	24.7 ± 26.6	
		REM: 10.6 ± 5.5	10.8 ± 15.0	
	BtB	W: 29.7 ± 8.6	53.0 ± 25.2	
		S1: 5.0 ± 2.2	0.7 ± 0.5	
		S2: 39.1 ± 11.7	67.9 ± 19.3	
		S3: 8.0 ± 2.7	2.1 ± 2.1	
		S4: 7.7 ± 6.1	14.0 ± 16.9	
		REM: 10.5 ± 5.2	5.6 ± 8.2	
diseased	RaK	W: 16.3	25.6	0.33
		S1: 4.7	0.0	0.00
		S2: 59.7	94.0	0.75
		S3: 8.8	0.0	0.00
		S4: 1.0	0.0	0.00
		REM: 9.6	2.1	0.04
	BtB	W: 18.5	25.2	0.32
		S1: 4.9	0.3	0.01
		S2: 57.6	93.5	0.73
		S3: 8.5	0.2	0.00
		S4: 1.0	0.0	0.00
		REM: 9.5	0.4	0.01

Table 10.20: Detailed sleep stage classification results for the ICA features. Further explanation is given in /7.4.8/.

10.8.9 Overall Shape: Spectral Transformations

		abs %	Class. Rate [%]	F-Measure
healthy	RaK	N: 97.4	99.9	0.99
		O: 0.2	0.0	0.00
		H: 2.3	0.0	0.00
		M: 0.0	(undefined)	0.00
		C: 0.0	(undefined)	0.00
		X: 0.2	0.0	0.00
	BtB	N: 97.2	99.8	0.99
		O: 0.2	0.0	0.00
		H: 2.3	6.5	0.11
		M: 0.0	(undefined)	0.00
		C: 0.1	0.0	0.00
		X: 0.1	51.2	0.67
∅	RaK	N: 76.3 ± 24.0	92.5 ± 9.8	
		O: 7.2 ± 8.3	21.8 ± 32.2	
		H: 14.0 ± 16.1	30.1 ± 34.8	
		M: 1.9 ± 4.1	17.6 ± 30.4	
		C: 0.2 ± 0.3	0.0 ± 0.0	
		X: 0.4 ± 0.4	19.2 ± 38.5	
	BtB	N: 79.3 ± 18.1	94.8 ± 6.5	
		O: 6.5 ± 7.4	28.9 ± 30.1	
		H: 12.2 ± 11.4	31.2 ± 22.3	
		M: 1.3 ± 2.7	17.3 ± 22.3	
		C: 0.5 ± 0.5	2.6 ± 1.8	
		X: 0.2 ± 0.3	53.8 ± 7.3	
diseased	RaK	N: 41.6	77.8	0.81
		O: 8.1	0.0	0.00
		H: 40.9	85.2	0.74
		M: 9.3	52.7	0.58
		C: 0.2	0.0	0.00
		X: 0.0	(undefined)	0.00
	BtB	N: 55.7	84.4	0.81
		O: 7.5	6.7	0.11
		H: 29.8	65.0	0.61
		M: 6.1	42.5	0.49
		C: 0.9	3.6	0.07
		X: 0.0	(undefined)	0.00

Table 10.21: Detailed SRBD event classification results for the spectral features. Further explanation is given in /7.4.9/.

		abs %	Class. Rate [%]	F-Measure
healthy	RaK	W: 27.3	91.3	0.91
		S1: 4.3	15.2	0.24
		S2: 29.9	86.1	0.82
		S3: 4.2	35.6	0.46
		S4: 14.3	92.8	0.88
		REM: 20.0	81.1	0.80
	BtB	W: 29.6	91.1	0.92
		S1: 4.3	31.7	0.43
		S2: 28.5	85.2	0.82
		S3: 4.2	29.8	0.40
		S4: 14.3	88.0	0.83
		REM: 19.1	81.9	0.81
∅	RaK	W: 28.2 ± 8.8	88.5 ± 5.9	
		S1: 5.1 ± 2.2	14.6 ± 6.7	
		S2: 40.3 ± 12.0	89.0 ± 2.1	
		S3: 8.1 ± 2.7	33.3 ± 10.5	
		S4: 7.8 ± 6.3	67.2 ± 38.9	
		REM: 10.6 ± 5.5	55.5 ± 21.2	
	BtB	W: 29.7 ± 8.6	85.7 ± 7.6	
		S1: 5.0 ± 2.2	22.9 ± 8.1	
		S2: 39.1 ± 11.7	86.3 ± 3.4	
		S3: 8.0 ± 2.7	27.9 ± 9.4	
		S4: 7.7 ± 6.1	61.3 ± 36.5	
		REM: 10.5 ± 5.2	54.9 ± 15.5	
diseased	RaK	W: 16.3	92.7	0.86
		S1: 4.7	19.1	0.28
		S2: 59.7	91.5	0.85
		S3: 8.8	38.6	0.43
		S4: 1.0	0.0	0.00
		REM: 9.6	30.2	0.44
	BtB	W: 18.5	88.3	0.86
		S1: 4.9	27.8	0.37
		S2: 57.6	92.4	0.85
		S3: 8.5	28.3	0.37
		S4: 1.0	1.3	0.03
		REM: 9.5	44.4	0.56

Table 10.22: Detailed sleep stage classification results for the spectral features. Further explanation is given in /7.4.9/.

10.8. Detailed Classification Results

10.8.10 Overall Shape: Differences of Spectral Transformations

		abs %	Class. Rate [%]	F-Measure
healthy	RaK	N: 97.4	100.0	0.99
		O: 0.2	0.0	0.00
		H: 2.3	0.0	0.00
		M: 0.0	(undefined)	0.00
		C: 0.0	(undefined)	0.00
		X: 0.2	0.0	0.00
	BtB	N: 97.2	99.9	0.99
		O: 0.2	0.0	0.00
		H: 2.3	2.5	0.05
		M: 0.0	(undefined)	0.00
		C: 0.1	0.0	0.00
		X: 0.1	31.7	0.48
∅	RaK	N: 76.3 ± 24.0	92.5 ± 10.1	
		O: 7.2 ± 8.3	23.7 ± 31.4	
		H: 14.0 ± 16.1	27.8 ± 32.7	
		M: 1.9 ± 4.1	9.3 ± 16.2	
		C: 0.2 ± 0.3	0.0 ± 0.0	
		X: 0.4 ± 0.4	15.4 ± 30.8	
	BtB	N: 79.3 ± 18.1	95.0 ± 6.1	
		O: 6.5 ± 7.4	21.2 ± 26.1	
		H: 12.2 ± 11.4	25.9 ± 21.6	
		M: 1.3 ± 2.7	5.1 ± 8.9	
		C: 0.5 ± 0.5	0.1 ± 0.3	
		X: 0.2 ± 0.3	37.0 ± 19.3	
diseased	RaK	N: 41.6	76.3	0.80
		O: 8.1	2.5	0.05
		H: 40.9	80.8	0.69
		M: 9.3	28.0	0.33
		C: 0.2	0.0	0.00
		X: 0.0	(undefined)	0.00
	BtB	N: 55.7	85.7	0.80
		O: 7.5	2.1	0.04
		H: 29.8	60.2	0.57
		M: 6.1	15.4	0.23
		C: 0.9	0.0	0.00
		X: 0.0	(undefined)	0.00

Table 10.23: Detailed SRBD event classification results for the differential spectral features. Further explanation is given in /7.4.10/.

		abs %	Class. Rate [%]	F-Measure
healthy	RaK	W: 27.3	92.7	0.90
		S1: 4.3	13.0	0.20
		S2: 29.9	81.1	0.76
		S3: 4.2	26.7	0.40
		S4: 14.3	86.8	0.83
		REM: 20.0	64.6	0.68
	BtB	W: 29.6	88.8	0.85
		S1: 4.3	3.2	0.06
		S2: 28.5	75.8	0.69
		S3: 4.2	2.4	0.04
		S4: 14.3	69.9	0.65
		REM: 19.1	50.5	0.55
∅	RaK	W: 28.2 ± 8.8	86.5 ± 6.0	
		S1: 5.1 ± 2.2	11.0 ± 4.9	
		S2: 40.3 ± 12.0	86.1 ± 4.0	
		S3: 8.1 ± 2.7	26.9 ± 6.7	
		S4: 7.8 ± 6.3	67.2 ± 38.5	
		REM: 10.6 ± 5.5	45.1 ± 20.6	
	BtB	W: 29.7 ± 8.6	81.4 ± 8.2	
		S1: 5.0 ± 2.2	8.0 ± 6.3	
		S2: 39.1 ± 11.7	82.3 ± 6.7	
		S3: 8.0 ± 2.7	12.1 ± 7.4	
		S4: 7.7 ± 6.1	48.8 ± 31.3	
		REM: 10.5 ± 5.2	34.9 ± 13.0	
diseased	RaK	W: 16.3	85.4	0.78
		S1: 4.7	8.5	0.14
		S2: 59.7	91.8	0.83
		S3: 8.8	28.4	0.39
		S4: 1.0	0.0	0.00
		REM: 9.6	13.5	0.22
	BtB	W: 18.5	82.2	0.77
		S1: 4.9	4.1	0.08
		S2: 57.6	92.8	0.81
		S3: 8.5	10.7	0.18
		S4: 1.0	0.0	0.00
		REM: 9.5	14.9	0.24

Table 10.24: Detailed sleep stage classification results for the differential spectral features. Further explanation is given in /7.4.10/.

List of Figures

2.1 Typical hypnogram of a healthy subject 10
2.2 Iceberg representing the different types of SRBD events 12
2.3 Genesis of obstructive apnea 14
2.4 Comparison of central and obstructive sleep apneas on the basis of respiratory flow and effort 15
2.5 The vicious cycle of sleep apnea 16
2.6 Typical hypnogram of an unhealthy subject 17
2.7 Clinical algorithm for diagnosing sleep disorders 20
2.8 CPAP mask (Product Image from `Weinmann.de`) 25

3.1 Human blood circulation 28
3.2 Cardiac conduction system 28
3.3 Placement of the ECG electrodes for Einthoven 30
3.4 Principal morphology of an ECG wave 31
3.5 Bradycardia during an apnea event 32
3.6 Heart rate and autonomous nervous activity 33
3.7 Heart rate variations during the course of sleep 33
3.8 Heart rate variations under the influence of an apnea 34
3.9 Balance of the ANS and the degree of activation 35
3.10 Repolarization and sympathetic activity 36
3.11 Diver reflex and heart rate variation 37
3.12 Dependency between HR and QT-time 40
3.13 AV-blocks under the influence of an apnea event 41
3.14 Blood pressure changes due to (artificial and deliberate) obstructions 43
3.15 ST-depressions in different common shapes 44
3.16 ST-elevations in different common shapes 45
3.17 Shapes of the T-wave under ischemia 46

4.1 Ratio of SNS and PNS activity levels during different sleep stages . . 48

4.2 Spectral analysis of HRV during NREM sleep in a healthy subject. In OSAS patients the SNS is activated to a higher extent resulting in a reduced power density in the high frequency range. The additional ordinate at 0.02 Hz indicates the "cyclic variation of the heart rate" during subsequent SRBD events which is evaluated by many approaches (see /3.2.2/ and Figure 3.11, original Figure taken from [Vano95]). 49
4.3 Evaluation of the heart rate to estimate the long-term ANS activity . 50

5.1 Sleep-Home-Monitoring device 60
5.2 Data flow chain from the recording to evaluation 61
5.3 Visual representation of the concordance of the annotations of the clinical partners 65

6.1 Comparison between a) the original ECG and b) the signal cleaned from the mains supply noise by the applied bandstop filter. 69
6.2 Amplitude and phase response of the 50 Hz bandstop filter 69
6.3 Comparison of the impact of the mains supply filter in the frequency domain 70
6.4 Compensation of DC-shifts by a highpass filter 70
6.5 Amplitude and phase response of the highpass filter compensating DC-shifts 71
6.6 Comparison of the ECG signal before and after the lowpass filtering . 71
6.7 Amplitude and phase response of the applied low pass filter 72
6.8 Delays of the ECG signal preprocessing filters 73
6.9 Labeling the distinctive points in the ECG 73
6.10 Results of the ECG distinctive points detection 75
6.11 Introduction to the Autonomous Model (Overview) 76
6.12 Stability of Body State and Spectrum of ANS Generators 78
6.13 Flow Chart of EVA ml processing the Autonomous Model 79
6.14 Expanded R-peak series 81
6.15 FM demodulation of the HR series 81
6.16 Computing the FM demodulated signal from HR series chunks 82
6.17 Comparison of different methods of FM demodulation 83
6.18 Spectra before and after Gaussian filtering 85
6.19 Local maxima for the template 85
6.20 Global histogram of maxima for all periods and the template 86
6.21 Approximation of the spectra by means of the EM algorithm 88

List of Figures

6.22 Interpolation of the missing values of the GMM 89
6.23 Spectrogram zoomed to reveal only the first 30 coefficients as the remaining coefficients are negligible. 90
6.24 Spectrum with template and the deleted ranges for the generator G_{Noise} 91
6.25 Energy of the generator G_{Noise} 92
6.26 Overall flow chart of the morphological functions 93
6.27 Mechanism of synchronizing the corresponding ECG points as detected by labelECGPoints() 94
6.28 Some features of the P-wave 95
6.29 P-wave feature results 96
6.30 Computing the "Increasing Load" feature 97
6.31 Some features of the R-peak 98
6.32 Amplitudes of the R-peaks in relation to the overnight and the floating mean reference, respectively 99
6.33 Total amplitudes A_{tot} and steepness of QR-segments 100
6.34 Some features of the ST-segment 101
6.35 Amplitudes and floating means $m_c(., \text{flmnLen})$ of the S-peaks and T-waves 102
6.36 Extracted ST-segment and its linear approximation 103
6.37 Extracted ST-segment and its gradient approximation 104
6.38 Computing the iso-electric potential from the PQ-segment 104
6.39 Some features of the T-wave as well as the funny current I_f 105
6.40 T-waves and the derived references 106
6.41 T-waves in respect to the derived references 107
6.42 Load based trends of the T-wave amplitude 108
6.43 Simple model for the funny current I_f and the measured amplitude of the T-wave. 109
6.44 Automatically extracted T-wave 110
6.45 Features to describe the repolarization period 111
6.46 Some features based on the timing of the ECG 112
6.47 Absolute durations of the PQ- and the QT-timing 113
6.48 Timing of the distinctive P-Q-T-points in relation to the current HR or its floating mean, respectively (see equation (6.10) for principle) . . 113
6.49 Principle of morphShape_Dev() 115
6.50 Template buffer for the complete recording 116
6.51 Template with markers 116
6.52 Histogram of the center values for the complete recording 117

List of Figures

6.53 Frequencies of ECG wave amplitudes for the complete recording . . . 118
6.54 Deviations of the ECG waves against the "weighted template" 119
6.55 Deviations of the ECG waves against the mean based template 120
6.56 Gradient Descent procedure failing and running into local minimum . 121
6.57 The idea of separating sleep induced components using the ICA . . . 122
6.58 ICA: Principle of retrieving the SRBD information 122
6.59 Results of running FastICA on "too many" components (some selected)123
6.60 Results of the FastICA algorithm run on few, i.e., three, ECG waves . 124
6.61 The IC with highest matching rank clearly represents the ECG wave. 126
6.62 ICs with lower matching rank 127
6.63 Spectrogram of the PNS component 128
6.64 Spectrogram of the noise component 128
6.65 Correlations between the ICA derived ECG component and the currently processed ECG signal or the overnight mean ECG signal, respectively. 129
6.66 Deviation of the current ECG wave from the overnight ECG and the two different ICs representing PNS and noise 130
6.67 Sums of ICs on signal without ECG wave 131
6.68 Dynamics of energies and their difference for the non-ECG components131
6.69 ICA: Deriving the number of differences 132
6.70 Creating the spectral transformations of the ECG wave 133
6.71 Centered buffer of ECG Waves 134
6.72 Estimating the minimal difference between two R-peaks 135
6.73 One ECG wave cut from the recording with different window lengths 136
6.74 An ECG wave and different fractions of the complete ECG wave length applied to delete the R-peak: in a) the deleting of the R-peak in the time domain and in b) the corresponding spectra. 137
6.75 Extinction methods of the R-peak 138
6.76 Original spectrum of the ECG wave and the spectra of the three different interpolation methods (On the abscissa, the coefficients are given, as the sample length does not equal the DFT length, i.e., sample length about 224 and sampling frequency 256 Hz, thus, one coefficient almost equals one Hertz.) 139
6.77 Different windowing functions and the their influence on the spectrum 141
6.78 Kaiser window function for some values of the scaling factor β 143
6.79 DFT spectrum from ECG signal with R-peak 143
6.80 DFT spectrum from ECG signal without R-peak 144

6.81 DCT spectrum from ECG signal with R-peak 144
6.82 DCT spectrum from ECG signal without R-peak 145
6.83 Number of DCT components and covered signal energy 145
6.84 Principle of `morphShape_SpecDiff()` 146
6.85 Remainders of an ECG wave after subtracting the overnight mean ECG wave 147
6.86 Magnitude of spectra for different spectral resolutions: in a) the resolution is 1 Hz and in b) it is half a Hz – accordingly the spectrum is stretched along the coefficients. 148
6.87 The phase of the signal 148

7.1 Different types of artifacts 152
7.2 Peak-like Artifact 154
7.3 R-peak misclassifications 155
7.4 ECG distinctive points detection remains stable during most artifacts 155
7.5 Case of a (possibly) unprecise S-peak and T-wave detection due to ischemic or chronic ST-depression in conjunction with a negative T-wave 156
7.6 Confusion Matrix 160
7.7 Distribution of the ST-elevation feature over the SRBD events 168
7.8 Feature values for $\frac{QT}{m_c(HR)}$ show a very high dynamic in REM. 170
7.9 Timing feature $\frac{QT}{m_c(HR)}$ for the different SRBD types 171
7.10 Distribution of the deviation features over the SRBD events 172
7.11 Comparision between annotations and evaluation period based single classifications 183

10.1 GUI of EVA ml having processed the morphological features of the P-wave 198
10.2 Flowchart of EVA ml 200
10.3 Deriving the respiration from the ECG signal 203
10.4 Superposition of different Gaussian distributions to approximate a given curve 205

List of Tables

1	Abbreviations used	viii
2.1	ICSD-2	8
2.2	AHI and severity of the SRBD according to ICSD-2	15
3.1	Cardiac pacemakers and their eigenfrequencies	29
5.1	The exported SRBD events and their ASCII coded markers	62
5.2	The results of Figure 5.3 in tabular presentation (in [%])	65
5.3	The MoC values for the two examples from Figure 5.3	66
5.4	The different Kappa coefficients	66
6.1	Overview of the successive processing steps and two feature extraction approaches	67
6.2	Properties of the 50 Hz bandstop filter: the very narrow transition range enables efficient filtering of the mains supply influences, while keeping as much of the morphological information as possible.	70
6.3	Properties of the applied high pass filter	71
6.4	Properties of the applied low pass filter	72
6.5	Distinctive ECG points and their corresponding search boundaries	75
6.6	SNR values for the 'chunk-wise' FM demodulation	82
6.7	The morphological processing functions and the number of extracted parameters	92
7.1	Best classifiers with respect to feature set and classification target	159
7.2	Classification rates for the grouped SRBD events	161
7.3	Classification rates for the grouped sleep stages	162
7.4	Artifact detection rate over the feature sets	176
7.5	Condensed classification rates for the SRBD events	177
7.6	Condensed classification rates for the sleep stages	177

7.7 Absolute occurrences of the SRBD events and the sleep stages in the test patient 179
7.8 Classification rates of the patient-independent evaluation (part 1) . . 180
7.9 Classification rates of the patient-independent evaluation (part 2) . . 181

10.1 Permutation matrix of a two-class-problem 196
10.2 Raters' concordance and the corresponding κ value 197
10.3 The processing functions and their numbers of processing parameters 199
10.4 Properties of the different (exemplary) Gaussian distributions 205
10.5 SRBD event classification results for the Autonomous Model features 212
10.6 Sleep stage classification results for the Autonomous Model features . 213
10.7 SRBD event classification results for the P-wave features 214
10.8 Sleep stage classification results for the P-wave features 215
10.9 SRBD event classification results for the R-peak features 216
10.10 Sleep stage classification results for the R-peak features 217
10.11 SRBD event classification results for the ST-segment features 218
10.12 Sleep stage classification results for the ST-segment features 219
10.13 SRBD event classification results for the T-wave features 220
10.14 Sleep stage classification results for the T-wave features 221
10.15 SRBD event classification results for the Timing features 222
10.16 Sleep stage classification results for the Timing features 223
10.17 SRBD event classification results for the deviation features 224
10.18 Sleep stage classification results for the deviation features 225
10.19 SRBD event classification results for the ICA features 226
10.20 Sleep stage classification results for the ICA features 227
10.21 SRBD event classification results for the spectral features 228
10.22 Sleep stage classification results for the spectral features 229
10.23 SRBD event classification results for the differential spectral features 230
10.24 Sleep stage classification results for the differential spectral features . 231

Bibliography

[Air 06] Air Liquide. *Schlafapnoetherapie mit individuellen Therapieangeboten von VitalAire*. VitalAire, 2006.

[Altu 09] M. Altuve, G. Carrault, J. Cruz, A. Beuchee, P. Pladys, and A. Hernandez. "Analysis of the QRS Complex for Apnea-Bradycardia Characterization in Preterm Infants". *Proceedings of the Annual International Conference of the IEEE Engineering in Medicine*, 2009.

[Bell 09] R. Bellman. "Curse of Dimensionality". http://en.wikipedia.org/wiki/Curse_of_dimensionality (last visited 10/16/2006), January 2009.

[Bish 95] C. Bishop. *Neural Networks for Pattern Recognition*. Clarendon Press, 1995.

[Blas 03] A. Blasi, J. Jo, E. Valladares, B. J. Morgan, J. B. Skatrud, and M. C. K. Khoo. "Cardiovascular variability after arousal from sleep: time-varying spectral analysis". *Journal of Applied Physiology*, No. 95, pp. 1394–1404, 2003.

[Bonn 97] A. Bonnet. "heart rate variability: sleep stage, time of night, and arousal influences". *Electroencephaloger Clin Neurophysiol*, 1997.

[Bouc 08a] R. R. Bouckaert. "Bayesian Network Classifiers in Weka for Version 3-5-7". *University of Waikato*, 2008.

[Bouc 08b] R. R. Bouckaert, E. Frank, M. Hall, et al. *WEKA Manual for Version 3-6-0*. The University of Waikato, December 2008.

[Bren 02] M. Brennan, M. Palaniswami, and P. Kamen. "Pointcare Plot Interpretation using a physiological Model of HRV based on a Network of Oscillators". *American Journal of Physiology*, 2002.

[Brin 02] H.-U. Brinkmann. *Einfluss der obstruktiven Schlafapnoe auf Blutdruck und Herzfrequenz im Wachzustand, im NREM- und REM-Schlaf*. PhD thesis, Philipps-Universität Marburg, 2002.

[Bund 00] A. Bunde, S. Havlin, J. Kantelhardt, T. Penzel, et al. "Correlated and uncorrelated Regions in Heart Rate Fluctuations". *Phys Rev Lett*, 2000.

[Byst 04] W. Bystricky and A. Safer. "Identification of Individual Sleep Apnea Events from the ECG Using Neural Networks and a Dynamic Markovian State Model". *Computers in Cardiology (IEEE)*, 2004.

[Char 89]   F. Charon, M. Dramaix, and J. Mendlewicz. "Epidemiological survey of insomniac subjects in a sample of 1,761 outpatients". *Neuropsychobiology*, 1989.

[Char 91]   E. Charniak. "Bayesian Networks without Tears". *AI MAGAZINE*, 1991.

[Clif 06]   G. D. Clifford, F. Azuaje, and P. E. McSharry. *Advanced Methods and Tools for ECG Data Analysis*. ARTECH HOUSE, INC., 685 Canton Street, Norwood, MA 02062, 2006.

[Cole 82]   R. Coleman, H. Roffwarg, S. Kennedy, et al. "Sleep-wake disorders based on a polysomnographic diagnosis. A national cooperative study.". *The Journal of the American Medical Association*, February 1982. http://jama.ama-assn.org/ (last visited 01/14/2005).

[Dank 01]   H. Danker-Hopfe and W. Herrmann. "Interrater-Reliabilität visueller Schlafstadienklassifikationen nach R-K". *Klin. Neurophysiol.*, No. 32, 2001.

[Davi 07]   M. Davies and C. James. "Source separation using single channel ICA". *Signal Processing*, Vol. 11, No. 87, pp. 1819 – 1832, January 2007.

[Farn 96]   R. Farney, L. Walker, R. Jennen, and J. Walker. "Ear oximetry to detect apnea and differentiate rapid eye movement (REM) and non-REM-sleep". *Chest*, 1996.

[Fisc 05]   J. Fischer, G. Mayer, T. Penzel, D. Riemann, and H. Sitter. *Nicht erholsamer Schlaf (Leitlinie S2 der DGSM, Kurzfassung)*. Thieme, 2005.

[Fuhr 04]   A. Fuhrmann. *Sleep Apnea Diagnosis based on an ECG Signal*. Master's thesis, Fraunhofer IIS, 2004.

[Grot 96]   L. Grote and H. Schneider. *Schlafapnoe und kardiovaskuläre Erkrankungen*. Georg Thieme Verlag, Stuttgart, New York, 1996.

[Grou 07]   U. Grouven, R. Bender, A. Ziegler, and S. Lange. "Der Kappa-Koeffizient". *Dtsch Med Wochenschr*, Vol. 132, No. 23, 2007.

[Habe 03]   R. Haberl. *EKG pocket*. Börm Bruckmeier Verlag, 4 Ed., 2003.

[Hade 04]   C. Hader, B. Sanner, and K. Rasche. "Das obstruktive Schlafapnoe-Syndrom - Diagnostik". *Dtsch Med Wochenschr*, Vol. 129, pp. 566–569, 2004.

[Hamm 01]   C. W. Hamm and S. Willems. *EKG Checkliste. Checklisten der aktuellen Medizin*, Thieme, 2. ausgabe Ed., 2001.

[Hofe 06]   A. K. Hofer. *Reliabilität und Validität eines Fragebogens zum Screening von Schlafstörungen*. PhD thesis, Ruprecht-Karls-Universität Heidelberg, 2006. http://www.ub.uni-heidelberg.de/archiv/6492.

[Hora 98]   T. Horacek. *Der EKG-Trainer*. Thieme, 1998.

[HUK 94]   HUK-Verband, Büro für Kfz-Technik München. "Struktur der Unfälle mit Getöteten auf Autobahnen im Freistaat Bayern im Jahr 1991". 1994.

Bibliography

[Hyvr 01] A. Hyvärinen, J. Karhunen, and E. Oja. *Independent Component Analysis*. John Wiley & Sons, Inc., Electronic, ISBN: 0-471-22131-7 Ed., 2001.

[Hyvr 07] A. Hyvärinen. "The FastICA Package for Matlab". http://www.cis.hut.fi/projects/ica/fastica/, 2007. Helsinki University of Technology.

[Jasc 08] H. Jaschinski. "Hochgenaue Drucksensoren in CPAP-Atemtherapiegeräten". *elektronik industrie*, Vol. 11, 2008.

[Jo 04] J. A. Jo, A. Blasi, E. Valladares, R. Juarez, A. Baydur, and M. C. K. Khoo. "Determinants of Heart Rate Variability in Obstructive Sleep Apnea Syndrome during Wakefulness and Sleep". *American Journal of Physiology*, 2004.

[Kama 07] J. Kamarainen and P. Paalanen. "EM estimated GMM parameters". Tech. Rep., Lappeenranta University of Technology, www.lut.fi, 2007.

[Kemp 05] B. Kemp. "European Data Format". http://www.edfplus.info/ (last visited 07/11/2005), 2005.

[Khoo 01] M. C. K. Khoo, V. Belozeroff, R. B. Berry, and C. S. H. Sassoon. "Cardiac Autonomic Control in Obstructive Sleep Apnea". *American Journal of Respiratory and Critical Care Medicine*, Vol. 164, pp. 807 – 812, 2001.

[Khoo 99] M. C. K. Khoo, T.-S. Kim, and R. B. Berry. "Spectral Indices of Cardiac Autonomic Function in Obstructive Sleep Apnea". *SLEEP*, Vol. 22, No. 4, pp. 443 – 451, 1999.

[Kirs 02] W. Kirsch. "Tauchreflex". *ZO-Glunggehüpfer*, No. 43, 2002.

[Koep 58] H. Koepchen and K. Thurau. "Über die Entstehungsbedingungen der atemsynchronen Schwankungen des Vagustonus (Respiratorische Arrhythmie)". *Pflügers Archiv*, 1958.

[Kram 01] G. Krammer. "Approximation der Negentropie durch Funktionen G(y)". Tech. Rep., TU Graz, 2001.

[Kryg 05] M. H. Kryger, T. Roth, *et al. Principles and Practice of Sleep Medicine, 4th e-dition*. Elsevier, 4th edition Ed., Apr 2005.

[Kuts 05] M. Kutschmann and G. Rippin. "Der Kappa-Koeffizient: Diskussion eines Missverständnisses und ein Modifizierungsvorschlag". Presentation, Institut für Rehabilitationsforschung (Norderney), 2005.

[Lasc 06] A. Laschober. "Schlafapnoe". http://www.gesundheitpro.de/Schlafapnoe-Schlaf-A050829ANONI (last visited 11/22/2006), 2006.

[Lee 02] J.-W. Lee, K.-S. Kim, B. Lee, B. Lee, and M.-H. Lee. "A Real Time QRS Detection Using Delay-Coordinate Mapping for the Microcontroller Implementation". *Annals of Biomedical Engineering*, Vol. 30, 2002.

[Mali 97] M. Malik. "Heart rate variability". *European Heart Journal*, Vol. 17, pp. 354 – 381, 1997.

[Mend 07] M. O. Mendez, D. D. Ruini, O. P. Villantieri, M. Matteucci, T. Penzel, S. Cerutti, and A. M. Bianchi. "Detection of Sleep Apnea from Surface ECG based on Features extracted by an Autoregressive Model". *Proceedings of the 29th Annual International Conference of the IEEE EMBS*, 2007.

[Mend 10] M. O. Mendez, J. Corthout, S. Van Huffel, M. Matteucci, T. Penzel, S. Cerutti, and A. M. Bianchi. "Automatic Screening of Obstructive Sleep Apnea from the ECG based on Empirical Mode Decomposition and Wavelet Analysis". *Physiol. Meas.*, 2010.

[Miet 00] J. E. Mietus, C.-K. Peng, P. C. Ivanov, and A. L. Goldberger. "Hilbert Transform based Sleep Apnea Detection using a Single Lead Electrocardiogram (apdet)". *www.physionet.org (last visited 07/23/2010)*, 2000.

[Miet 06] J. E. Mietus. "HRV in Sleep Apnea Detection and Sleep Stability Assessment". Tech. Rep., Beth Israel Deaconess Medical Center, Harvard Medical School, Boston, 2006.

[Miet 10] J. Mietus, C.-K. Peng, P. C. Ivanov, and A. L. Goldberger. "Detection of Obstructive Sleep Apnea from Cardiac Interbeat Interval Time Series". *Physionet.org*, 2010.

[Moor 01] A. W. Moore. "Bayes Nets for representing and reasoning about uncertainty". Presentation Slides, 2001. Carnegie Mellon University.

[Niem 03] H. Niemann. *Klassifikation von Mustern*. Springer Verlag, Berlin, Heidelberg, New York, Tokyo, 2 Ed., 2003.

[Noel 97] E. Noelle-Neumann and R. Köcher. *Allensbacher Jahrbuch der Demoskopie 1993 - 1997*. Verlag für Demoskopie, Allensbach, 1997.

[None 05] P. Nonell. *Subjektive Schlafqualität, Traumerinnerung und Alptraumhäufigkeit bei Patienten mit Panikstörung*. PhD thesis, Ruprecht-Karls-Universität Heidelberg, 2005.
http://www.ub.uni-heidelberg.de/archiv/5239
(last visited 01/03/2007).

[Olsh 96] K. von Olshausen and H. H. Börger. *EKG Information*. SteinKopff, 7 Ed., 1996.

[Penz 02a] T. Penzel, R. Fricke, U. Brandenburg, H. Becker, and C. Vogelmeier. "Peripheral Arterial Tonometry monitors Changes of Autonomous Nervous System in Sleep Apnea". *Proceedings of the Second Joint EMBS/BMES Conference*, Vol. 1, pp. 1552 – 1553, 2002.

[Penz 02b] T. Penzel, J. McNames, P. de Chazal, B. Raymond, A. Murray, and G. Moody. "Systematic Comparison of Different Algorithms for Apnea Detection based on Electrocardiogram Recordings". *Medical & Biological Engineering & Computing*, Vol. 40, 2002.

[Penz 05] T. Penzel, H. Peter, and J. H. Peter. *Schlafstörungen (Gesundheitsberichterstattung des Bundes)*. Vol. Heft 27, Robert Koch-Institut, 2005.

[Penz 06] T. Penzel, M. Nottrott, S. Canisius, T. Greulich, H. F. Becker, and C. Vogelmeier. "ECG Morphology Changes improve Detection of Obstructive Sleep Apnea". *Sleep Medicine*, Vol. 7, 2006.

Bibliography

[Pete 87] J. H. Peter, T. Podszus, and P. von Wichert. *Sleep Related Disorders and Internal Diseases*. Springer, Berlin, 1987.

[Pete 91] J. Peter, T. Penzel, T. Podszus, and P. von Wichert. *(Sleep and Health Risk) Nocturnal Myocardial Ischaemia and Cardiac Arrhythmias in Patients with Coronary Heart Disease and Sleep-Related Breathing Disorders*. Springer-Verlag, Berlin, 1991.

[Pete 95] J. Peter, U. Koehler, L. Grote, and T. Podszus. "Manifestations and consequences of obstructive sleep apnea". *European Respiratory Journal*, 1995.

[Phys 04] PhysioNet.org. 2004. www.physionet.org (last visited 06/11/2004).

[Psch 98] W. Pschyrembel (Editor). *Pschyrembel Klinisches Wörterbuch*. Walter de Gruyter, Berlin, New York, 258 Ed., 1998.

[Rech 68] A. Rechtschaffen and A. Kales. "A manual of standardized terminology, techniques and scoring system for sleep stages of human subjects". *National Institute of Health Publications*, Vol. 204, 1968.

[Rich 78] C. Richardson, M. Carskado, W. Flagg, J. Van den Hood, W. Dement, and M. Mitler. "Excessive daytime sleepiness in man: Multiple sleep latency measurements in narcoleptic and control subjects". *Electroencephaloger Clin Neurophysiol*, Vol. 53, pp. 658 – 661, 1978.

[Roch 99] F. Roche, J.-M. Gaspoz, I. Court-Fortune, P. Minini, V. Pichot, D. Duverney, F. Costes, J.-R. Lacour, and J.-C. Barthelemy. "Screening of Obstructive Sleep Apnea Syndrome by Heart Rate Variability Analysis". *Circulation - Journal of the American Heart Association*, 1999.

[Schl 07] Schlaf.de. "Machen Sie jetzt den Schlaftest". http://www.schlaf.de/schlaf_gestoert/2_50_10_epworth.php, 2007. (last visited 09/07/2007).

[Schu 06] B. SchultheiSS, A. Möller, and E. Schmittendorf. "Technische Untersuchungen zur Qualität von Pulsoximetriedaten im Schlaflabor". Tech. Rep., Fachhochschule Oldenburg, Ostfriesland, Wilhelmshaven, 2006.

[Schu 95] E. G. Schukat-Talamazzini. *Automatische Spracherkennung*. Vieweg Verlag, 1995.

[Shio 97] T. Shiomi, C. Guilleminault, R. Sasanabe, K. Usui, M. Maekawa, and T. Kobayashi. "Heart Rate Variability in Obstructive Sleep Apnea Syndrome before and during Treatment with Nasal Continuous Positive Airway Pressure". *NAPS*, 1997.

[Shou 04] R. Shouldice, S. Ward, L. M. O'Brian, C. O. Brien, S. Redmond, D. Gozal, and C. Heneghan. "PR and PP ECG Interval Variation during Obstructive Apnea and Hypopnea". *Proceedings of the 30th IEEE Annual Northeast Bioengineering Conference*, 2004.

[Smit 99] S. W. Smith. *The Scientist's and Engineer's Guide to Digital Signal Processing*. California Technical Publishing, P.O. Box 502407, San Diego, CA 92150-2407, second edition Ed., 1999. DSPguide.com.

[SOMN 06a] SOMNOmedics. *SOMNOscreen - Vom Screener bis zum vollständigen PSG-System*. SOMNOmedics, Nonnengarten 8, D-97270 Kist, 2006.

[SOMN 06b] SOMNOmedics. *SOMNOwatch - Das Multitalent.* SOMNOmedics, Nonnengarten 8, D-97270 Kist, 2006.

[Tels 04] S. Telser, M. Staudacher, and Y. Ploner. "Can One Detect Sleep Stage Transitions for On-Line Sleep Scoring by Monitoring the Heart Rate Variability?". *Somnologie*, Vol. 8, pp. 33–41, 2004.

[Temm 06] A. Temmel. "Gefahr im Schlaf". *ärztemagazin*, Vol. 19, 2006.

[The 10] The University of Waikato. "WEKA – The University of Waikato". http://www.cs.waikato.ac.nz/ml/weka/, 2010. (last visited 04/09/2010).

[Thom 03] R. J. Thomas. "Arousals in Sleep-disordered Breathing: Patterns and Implications". *SLEEP*, Vol. 26, No. 8, p. (no pagination), 2003.

[Trol 05] Trolltech. "Qt - A cross-platform application and UI framework". http://www.qtsoftware.com/, 2005.

[Vano 95] E. Vanoli, P. B. Adamson, B. Lin, G. D. Pinna, R. Lazzara, and W. C. Orr. "Heart Rate Variability during Specific Sleep Stages". *Circulation - Journal of the American Heart Association*, 1995.

[Virc 04] J. C. Virchow, R. Staats, and H. Matthys. *Handbuch Schlafmedizin*. Dustri-Verlag Dr. Karl Feistle, München - Orlando, 3 Ed., 2004.

[Voss 08] A. Voss. *Methoden zur Kompensation von Bewegungsartefakten in ambulanten EKG-Signalen*. Master's thesis, Friedrich-Alexander-Universität Erlangen-Nürnberg, Lehrstuhl für Informationstechnik mit dem Schwerpunkt Kommunikationselektronik (Stiftungslehrstuhl), 2008.

[Weib 04] C. T. Weiberle. *Implementierung und Untersuchung von Verfahren zum objektiven Vergleich von Segmentierungs- und Klassifikationsergebnissen*. Master's thesis, Friedrich-Alexander-Universität Erlangen-Nürnberg, Lehrstuhl für Mustererkennung, 2004.

[Wenk 05] S. Wenk. *Kardiovaskuläre Erkrankungen - Symptome, Messwerte und deren Auswertung*. Master's thesis, Universität Erlangen-Nürnberg, 2005.

[Witt 05] I. H. Witten and E. Frank. *Data Mining*. Elsevier, 2 Ed., 2005.

[Xu 08] W. Xu, X. Liu, and Z. Pan. "Definition of Sleep Apnea Events by one minute HRV Spectrum Analysis". *IEEE*, 2008.

[Zwil 82] C. Zwillich, T. Devlin, D. White, N. Douglas, *et al.* "Bradycardia during Sleep Apnea: Characteristics and Mechanism". *J Clin Invest*, 1982.

[Zywi 02a] C. Zywietz, B. Widiger, R. Fischer, and G. Joseph. "A System for Comprehensive ECG Waveform and Trend Analysis Accompanying Polysomnographic Sleep Apnea Detection". *Computers in Cardiology*, 2002.

[Zywi 02b] C. Zywietz, B. Widiger, and T. Penzel. "Polysomnographic Sleep Recordings with Simultaneously Acquired 12 Lead ECGs: A Study for Detection and Validation of Apnea Related ECG Changes". *Computers in Cardiology*, 2002.

[Zywi 04]   C. W. Zywietz, V. von Einem, B. Widiger, and G. Joseph. "ECG Analysis for Sleep Apnea Detection". *Methods Inf Med*, 2004.

Index

AASM, 7
AHI, 15
ANS, 34
Apnea
    central, 13
    mixed, 14
    Risk Factors, 18
    Symptoms, 18
ARFF, 63, 198, 201
Arousal, 17, 33
    Sleep Interruption, 9
ASDA, 7
AV-Node, 29

BMI, 18
bpm, 29, 32
BtB, 201

Cardiac Conduction System, 27
Central Limit Theorem, 207
CHD, 19
CiC, 50
COPD, 18
CPAP, 19
CSAS, 13
Curse Of Dimensionality, 145
CVHR, 53

DCT, 132
DFT, 132, 139
DGSM, 19, 26
diastole, 27
Diver Reflex, 36

DWT, 53

ECG, 22, 27
EDF, 62
EDR, 53
EEG, 9, 21
EM, 87, 205
EMD, 51
EMG, 9, 22
EOG, 9, 22
Euler-Liljestrand-Reflex, 33
EVA
    ml, 197
    Plausibility Check, 198
    qt, 62

FastICA, 120, 207
FIR, 68
Funny Channel, 36

GMM, 87, 187
Gradient Descent Procedure, 120

HD Buffering, 198
Hilbert Transformation, 54
HR, 31
HRV, 31, 76
Hypoxemia, 36

IC, 121
ICA, 119, 205
    Non-Gaussianity, 206
    Overlearning, 121
    underdetermined, 208

ICSD, 7
Incidence, 5
Ischemia, 43

Kales, 198
Kappa
    Paradox, 196

Leakage, 139

NIH, 19

OSAS, 13
pdf, 206
PLS, 50
PNS, 34
Poincare Plot, 50
Prevalence, 5
Processing Configuration, 199
PSD, 47
PSG, 21

Rechtschaffen, 198
Respiratory Arrhythmia, 37
    Bainbridge Reflex, 38
    Central Theory, 38
    Lungs Reflex, 38
    Pressoreceptor Theory, 38
Respiratory Effort, 14

SA, 27
SAS, 13
SFS, 52
SHS, 13
SIDS, 7, 56
Sinus Arrhythmia, 37
Sleep
    Architecture, 10
    REM, 9
    Slow Wave, 9
    Stages, 9
Sleep Hygiene, 19, 24
SMZ, 21
SNS, 34
SRBD, 1, 5
systole, 27

TST, 10

VCO, 76
Vigilance, 1

WEKA
    Experimenter, 151
    Explorer, 151
    Windowing, 139

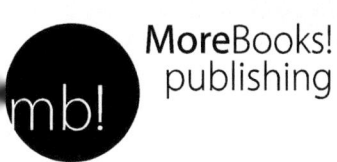

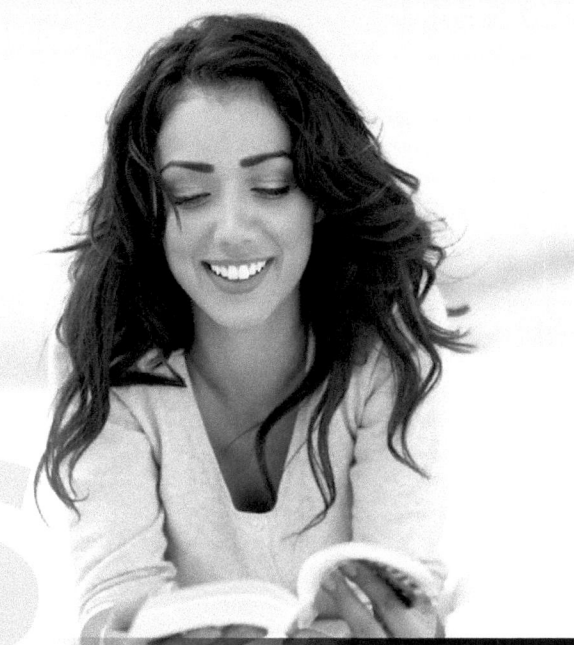

i want morebooks!

Buy your books fast and straightforward online - at one of world's fastest growing online book stores! Environmentally sound due to Print-on-Demand technologies.

Buy your books online at
www.get-morebooks.com

Kaufen Sie Ihre Bücher schnell und unkompliziert online – auf einer der am schnellsten wachsenden Buchhandelsplattformen weltweit! Dank Print-On-Demand umwelt- und ressourcenschonend produziert.

Bücher schneller online kaufen
www.morebooks.de

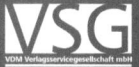

VDM Verlagsservicegesellschaft mbH
Heinrich-Böcking-Str. 6-8   Telefon: +49 681 3720 174   info@vdm-vsg.de
D - 66121 Saarbrücken   Telefax: +49 681 3720 1749   www.vdm-vsg.de

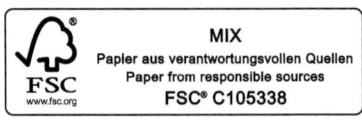

Printed by Books on Demand GmbH, Norderstedt / Germany